THE GOVERNANCE OF]
The Romanow Papers, Volume 3

MW01579005

Edited by Tom McIntosh, Pierre-Gerlier Forest, and
Gregory P. Marchildon

The papers in this third volume of the research program for the
Romanow Commission look at the nature of Canadian federalism
and the politics of intergovernmental relations and how they relate
to questions concerning the governance of the Canadian health care
system.

In the first section, the papers discuss the formal division of powers
regarding health care as outlined in the Canadian Constitution and
the Charter of Rights and Freedoms. The second section is devoted to
an examination of intergovernmental relations with respect to health
care. Finally, the third section focuses on the social and legal context
of health care. It was evident to the commission that intergovernmental relations in the health care sector had become increasingly acrimonious and dysfunctional. The essays in this collection examine the
causes of this dysfunction from a variety of perspectives, and offer concrete solutions to managing intergovernmental conflict in regard to
health care.

TOM MCINTOSH is assistant professor of political science and a member
of the research faculty at the Saskatchewan Population Health and
Evaluation Research Unit at the University of Regina.

PIERRE-GERLIER FOREST is professor of public policy and management
in the department of political science at Université Laval. He currently
holds the G.D.W. Cameron Chair with Health Canada.

GREGORY P. MARCHILDON holds a Canada research chair in public policy and economic history, and is professor of public administration at
the University of Regina.

THE ROMANOW PAPERS: VOLUME III

The Governance of Health Care in Canada

Edited by

Tom McIntosh,

Pierre-Gerlier Forest, and

Gregory P. Marchildon

UNIVERSITY OF TORONTO PRESS
Toronto Buffalo London

ISBN 0-8020-8619-5

Printed on acid-free paper

National Library of Canada Cataloguing in Publication

Romanow papers / edited by Gregory P. Marchildon, Tom McIntosh and
Pierre-Gerlier Forest.

Contents: v. 1. The fiscal sustainability of health care in Canada   v. 2.
Changing health care in Canada   v. 3. The governance of health care in
Canada.
ISBN 0-8020-8626-8 (set).   ISBN 0-8020-8617-9 (v. 1).
ISBN 0-8020-8618-7 (v. 2)   ISBN 0-8020-8619-5 (v. 3)

1. Medical care – Canada.   2. Medical policy – Canada.   3. Public health –
Canada.   I. Marchildon, Gregory P., 1956–   II. McIntosh, Thomas A.
(Thomas Allan), 1964–   III. Forest, Pierre-Gerlier   IV. Title: The fiscal
sustainability of health care in Canada.   V. Title: Changing health care in
Canada.   VI. Title: The governance of health care in Canada.

RA449.R65 2003   362.1'0971   C2003-904073-9

University of Toronto Press acknowledges the financial assistance to its
publishing program of the Canada Council for the Arts and the Ontario
Arts Council.

University of Toronto Press acknowledges the financial support for its
publishing activities of the Government of Canada through the Book
Publishing Industry Development Program (BPIDP).

Contents

Part III. The Social and Legal Context

Acknowledgments

The papers in this volume, and its two companion volumes, were originally commissioned as part of the research activities of the Commission on the Future of Health Care in Canada headed by Roy J. Romanow and were first issued on the commission's website during the summer and fall of 2002. From the outset of the commission's work, Mr Romanow made it clear to us that we had a mandate to ensure that the Report's recommendations were based on the best available evidence and analysis. His support for our contention that there were still important gaps in our knowledge about health care in Canada that needed to be filled was unwavering. As, respectively, the commission's executive director, director of research, and research coordinator, we were given an opportunity that few academics ever get and the commissioner's trust in, and support of, our work on behalf of the commission is deeply appreciated.

We want also to acknowledge Steven Lewis's contribution to the development of the terms of reference for the authors and in helping us matching the right author with the right research assignment. Morris Barer, Diane Watson, Donna Shilds-Poe, and Rob Courchene of the Institute of Health Policy and Services Research of the Canadian Institutes of Health Research managed the often time-consuming independent peer-review process of the papers during the commission's work. The comments provided by the anonymous reviewers contributed greatly to the quality of the papers and their efforts on behalf of the commission are appreciated. Louise Séguin-Guenette provided invaluable services in coordinating the tranlsation and publication of the

University of Toronto Press, was especially helpful in assisting us in turning a set of separate studies into three thematic volumes.

We also want to thank the staff of the University of Toronto Press and the University of Ottawa Press, especially Virgil Duff (who acted as our experienced sherpa from the beginning), Bill Harnum, and Lynn Mackay, for their assistance in creating a more permanent legacy for these papers and for the work of the commission.

Finally, we want to thank our contributors who approached their respective papers with enthusiasm and who so clearly shared the import of the overall project in which we were engaged.

TOM McINTOSH
PIERRE-GERLIER FOREST
GREGORY P. MARCHILDON

March 2003

Contributors

André Braën is a professor of law at the University of Ottawa.

Kina Chenard is a doctoral candidate in political science at Université Laval.

Sujit Choudhry is an assistant professor of law at the University of Toronto.

Adriana Dudas is a doctoral candidate in political science at Université Laval.

Colleen M. Flood is an associate professor of law at the University of Toronto.

Pierre-Gerlier Forest is professor of public policy and management with the department of political science at Université Laval. He currently holds the G.D.W. Cameron Chair with Health Canada.

Donna Greschner is a professor of law at the University of Saskatchewan.

Louis M. Imbeau is a professor of political science at Université Laval.

Candace Johnson is an assistant professor of political science at the University of Guelph.

John N. Lavis is an associate professor in the Department of Clinical

Epidemiology and Biostatistics and Canada Research Chair in Knowledge Transfer and Uptake at McMaster University.

Howard Leeson is a professor of political science at the University of Regina.

Pascale Lehoux is an associate professor in the Department of Health Administration at the University of Montreal and a researcher in the Groupe de recherche interdisciplinaire en santé.

Antonia Maioni is director of the McGill Institute for the Study of Canada, an associate professor of political science, and William Dawson Scholar at McGill University.

Gregory P. Marchildon holds a Canada research chair in public policy and economic history, and is professor of public administration at the University of Regina.

Tom McIntosh is an assistant professor of political science and research faculty at the Saskatchewan Population Health and Evaluation Research Unit at the University of Regina.

Réjean Pelletier is a professor of political science at Université Laval.

Stephen Tomblin is an associate professor of political science at the Memorial University of Newfoundland.

THE GOVERNANCE OF HEALTH CARE IN CANADA

Introduction: Restoring Trust, Rebuilding Confidence – The Governance of Health Care and the Romanow Report

TOM McINTOSH

It should come as no surprise that the research program of the Romanow Commission on the Future of Health Care in Canada paid a significant amount of attention to the nature of Canadian federalism and the politics of intergovernmental relations, and how these relate to questions concerning the governance of the Canadian health care system. Try as one might to focus exclusively on the financing, organization, and delivery of actual health care services to Canadians, one cannot avoid running up against contending and contentious disagreements over the relative role of federal, provincial, and territorial governments in each of these activities. In all aspects of the so-called health care debate, the politics of Canadian federalism not only dares to speak its name, but shouts it so loudly as to often drown out all other discussions.

The prominence of intergovernmental politics within the health care debate in Canada may be lamentable for some (and there is no doubt that intergovernmental conflict often obscures and distracts from other important debates about health care in Canada), but it is unavoidable. Canada is not only a federal state – with all the advantages and disadvantages that this implies (Watts 1999) – but also a federal society. That is to say, Canadians, both individually and collectively, wrestle with multiple identities and attachments to locality, province, region, and country.

What E.R. Black (1975) referred to as Canada's 'divided loyalties,' Banting and Boadway (2001) more recently characterized as the possession of multiple, sometimes cross-cutting and sometimes conflictual, notions of different 'sharing communities' around which they coalesce to achieve particular economic, social, and political goods. These sharing communities can find their political articulation in the formal institutional divisions that characterize a federal state whereby a number of political and economic considerations contribute to decisions to 'share' risk or redistribute resources at the level of the provincial or national community. Thus, to the extent that the provision of health care is a 'public good' about which Canadians care, this can lead to intense debate within the country about the relative role of federal, provincial, and territorial political institutions in the articulation and protection of this particular public good.

In some areas of public policy the definition of the sharing community within Canada can be relatively free of conflict. For example, there is no serious debate about the relative role of the federal versus provincial governments in the area of defence. The constitutional authority of the federal government is unambiguous and, while some may argue that the federal government should dedicate more resources to the armed forces, there is no contending argument for a provincial role in defence matters.

But it is evident to even the most casual observer of the debate over health care in Canada that there is considerable disagreement over whether the community responsible for the financing, organization, and delivery of health care can or should exist at the provincial/territorial or federal level or, more precisely, which community is responsible for which aspects of that financing, organization, and delivery. What is clear from analyses such as Banting and Boadway's work and from many of the essays collected here is that health care is politically contentious not only because it is Canada's most expensive (and expansive) social program but because it mirrors the tensions inherent in any federal system. Public opinion data consistently show that Canadians in all parts of the country see medicare as having both national and provincial/local dimensions (Mendelsohn 2002). They want both a degree of similarity across the country, such that all Canadians have access to comparable services as needed, and a degree of specificity, such that the services delivered in their community reflect the specific health needs in that community. In short, they want a health care system that does not require them to choose either the system's national or its provincial/local dimensions at the expense of the other.

The governance of specific policy sectors in federal states can be said to exist along a continuum, ranging from those sectors marked by a high degree of 'federal unilateralism' (i.e., where the federal government uses its superior fiscal or political resources to operate in areas of provincial jurisdiction without consent or consultation) at one end, to those characterized as 'disentangled' where each order of government operates independently in its own areas of competence at the other end. Between these extremes lies various forms and degrees of both federal-provincial and interprovincial collaboration. The success of any particular governance regime depends on its ability to balance three key components: (1) policy goals and outcomes (e.g., redistributive equity, equality of access, and opportunity), (2) democratic goals and values (e.g., citizen engagement, transparency), and (3) federalism considerations (e.g., respect for the legal and political sovereignty of both orders of government). The functionality or dysfunctionality of any specific governance regime is reflective of how that regime resolves the tensions that exist within and between each of these three components (Lazar and McIntosh 1998; McIntosh 2000).

Thus, the governance of health care in Canada requires a set of institutions and relationships that simultaneously promote some set of shared values and goals at the macro-level while also promoting some degree of divergence and respect for provincial differences in a manner that allows for the kind of provincial policy innovations that have traditionally been the hallmark of Canadian public health care. Building such relationships and institutions will necessarily involve conflict and disagreement over how these broadly stated values and goals are operationalized in policy terms and over the roles and responsibilities of each set of actors. Conflict in and of itself is neither positive nor negative, but the ability of governments to resolve conflicts in a manner that respects the equality of the partners involved and that harnesses the creative tensions inherent in such a relationship will determine whether this relationship – despite the conflicts – is functional or dysfunctional.

It was evident to the commission that the very nature of the intergovernmental debate over health care in Canada had become, since at least the mid-1990s, increasingly acrimonious and dysfunctional. In its Interim Report, released in February 2002, the commission made it clear that 'Canadians are tired of the finger-pointing and "hollering from a distance" while both parties squabble over fundamental directions and funding' (Commission 2002b, 40). As a number of essays collected in this volume attest, the source and causes of this dysfunction are many and varied – and neither order of government can be absolved of some responsibility for this state of affairs.

This acrimony had, to a very great extent, poisoned the atmosphere around health care policy-making and, as a consequence, not only hindered the ability of both orders of government to engage in serious debate around potential reform of the system but had served to undermine the confidence of the Canadian public that the health care systems in the provinces were capable of providing quality services to people when and where they were needed. The frustration of the Canadian public with the intergovernmental conflict over health care was made evident to the commission not only during the public hearings but also during the 'Citizens' Dialogue' events held in communities across the country (Commission 2002a).

Thus, it was because the commission believed that intergovernmental relations in the health care sector were increasingly dysfunctional that it chose to dedicate a significant portion of its research agenda to examining the source of that dysfunction. Was there a significant constitutional ambiguity that led to intergovernmental competition in this area? Was there public ambivalence about the relative role of each order of government that fuelled intergovernmental conflict, fingerpointing, and blame-avoidance? What are the political dynamics involved in the intergovernmental relations around health care and to what extent is this influenced by the fiscal context of contemporary health care funding? How do other non-governmental actors with governance responsibilities fit into these dynamics? What role does the enforcement or non-enforcement of the Canada Health Act play in those political dynamics and what role will the Charter of Rights and Freedoms play in future intergovernmental dynamics in this sector? What mechanisms exist or could be created to facilitate more functional intergovernmental relations?

The essays collected here provide, as expected from such a diverse collection of scholars, a variety of answers from a variety of perspectives. But they share a few consistent themes. In the first instance, there is little prospect of eliminating intergovernmental conflict over health care – it is simply too important a policy area both in terms of its level of public support and its proportion of public spending to not engender serious and principled disagreements about how it should best be financed, organized, and delivered. The goal is not to eliminate intergovernmental conflict but to find processes that manage that conflict in a more functional manner.

The Constitutional Context

If it is true that much of Canadian politics is dominated, for good and for ill, by the politics of federalism and intergovernmentalism, then it is also true that those debates are conditioned by our understanding of the constitutional arrangements that set out the division of powers in the Canadian federation. Specifically, the terms of sections 91 and 92 of the Constitution Act, 1867, and the body of constitutional interpretation surrounding them are the basis of each order of government's claim to have an active and ongoing role in the provision of health care services to Canadians. More recently, the adoption of the Canadian Charter of Rights and Freedoms as part of the Constitution Act, 1982, has added an entirely new dimension to public policy debates by allowing individuals and groups to use the courts in an attempt to hold governments to account for policy choices by claiming any number of rights enumerated in the Charter. Thus, for the commission, it became important to try to shed some light on the constitutional context of the current debates over health care, both in terms of the relative role of each order of government and in terms of the possible role that the Charter might play in allowing individuals to claim a constitutional right to specific health services that governments may choose to deny or ration in some manner.

As the commission notes in its Final Report, neither 'health care' generally nor the specifics of the universal, publicly administered single-payer system that has evolved in Canada is enumerated as a responsibility of either the federal or provincial government (Commission 2002c). While sections 91 and 92 of the Constitution Act, 1867, might first appear to provide an exhaustive listing of the exclusive and shared responsibilities of each order of government, such has never really been the case. New policy areas have emerged over time while others have fallen into disuse. Nearly all the health and social services Canadians currently see as a legitimate area of State activity – either in terms of actual delivery or of regulation – were seen to be private concerns that were undertaken by charitable or religious organizations in nineteenth-century Canada. But as the role of the State in these areas grew, it fell to the courts to interpret whether specific policy initiatives were the responsibility of either the federal or provincial government. For example, when the federal government, in an effort to provide relief from the effects of the Great Depression, attempted to introduce legislation similar to the Roosevelt New Deal in the United States, the legislation was ruled ultra vires, or beyond the jurisdiction of the federal government. Indeed, it took an amendment to the Constitution in 1940 to allow the federal government to introduce a national unemployment insurance program.

As both André Braën and Howard Leeson point out in their contributions to this volume, neither the federal nor the provincial governments has exclusive constitutional responsibility for health care. The two contributors, one a constitutional law professor and the other a political scientist specializing in federalism and intergovernmental relations, come to remarkably similar conclusions about the specifics of the relative roles played by each order of government. In short, provincial governments have the primary authority for the organization, administration, and delivery of the vast majority of health care services. As Braën asserts, 'When it comes to health, the provinces man the front lines.' While provincial authority over 'hospitals, asylums, charities and eleemosynary institutions' as outlined in section 92(7) of the Constitution Act, 1867 provides the key basis for the provincial authority over the administration and delivery of health care services, this is only one of a number of constitutional provisions that legitimize the provinces' primary role in health care and the delivery of health care services. In contrast, the federal government has a more limited role that rests, in part, on its authority over the criminal law, patents, and, most controversially, the federal spending power.

What both authors make clear is that the source of the intergovernmental conflict over health care lies in the transformation of health care from a private matter to a public matter. As the role of the State as a regulator and later an insurer and deliverer of health care services grew, so did the intergovernmental conflict over which order of government was responsible for which specific elements of what we commonly refer to as 'the health care system.' Thus, we are left with something of a constitutional conundrum.

When the federal government used its financial resources to encourage provinces to develop and then expand publicly insured health services, first through the Hospital Insurance and Diagnostic Services Act (HIDSA) then through the Medical Care Act and the Canada Health Act, it was clearly exercising a legitimate federal prerogative. But at the same time, the increased federal role within the health system – especially in terms of the system's financing – inevitably set the stage for increased intergovernmental conflict over which order of government's priorities would drive the development of public health care in the country.

Thus, the manner in which the Canadian Constitution divides authority over the financing, organization, and delivery of health care services reinforces the political competition between the federal and provincial governments on the so-called health file. Claims by some provincial governments that they hold 'exclusive' jurisdiction over health care are not in accordance with either the terms of the Constitution Act, 1867, or the jurisprudence that stems from it. At the same time, the claim that the federal government is the 'guarantor' or 'protector' of the national dimensions of the health care system rests not so much on a clearly defined constitutional role assigned to it as on the political commitment of the federal government to contribute significantly to off-setting the costs incurred by the provinces for the delivery of health care services.

The modernization of the Canadian constitutional order in 1982 introduced yet another set of priorities into the federal-provincial mix. The adoption of the Canadian Charter of Rights and Freedoms as the cornerstone of the Constitution Act, 1982, has irretrievably altered both Canadian politics and Canadian federalism by providing citizens – both individually and collectively – the right to seek redress from the courts for government action (or inaction) that violates the now constitutionally entrenched rights of citizens. Since its adoption, the Charter has enjoyed tremendous support among the public, and it remains very much in line with the post–Second World War 'rights revolution' in liberal-democratic states.

But the Charter also raises some very important questions about how governments and the courts will be asked to balance the rights of individual citizens with public policy decisions aimed at – to put it in strictly utilitarian terms – maximizing the benefits of public health care for the greatest number of people. All governments have limited resources that can be dedicated to health care and these limits necessitate that choices be made – what services to insure, what prescription drugs to cover, what facilities to operate, and so on. Again, the tension between the protection of individual rights and sound policy-making, based on allocating limited resources by weighing the trade-offs for different courses of action, can be either creative or destructive.

If a government chooses not to insure a particular drug because it is too expensive, does an individual have a right to that drug regardless of its cost? If the same drug is excluded because it is deemed to be only effective in a minority of cases, does the individual have a right to the drug even though it is not clear he or she would benefit from it? The dilemma of the Charter is that its guarantees may not lend themselves to the kind of priority-setting that is at the heart of social policy-making through the formal democratic process. The courts are ill-equipped (and likely ill-prepared) to make the kind of choices that governments regularly make. At the same time, the Charter embodies many of the key values – equality, universality, and accessibility – that drove the creation and expansion of publicly administered health care in Canada; there need not be a fundamental conflict between respect for an individual's right to health care and sound choices in public policy.

Donna Greschner's essay tackles the current and likely future effect the Charter will have on the Canadian health care system, with specific emphasis on the Charter's potential as a 'cost-driver' within the health care system (i.e., the possibility of court decisions to increase overall health care costs without reference to the competing policy priorities of governments both within and outside the health care system). Greschner's analysis demonstrates that, to date, the Charter has had little direct influence on the costs of the health care system and that the judiciary has been reluctant to cavalierly override the decisions taken by policy-makers with regard to the organization of the health care system. The one exception to this is the successful challenge to the British Columbia government's attempt to restrict access to billing numbers for physicians in an attempt to encourage a greater number of doctors to practise in smaller communities. But the Supreme Court of Canada has itself rejected the reasoning presented in those cases by the B.C. Supreme Court.

It is clear, however, that the Charter's impact on health policy decision-making has only begun to be felt. As is the case in other areas of public policy, it will be increasingly incumbent upon policymakers to perform a 'Charter-check' on proposed reforms or restructuring of the health care system to insure that such proposals do not run contrary to the existing body of Charter jurisprudence. In particular, governments that attempt to 'delist' previously insured services could find themselves subject to review by the courts. This could pose significant political problems for processes such as that initiated by the Government of Alberta following the release of the Mazankowski Report (Alberta 2001), which called for a systematic review of insured services with an eye to identifying presumably some range of services that could be de-insured.

As Greschner herself argues, the potential for Charter-based challenges to health policy decisions should force governments to be very clear about the rationale for future decisions concerning which facilities to continue to operate, which services might be delisted, or, perhaps more importantly, which services and therapies are to be added to provincial health care insurance plans. For example, a decision to not list a specific drug on a provincial formulary will need to be based on scientifically sound evidence concerning the effectiveness and efficiency of that drug such that the decision can be seen as a reasonable limit on a person's perceived right to the drug of their choice at public expense. As the Commission itself pointed out in its final report, the capacity of governments to make these kinds of evidence-based decisions is, in many instances, clearly lacking and raises the question of whether, in the absence of such evidence, that the language of rights will, by default, become the trump card in future health care debates.

The Intergovernmental Context

The four essays in this section of the volume cover a great deal of ground in their examination of Canadian intergovernmental relations as it relates to health care. Réjean Pelletier's essay examines the kinds of intergovernmental relations that can be deemed the most productive in a federation like Canada, where intrastate federalism has clearly failed to accommodate the provincial and regional variations that are themselves a key rationale for a federal state. Antonia Maioni's historical and contemporary overview of how governments have exercised their responsibilities with regards to health care provides further insight into how the divided authority over health care outlined by Braën and Leeson can be better managed on the political front. Candace Johnson's essay serves as an important bridge between Donna Greschner's examination of Charter jurisprudence and the essays that follow on the future governance of the system. Johnson examines how contemporary intergovernmental relations must confront the dynamics of rights, civil society, and bioethical reflection on both what the health care system can and should do for citizens. Finally, Louis Imbeau, Kina Chenard, and Adriana Dudas examine the current intergovernmental debate on the sustainability of the health care in terms of the short-sighted nature of governments' current preoccupation with

deficit reduction and debt repayment and the limitations of neo-classical economics to insure the intergenerational equity that is a hallmark
of the health care system.

As Pelletier notes, federalism rests on the division of sovereignty
between the national and subnational states which, in turn, requires
some set of processes and mechanisms to be put into place to manage
the relations between each order of government. These mechanisms
can take the form of providing the subnational units with formal or
informal representation in the political institutions of the central state
(known as intrastate federalism) as in the German federation, or
through either formal or informal negotiations on a government-to-
government basis (known as interstate federalism), which has tended
to be the Canadian approach. Although the Senate was intended to be
a vehicle to promote intrastate federalism in Canada, Pelletier is hardly
alone in noting that it has failed to play that role in any effective manner and, as such, he focuses primarily on Canada's recent history of
interstate federalism.

What makes Pelletier's essay important is the significant attention
he pays to comparing and contrasting the different kinds of intergovernmental mechanisms that exist not only in the health care field but
also in different policy areas. The ability of governments in Canada to
reach agreements that commit them to common goals while preserving
provincial and regional differences can be seen in Pelletier's examination of both the 1997 agreement on labour training, which he character-
izes as a prime example of asymmetric federalism, and the Internal
Trade Agreement of 1994, which exemplifies as an essentially interprovincial federalism. He is, however, highly critical of the Social Union
Framework Agreement (SUFA) to which the government of Quebec is
not a party. While the SUFA is virtually unknown by the Canadian
public, it has been the subject of significant academic interest – but
little consensus – on whether it embodies a workable framework to
guide governmental and intergovernmental social policy making
and its articulation of a particular kind of federalism (Robson and
Schwanen 1999; Gagnon and Segal 2000; Lazar 2000; Marchildon 2000;
McIntosh 2002). In the final analysis, Pelletier points to the need for the
rhetoric around 'cooperative federalism' to move away from merely
the gaining of provincial assent for Ottawa's policy priorities towards
the development of intergovernmental mechanisms that recognizes the
equality of the participants and that incorporates substantive negotiation about priorities and policy directions.

Maioni's essay provides a detailed analysis of the historical and contemporary intergovernmental dynamics in the health care field. Indeed, for Maioni, federalism and intergovernmental relations prove to be double-edged swords. On the one hand, Canada's federal system was a source of innovation in health policy while, on the other hand, the dynamics of Canadian intergovernmental relations has also delayed needed health policy reforms. Like Pelletier, Maioni points to a reaffirmation of those positive aspects of federalism that created Canada's public health care system – a respect for regional and provincial autonomy and innovation coupled with a national vision of health care as a public good to be protected from coast to coast to coast – as key to insuring the system's political sustainability. In particular, the federal government's role needs to change from its current stance of being the enforcer of the 'rules' laid out in the Canada Health Act, to one where its focus is on enabling necessary reforms within provincial systems that are consistent with a vision of health care as a national public good to be preserved. The temptation of the federal government to micromanage provincial health policy needs to be resisted, in Maioni's view, if the dynamism and innovation that characterized the first decades of Canada's public health care system are to be recaptured.

Interestingly, Candace Johnson reaches similar conclusions in her essay, but she launches her analysis from a vantage point outside the federal-provincial dynamics explored by Pelletier and Maioni. Johnson focuses on changes underway outside the federal-provincial arena – within the health care system proper and within society more generally – to argue that the current structure of intergovernmental relations is proving itself unable to cope with the kinds of changes underway in the external environment and that this inability to cope with change poses a threat to the system's operation. The upshot for Johnson is that the current intergovernmental regime – characterized by federal unilateralism and ongoing debates over the federal government's relative share of provincial health care costs – has hindered the health care system's ability to effectively incorporate a respect for the increased diversity of Canadian society and address the health care needs of diverse citizenship. It has also prevented the system from responding to the increased demands for citizen participation in health care decision-making and from engaging in the kinds of serious bioethical debates that medical and scientific advances necessitate. Following Tuohy (1999), Johnson demonstrates that while the system, by some accounts, can be seen as 'stable,' it is probably more aptly characterized as 'static.' And this stasis results in the system's inability to respond to the need for real innovation and change in light of societal, medical, and technological transformations. The problem, Johnson asserts, lies with an intergovernmental dynamic that has become increasingly dysfunctional and that is unable to deal with the dynamic nature of health care in the twenty-first century.

Imbeau, Chenard, and Dudas provide a complementary but very different line of analysis to the current state of intergovernmentalism articulated by Johnson, Pelletier, and Maioni. Moving away from a focus on the formal and informal mechanisms of intergovernmental relations in Canada, Imbeau, Chenard, and Dudas examine the sustainability of Canada's health care system from the perspective of the changing domestic and international political economy, and look at how changes in these realms have played themselves out in the Canadian political and intergovernmental arenas with regard to health care. The authors argue that the current focus on deficit reduction and debt repayment – at the provincial, federal and international level – has undermined the health care system's ability to meet the current health needs of citizens and, perhaps more importantly, has compromised intergenerational equity (i.e., the system's ability to meet the health needs of future generations), which is itself an often neglected component of the health care bargain. The political emphasis on budgetary restraint at the provincial level has increased calls for wider-scale private sector involvement in provincial health care systems which, when coupled with similar cuts to federal transfers to the provinces in the 1990s (themselves a result of a desire to impose 'fiscal discipline' on federal and provincial budgets), have stymied those health care reform proposals aimed at improving quality and equity within the system.

Taken together, these four essays present a troubling picture of Canadian intergovernmental relations, especially in regard to the governance of health care. Whatever the differences in interpretation and emphasis between the essays, it is clear that they share a consensus that the current mechanisms lack the capacity to cope with the overall management and direction-setting for the system and with the design and implementation of the kinds of reforms that have been proposed for the system of late. In effect, the essays point to a kind of intergovernmental dead end whereby debates over roles, responsibilities, and funding have crowded out serious discussion about the system's reform, its future structure, and its ability to integrate new and important social and economic transformations.

The Social and Regulatory Context

The final grouping of contributions to this volume explores the governance of the health care system from outside the constitutional and intergovernmental contexts described above. Although their focus is much more on the health care system itself, the authors do not ignore the intergovernmental dynamics in their analyses nor, as is the case in Colleen Flood and Sujit Choudhry's essay, do they fail to recognize that changes to the governance of the health care system must take into account the overall health of the intergovernmental regime in which it exists.

John Lavis's examination of the role that particular political elites have on the process of health care reform fills a significant gap in our understanding of the dynamics that surround health reform initiatives. While much is made in both the popular press and in some academic literature of the influence that some organized interests play in the health reform debate, there has been little sustained analysis of how some of these groups interact to facilitate or to derail health reform initiatives in Canada.

Lavis focuses on the role that federal government officials, physicians associations, and hospital associations play in the making of the 'core' political bargains that underpin the publicly financed and administered health care system – namely, the 'private practice/public payment' system for physician services and the 'private-not-for-profit/public payment' system for hospital services. His thorough analysis of the existing case-study literature about the influence these officials and organizations have demonstrates that all three have the ability to effectively prevent any proposed change to those core political bargains that would conceivably threaten their autonomy or decision-making capacity. Interestingly, hospital organizations, except perhaps in Ontario, have seen their influence on the health reform debate weakened considerably through the process of regionalizing the governance of health service delivery over the past few decades. It should be pointed out, though, that this process may itself create a new locus of influence centred on the larger regional health authorities within a given province that, over time, may organize to protect a self-defined set of economic and political interests.

At the same time, neither the officials nor the organizations under examination has, either individually or collectively, an absolute veto over health reform. And as Lavis himself warns, the organizations themselves are influenced by public opinion, research knowledge, and political dynamics that both limit and change their influence over time. The future for health care reform rests not only on establishing a renewed commitment to the core political bargains that underpin the system but also, Lavis argues, on ensuring that other groups have access to the knowledge, expertise, and organizational capacity necessary to balance the influence of these political elites.

Indeed, this is the theme picked up by Steven Tomblin in his esssay about the role of public participation and citizen engagement in the design and implementation of future health reform initiatives. Tomblin recognizes the past constraints that have been placed on effective citizen participation in health reform debates – including the influence of the political elites identified by Lavis – and articulates concrete proposals that would, in his view, facilitate the empowerment of new actors within the health reform debate who could provide effective vehicles for the democratization of health reform decision-making. In short, Tomblin's analysis rests on the development of a new Canada-wide commission that would provide better and more complete information and evidence to actors within the health care system and encourage citizen participation in and oversight of health policy decisions.

But as Pascale Lehoux ably demonstrates, the need for rethinking the governance of health policy decision-making is not limited to the need for a more open and democratic process. Governments themselves have to give serious thought to reconceptualizing their own regulatory regimes that control specific aspects of the system, which are linked to the kind of evidence and information dissemination identified by Lavis and Tomblin. In tackling the complex manner in which governments in Canada identify and evaluate new technology within the health care system, Lehoux identifies the deficiencies of the current regulatory regimes in place and argues that these deficiencies leave governments with little ability to identify the relative costs and benefits of new technologies. The problem for both governments and citizens, of course, is that these new technologies are important cost-drivers within the contemporary system and that without an effective means of evaluating and regulating their integration into the system then both governments and citizens are at the mercy of those who develop technological innovations for the assessment of their effectiveness. Indeed, the development of a more critical perspective about the efficacy of technological developments by both citizens and governments is key, for Lehoux, to the rational integration of new technologies within the ever-changing health care landscape.

The final essay in the volume returns, in some respects, to the kinds of governance questions raised by the earlier essays insofar as it provides a sustained argument for a 'modernized' Canada Health Act as the legislative basis for a reformed health care system. Recognizing the important symbolic and substantive role that the CHA plays in the governance of health care system, Flood and Choudhry provide a series of recommendations designed to take into account changes that have occurred within the system since its introduction in the 1980s and to facilitate future health care reforms. Of particular importance is the need for the system to restore confidence in the public that they will receive treatment in a timely manner – the provision of which will itself forestall pressures to further privatize both the financing and delivery of health care services. As with Tomblin, the authors argue for a permanent national commission to act as both an information clearing-house and to deal with intergovernmental disputes over the interpretation and enforcement of the principles of the CHA.

Despite the very different subjects covered by each of the essays in this section, they share a common concern with finding concrete vehicles for restructuring the governance of the health care system in a manner that would not only serve to break the log-jam that currently exists within the intergovernmental arena but would also seek to do so in a manner that, while sensitive to the realities of the federal-provincial dimension of health care reform, is more concerned with elevating the role of the citizen in the decision-making processes.

Governance and the Romanow Commission

As was noted at the outset, the final report of the Romanow Commission highlighted the need to rethink and restructure the governance of the health care system in some very fundamental ways. Indeed, it would be fair to say that it was the inability of the current intergovernmental regime to tackle some of the more pressing problems of the health care system and growing public dissatisfaction with the intergovernmental disputes that was a key motivation for the appointment of the commission in the first instance. For some, however, the key problem has not been one of governance, but rather one of financing the system. The acrimonious debate between the federal and provincial governments in recent yeas has been a result of federal underfunding of the system in the years since the creation of the Canada Health and Social Transfer (CHST).

Although it is true that the unilateralism that characterized the introduction of the CHST did a great deal to damage intergovernmental relations in Canada and has, as the commission recognizes, created a dynamic whereby provinces are put in the position of arguing for annual increases in the transfer (Commission 2002c, 39), there is an even more fundamental concern that needs to be addressed. The inability of the intergovernmental and other governance mechanisms to find effective means to manage the inevitable conflicts that is part and parcel of a diverse federal state points clearly to the shortcomings of the governance regime itself.

The commission's recommendations begin quite clearly with an acceptance of the basic premises put forward by Braën and Leeson. In short, there is no 'exclusive' jurisdiction over either health or health care and both orders of government have legitimate and important roles to play. At the same, it is clear that the primary responsibility for the delivery of health care services lies with the provincial governments and that the federal government's legitimate exercise of its spending power as a lever used in the creation and maintenance of certain national elements across the system does not translate into a legitimate right (or even the ability) to micromanage provincial health care systems.

That being said, the financing of the system (and especially the size and nature of the federal transfer) and the dysfunction of the governance regime are inextricably linked. Thus, in restructuring the financing of the system the commission needed to simultaneously rethink both the intergovernmental relationship around health care and to take seriously the need to make all aspects of the system's governance both more accountable and more democratic. As both Mendelsohn (2002) and the Citizen's Dialogue processes (Commission 2002a) demonstrated, the Canadian public is increasingly concerned about the sustainability of the health care system as well as that system's ability to provide timely access to necessary health care services. There is an increasing unease among Canadians that the system is falling further and further behind in meeting their health care needs, that the reforms that have been recommended time and again over the past decades have not been implemented, and that the response of each order of government has been to blame the other for the system's ills.

For the commission then, a first step in restoring public confidence and setting a new tone for the governance regime within the system was the proposed Health Covenant – a declaration on the part of governments which articulated the entitlements and responsibilities of governments, citizens, and actors within the system. The Covenant will not, in all likelihood, solve the kinds of democratic and participatory problems identified by people like Johnson and Tomblin. It was designed as a formal statement to Canadians to recognize that they have both entitlements and responsibilities within the system and that the preservation (and the expansion) of the system is ultimately a political act that will depend on their ability and willingness to hold governments, managers, and health professionals accountable for the system's operation.

At the same time, the commission avoided positing the Covenant in a manner that would make it justiciable by the courts. As such, the Covenant will undoubtedly be criticized as being more symbolic than substantive insofar as it does not articulate a formal process by which citizens can hold governments (or health providers) accountable for the system's shortcomings. The commission's caution reflects the kinds of concerns noted above about the capacity of the judiciary to make the kinds of resource-allocation decisions normally left to elected officials. But it must also be admitted that, as Greschner argues, there is a strong connection between the values embodied in the Charter and those embodied in the health care system. That there may be risks in recognizing a constitutional 'right' to health care that is enforceable by the courts is undeniable, but insofar as the courts recognize the congruity between the values of the Charter and the health care system itself there could also be significant benefits to such an entrenchment.

In the era of the Charter and the growing reliance on the courts to resolve public policy disputes that governments are unwilling or unable to tackle themselves, it remains to be seen whether a document like the Covenant will either resonate with Canadians or be respected by governments or health care providers. There is, unarguably, a need to restore public confidence and a sense of public ownership or stewardship over the system. The courts can protect a person's rights and can presumably insure that particular services are delivered in particular instances. In this manner, at least, the courts can insure some accountability. And there is no doubt that Canadians have embraced the Charter as a key means by which to protect their rights from government infringement. But the Covenant is an attempt to articulate a different kind of accountability and to inculcate, for want of a better word, a healthier relationship between citizens, providers, and governments that rests on the values of solidarity and a shared sense of purpose. Emmett Hall proposed a similar document in the report that led to the development of medicare (Canada 1964), and it is worth pondering whether things would be different now if governments had taken up that particular recommendation.

Linked to the Covenant is the commission's recommendation to create a national Health Council that would provide analysis and advice to governments on an ongoing basis. The council would be explicitly designed as an intergovernmental body with a large majority of its membership coming from the provinces. This would differentiate it from the similar body proposed by the recent Senate committee report (Senate 2002). In assuming responsibility for much of the ongoing and ad-hoc intergovernmental activity already being undertaken around health care and building on existing intergovernmental bodies such as the Canadian Institute of Health Information (CIHI) and the Canadian Coordinating Office for Health Technology Assessment (CCOHTA), the council would not act as a federal body to 'watch over' the provinces and insure their observance of the 'rules of the game' but as a forum for the kinds of intergovernmental collaboration and cooperation that Pelletier, Maioni, and Johnson feel is necessary for the restoration of public confidence in the system.

Given the constitutional reality of the provinces' central role in the design and delivery of health services, the council could be an effective means of intergovernmental collaboration if its very structure (and indeed its future mandate) was designed to reflect that reality. This is not to remove the federal government from the equation but to insure that the council operates on a premise of greater equality among the partners involved.

In the final analysis, the recommendations presented by the commission probably do not create the fully participatory governance regime envisioned by some of the contributors to this volume. Although the commission refers to the potential for the council to act as a facilitator for increased citizen engagement in health care decision-making and to the role the council could play in providing reliable and objective evidence about the system to aid citizens in making health-related choices, neither of these functions is fully fleshed out in the body of the report. For obvious reasons, the commission's report focuses on laying the groundwork for what will be a much larger process of changing the dynamics currently at work within the intergovernmental arena.

As many of the contributors make clear in their essays, the current governance regime, in both its intergovernmental and citizen-state dimensions, is deeply flawed. Neither the formal nor informal intergovernmental mechanisms currently in place appear capable of focusing the necessary attention on making significant reform to the manner in which the system is organized, financed, or governed. Citizens are feeling increasingly shutout of the decision-making process at a time when their concern about the future viability of the system is growing.

If there is a single theme that resonates through the contributions to this volume – and which is itself a call for more and deeper analysis – it is that the governance of the system has become locked in a cycle of mutual recrimination, blame-assigning, and blame-avoidance. This applies not only to the actions of the federal and provincial governments (where it is, however, most visible) but also to the managers and health professionals within the system who jealously guard their traditional perquisites and roles while demanding that the other actors change their behaviour. And it applies to citizens who must accept not only their entitlements within the system but also their responsibility to use the system wisely, and who must exercise their democratic responsibility to hold managers, health professionals, governments, and their fellow citizens accountable for the system's sustainability.

REFERENCES

Alberta. 2001. *A Framework for Reform: Report of the Premier's Advisory Council on Health*. Edmonton: Premier's Advisory Council on Health.

Banting, Keith, and Robin Boadway. 2001. 'Dimensions of Choice: The Role of the Federal Government in Health Care.' Background paper prepared for the Commission on the Future of Health Care in Canada as part of the Fiscal Federalism and Health Research Project. Kingston: Institute of Intergovernmental Relations, Queen's University.

Black, Edwin R. 1975. *Divided Loyalties*. Montreal: McGill-Queen's University Press.

Canada. 1964. *Royal Commission on Health Services*. Volumes 1 and 2. Ottawa: Royal Commission on Health Services.

Commission. 2002a. *Report on Citizens' Dialogue on the Future of Health Care in Canada*. Prepared for the Commission on the Future of Health Care in Canada by J. Maxwell, K. Jackson and B. Legowski (Canadian Policy Research Networks), S. Rosell and D. Yankelovich (Viewpoint Learning) in collaboration with P.-G. Forest and L. Lozowchuk (Commission on the Future of Health Care in Canada). Saskatoon: Commission on the Future of Health Care in Canada.

– 2002b. *Shape the Future of Health Care: Interim Report*. Saskatoon: Commission on the Future of Health Care in Canada.

– 2002c. *Building on Values: The Future of Health Care in Canada – Final Report*. Saskatoon: Commission on the Future of Health Care in Canada.

Gagnon, Alain, and Hugh Segal, eds. 2000. *The Canadian Social Union without Quebec: Eight Critical Analyses*. Montreal: Institute for Research on Public Policy.

Lazar, Harvey. 2000. 'The Social Union Framework Agreement and the Future of Fiscal Federalism.' In *Toward a New Mission Statement for Canadian Fiscal Federalism, Canada: The State of the Federation, 1999–2000*, Harvey Lazar, ed., 99–128. Kingston: SPS/McGill-Queen's University Press.

Lazar, Harvey, and Tom McIntosh. 1998. *Federalism, Democracy and Social Policy: Towards a Sectoral Analysis of the Social Union*. Kingston: Institute of Intergovernmental Relations, Queen's University.

Marchildon, Gregory P. 2000. 'Reply to Ryan and Burelle: A Step in the Right Direction.' *InRoads* 9: 124–33.

McIntosh, Tom. 2000. 'Governing Labour Market Policy: Canadian Federalism, The Social Union and a Changing Economy.' In *Federalism, Democracy and Labour Market Policy*, Tom McIntosh, ed., 1–28. Kingston: SPS/McGill-Queen's University Press, 2000.

– ed. 2002. *Building the Social Union: Perspectives, Directions and Challenges*. Regina: Canadian Plains Research Center.

Mendelsohn, Matthew. 2002. *Canadians' Thoughts on Their Health Care System: Preserving the Canadian Model through Innovation*. Saskatoon: Commission on the Future of Health Care in Canada.

Robson, William B.P., and Daniel Schwanen. 1999. 'The Social Union Framework Agreement: Too Flawed to Last.' C.D. Howe Backgrounder. Toronto: C.D. Howe Institute.

Senate. 2002. *The Health of Canadians: The Federal Role. Final Report on the Health Care System in Canada*. Volume 6: *Recommendations for Reform*. Ottawa: Senate Standing Committee on Social Affairs, Science and Technology.

Tuohy, Carolyn Hughes. 1999. *Accidental Logics: The Dynamics of Change in the Health Care Arena in the United States, Britain and Canada*. New York: Oxford University Press.

Watts, Ronald L. 1999. *Comparing Federal Systems*. 2d ed. Kingston: Institute of Intergovernmental Relations, Queen's University.

PART I

THE CONSTITUTIONAL CONTEXT

1 Health and the Distribution of Powers in Canada

ANDRÉ BRAËN

When the Canadian union was formed in 1867, health care was primarily the concern of religious or charitable organizations and individuals. It was only gradually, and in particular after the Second World War, that the role of the State – both federally and provincially – began to expand in the field of social health. With the cost of health services on the rise, governments appeared to be a good way to provide Canada with a system of publicly accessible health services. Today, the implementation and especially the maintenance of a viable and accessible public system of quality health care remain priorities for Canadian society. Against the backdrop of an aging population, rapidly escalating costs, the remarkable growth of scientific research and medical technology, and rising expectations, crucial questions are being raised that deal with the need for sufficient and sustainable funding, the availability and universality of care, and the development of related human resources.

In Canada, federal and provincial governments are important actors in this field. Needing to reflect on the various issues involved and determined to play an important role, the federal government established the Commission on the Future of Health Care in Canada. The Commission's mandate is to recommend to the Canadian government the policies and measures needed to ensure the long-term viability of a publicly funded, universally accessible health care system. However, this exercise must take into account the distribution of powers and jurisdiction in Canada. Accordingly, four main research themes were identified by the Commission: (1) Canadian values; (2) viability; (3)

cooperation among the main public and private stakeholders in the field of health; and (4) management of change.

This was the context in which I was invited to prepare a study on the constitutional distribution of powers in the area of health and health services. The objective of my study was to inform the Commission about the legal principles underlying the role of each level of government in this area and about their development and transformation. Generally, this involved verifying the historical and legal origins of the assignment and distribution of powers among the various levels of government in Canada in the field of health. Specifically, I was required to verify (a) the constitutional bases of both the provincial and federal roles in the area of health; (b) the constitutional basis of the federal spending power as it relates to health; (c) the effect, if any, which the Charter of Rights and Freedoms has had on the distribution of powers; and (d) changes in the role played by both the federal and provincial governments in the field of health. For comparative purposes, I was also asked to look at the situation in other federations.[1]

Canadian constitutional law, and, in particular, the Constitution Act, 1867, distributes legislative authority between the Parliament of Canada and the legislature of each province. Generally, it is the provinces that play the primary role in the field of health services; thus, I will analyse the constitutional provisions that authorize this role before considering those that form the basis of the federal role. In Canada, the courts are the guardians of the constitutional order. Consequently, my analysis of the constitutional enactments takes into account the judicial decisions rendered in this field. I also consider the situation in other federations. But to begin with, I take a detailed look at the difficulties in defining our subject, namely 'health,' and the consequences from a legal analysis standpoint. I also examine the historical context in which Canada's public health care system developed and, for introductory purposes, the principal rules of interpretation that should be adopted concerning the constitutional enactments. Finally, I look at the impact that the Charter might have on the assignment of powers in the field.

Constitutional Distribution of Powers

Difficulties Defining Our Terms

The Canadian Constitution assigns, exclusively in most cases, to the Parliament of Canada or the legislature of a province the authority to make laws in all matters coming within the classes of subjects enumerated therein (Constitution Act, 1867, ss. 91, 92). The constitutional assignment of authority for health was not, as such, covered by a specific provision. In fact, nowhere in the Constitution is there mention of the authority to make laws in the matter of 'health,' 'health services,' or 'health care.' The word 'health,' as defined in *The Canadian Oxford Dictionary* (1988), refers to 'the state of being well in body or mind or a person's mental or physical condition.' In French the word 'santé' is also defined in relation to the state of being well in body and mind (*Petit Robert*, 10th ed.).

This amorphous nature of 'health' was not lost on the Supreme Court of Canada in *Schneider v. The Queen*:

> In sum 'health' is not a matter which is subject to specific constitutional assignment but instead is an amorphous topic which can be addressed by valid federal or provincial legislation, depending in the circumstances of each case on the nature or scope of the health problem in question. (142, Estey J.)

It is easy to see that actions taken in the public realm that could affect or change human welfare or equilibrium, either directly or indirectly, can take an infinite number of forms and rest on disparate constitutional foundations. For example, a measure aimed primarily at protecting the environment could ultimately have an impact on this welfare. As we will see, several federal initiatives in the field of public health are based first and foremost on the authority of the Canadian Parliament in the field of criminal law. In short, health has many facets, which can fall under different areas of jurisdiction. In this study, I confine myself, from a content standpoint, to the contemporary conception of a public health care system, be it in terms of the structure of health care institutions or the provision of health services.

Historical and Legislative Background

Although the State has long been involved in certain public health issues (the elimination of epidemics, for example), in 1867 its activities in the field of health care proper were limited and undertaken in concert with religious or charitable organizations (see Canadian Bar Association 1994, 2–14, Swartz 1993, 219; Lajoie and Molinari 1978, 579). The Constitution Act, 1867, is a reflection of the times in its provisions that the provinces have authority over 'the establishment, maintenance, and management of hospitals, asylums, charities, and eleemosynary institutions in and for the province, other than marine hospitals' (s. 92(7)) and that the federal government has authority over 'quarantine and the establishment and maintenance of marine hospitals' (s. 91(11)). Personal health was seen by society, and therefore politicians, as a purely private matter (Canadian Bar Association 1994, 3).

It was only as mind-sets began to change that the State gradually stepped in to adopt social measures, and that the idea for a health insurance program began to form in Canada's political consciousness (ibid.).[2] During the Second World War, a proposal for a provincial health insurance plan subsidized by the Dominion was put forth but rejected. A federal cost-sharing plan in this field was also rejected in 1945 (ibid.).[3] It was not until 1957 that the Canadian Parliament passed the Hospital Insurance and Diagnostic Services Act (S.C. 1957, c. 8). By 1961, all the provinces had climbed aboard with their own hospital insurance plans. In response to the Royal Commission on Health Services, Parliament passed the Medical Care Act in 1966 (S.C. 1966–7, c. 64).[4] Clearly, the purpose of both Acts was to share between the two levels of government the costs of implementing a public plan for hospitalization and medical care.

The federal government acted as a catalyst for the implementation in Canada of provincial health services plans, intervening through direct programs or, more often, transfer programs and conditional grants. It was within this system that the provinces put in place their public health care plans (Dupéré 1987, 2–3). The cost-sharing formula was amended a few times.[5] In 1984, the Canada Health Act (CHA; R.S.C. 1984, c. C-6) merged the 1957 legislation on hospital insurance with the 1966 legislation on medical care. Sections 7–12 of the CHA listed the eligibility criteria that provincial plans needed to meet in order to qualify for federal grant money: public administration, comprehensiveness, universality, portability, and accessibility. Subsequently, financial difficulties led the federal government to slash its financial contributions to the provincial plans. It should be pointed out that in moulding the provincial health care plans, the federal government did not alter the constitutional assignment or distribution of powers, and that it carved out for itself an active and very important role in this field (Canadian Bar Association 1994, 12).

Principles of Interpretation

The constitutional provisions dealing with distribution of powers are, in and of themselves, insufficient and too imprecise to allow a determination of the tasks that might fall to each level of government in the field of health. They must be supplemented with the decisions rendered by the courts that had to interpret them. Indeed, in the final analysis, it is the courts that are called on to interpret a legislative or constitutional provision and assign it meaning, content, and scope. In terms of distribution of powers, the courts have endeavoured to verify the true nature of legislative provisions whose validity was contested from a constitutional standpoint. To do so, they have set out several principles that we should touch on (see Brun and Tremblay 1997, 457–75; Hogg 2001, 387–99).

First, the constitutional provisions governing distribution of powers, in particular sections 91 and 92 of the Constitution Act, 1867, must be interpreted in the light of the federative intent underlying Canada's political and legal system. Second, these provisions must not be interpreted literally and in isolation, but in relation to one another by means of a correlative interpretation. It is the entire body of legislative jurisdiction that is distributed in this manner through the Constitution and, consequently, any matter can be governed by one or the other level of government. In theory, the jurisdiction assigned to a level of government is exclusive to that level and cannot be encroached on by the other, whether the incumbent government has exercised it or not.[6] There are, however, limits to this principle. A question can have two facets, with one coming under federal and the other under provincial jurisdiction. In addition, while exercising its powers in a valid manner, one legislature can produce an incidental affect on a matter that falls under the jurisdiction of the other. At the same time, as the distribution of legislative jurisdiction was explicitly set out, the distribution of the ensuing executive powers was also set out, implicitly.[7]

In order to confirm that a statute is valid in terms of division of powers, the courts examine its true nature. By analysing the actual objectives pursued by the statute under challenge and by taking into account – where appropriate but not necessarily – the effects it produces, the courts seek to verify the question to which the statute pertains and to identify which level of government holds the jurisdiction. If there is incompatibility between two constitutionally valid statutes, one federal and the other provincial, the federal statute prevails.

Impact of the Charter

The Charter guarantees the rights and freedoms it sets out. Exceptions to and limits on these rights and freedoms are possible only to the extent permitted.[8] Legislators, as well as the federal and provincial governments, are bound by it in all areas coming under their jurisdiction. On this level, the main effect of the Charter is to limit State sovereignty. That is why the federal or provincial State, in the exercise of its legislative and executive functions, cannot undermine it. Since it is a constitutional enactment, it applies to matters of both federal and provincial jurisdiction. Consequently, the distribution of powers between the two levels of government has no effect on the Charter, since the latter has no effect on the distribution of powers. One could not, for example, invoke the equality rights set out in section 15 of the Charter to contest before the courts a distinction that might exist between two provincial schemes.[9] Indeed, the Charter cannot be invoked in such a way as to amend the distribution of powers (Brun and Tremblay 1997, 886).

So we see that the Charter limits legislators' sovereignty and does not affect the distribution of powers as such. But it is in the exercise of these powers that its effects are felt. Thus, a legislative measure or the exercise of jurisdiction by a government entity may be challenged from the standpoint of its compatibility with the Charter. As in any other sector of activity, challenges based on the Charter can be the subject of legal proceedings. In terms of content, the Charter does not confer on individuals any right to health (Canadian Bar Association 1994, 21–9). But other provisions can be invoked. For example, the Supreme Court of Canada in *Eldridge v. British Columbia (A.G.)* ruled that a hospital, even if it is a private organization,[10] controlled by the provincial government and implementing the policies of this government, must comply with the Charter and can be required on the basis of the equality rights set out in section 15 to offer sign-language interpretation services to its patients who are hard of hearing. Similarly, if the federal government offers services to the public in the field of health, in so doing it must comply with section 20 of the Charter and make them accessible in both official languages. In its negotiations with the provinces on the public health care system, in accordance with the principle of linguistic duality (sec. 16 of the Charter), and in its commitments under the Official Languages Act (S.C. 1988, c. 38),[11] it must take all necessary measures in this regard to enhance the vitality of the official languages wherever they are found.

Constitutional Basis of the Provincial Role

When it comes to health, the provinces hold the front lines. If the constitutional enactments did not assign specific authority for health, it was because in 1867 health was seen as a private matter. Public authorities intervened only on an exceptional basis in response to emergencies caused by epidemics or by the need to undertake rudimentary public health measures in urban areas. Most of the time, these measures were ordered by city councillors. The Constitution Act, 1867, seemed to reflect this reality when some of its provisions assigned the province jurisdiction for hospitals (subsection 92(7)), matters of a local nature (subs. 92(16)), and municipal institutions (subs. 92(8)) (McKall 1975, 317–18). In fact, it was in making reference to these provisions that right from the start, case-law gave a very liberal interpretation to the provincial jurisdiction over health (Lajoie and Molinari 1978, 581–4). Thus, 'all matters concerning public health, with the exception of quarantine stations and marine hospitals, are within the exclusive purview of provincial legislation' (*Rinfret v. Pope*, 315).[12]

Relevant Provisions

Today, the exercise of provincial jurisdiction over health care is a multifaceted undertaking, with each of the provisions pertaining to a specific class of subjects listed in the Constitution Act, 1867. The most important are those which give the provinces exclusive authority to make laws in the following areas:

- 'the establishment, maintenance, and management of hospitals, asylums, charities, and eleemosynary institutions in and for the province, other than marine hospitals' (subs. 92(7));
- 'generally all matters of a merely local or private nature in the province' (subs. 92(16));
- 'property and civil rights in the province' (subs. 92(13)); and
- 'education' (sec. 93).

Taken individually or together, these provisions are seen as assigning the provinces primary authority for health, in the form of hospital or health care services, the practice of medicine, training of health professionals and regulation of their profession, hospital and health insurance, and occupational health (Beaudoin 1990, 509–12; Hogg 2001, 463–4; Gibson 1996, 1–5; Jackman 1996, 4; McKall 1975, 320–3; Brun and Tremblay 1997, 547; see also, in general, Lajoie and Molinari 1978).

Establishment and Management of Hospitals
Subsection 92(7) assigns the provinces specific jurisdiction over the establishment and administrative organization of the hospital system

(*In Re Shelley*). The public or private nature of an institution is of no import here; it is the provinces that determine their vocation and services. The only limit explicitly mentioned in this provision has to do with marine hospitals. The reason for this exception is that subsection 91(11) assigns the Parliament of Canada exclusive authority for quarantine and the establishment and maintenance of marine hospitals. It is on the basis of this jurisdiction that the courts have, among other things, confirmed the provinces' authority to make laws on detention of mentally ill persons (*Fawcett v. A.G. of Ontario & A.G. of Canada*), establishment of hospital therapeutic abortion committees (*Carruthers v. Therapeutic Abortion Committee*) and the right to strike and labour relations within a hospital (*C.E. Jamieson and Co. v. A.G. Canada*).

Matters of a Strictly Local or Private Nature

Some argue that subsection 92(16) is the basis on which the provinces are recognized as having general if not extensive jurisdiction over public health (Lajoie and Molinari 1978, 581, 597; Hogg 2001, 464). Indeed, it seems that health itself can be seen on the whole as a strictly local matter. If that is the case, it should be pointed out that such jurisdiction, as general as it is, cannot extend to the classes of subjects assigned exclusively to the federal domain.[13] In any event, in *Schneider v. The Queen*,[14] the Supreme Court of Canada upheld the constitutional validity of a British Columbia statute imposing drug treatment, basing its decision on, among other things, subsection 92(16). Drug dependency constitutes a local matter, even though, seen in a different light, it could come under criminal law.

Property and Civil Rights

It has already been determined that, from a constitutional standpoint, Canada's Parliament could not institute an unemployment insurance plan.[15] This program involves insurance and affected employers' and employees' civil rights. Consequently, subsection 92(13) was invoked to allow the provinces to establish a contributory health plan, be it a hospital, medical or drug insurance scheme, and to define its terms and conditions. In 1977, the Supreme Court of Canada in *Canadian Indemnity Co. v. A.G. British Columbia* upheld the provinces' authority to establish a compulsory, universal automobile insurance plan, basing its ruling on subsection 92(13). This applies as well to health insurance (Beaudoin 1990, 510). Also, the courts ruled very early on that, because they are based on contracts, trade and commerce within a province constitute a matter of private law coming under provincial jurisdiction, pursuant to subsection 92(13) (*Citizens Insurance Co. v. Parsons*). The provinces can, therefore, intervene in all the stages of the production and marketing of a product, and can also control its quality and quantity. For our purposes, this provincial jurisdiction comes into play for food products, drugs, and other health products.[16] But this authority is limited by the principle of extra-territoriality, which opens the door to federal intervention.[17] Last, and in a general sense, private law comes under provincial jurisdiction in accordance with subsection 92(13). Consequently, relations between a patient and a physician or with another health professional, and between a patient or physician and a hospital, constitute a matter coming under provincial authority, as do most questions of liability in contract and tort. The same is true of the establishment, regulation, and control of health professions, in particular the practice of medicine, as well as professional discipline and, in a general sense, the field of labour relations.[18]

Education
Section 93 of the Constitution Act, 1867, assigned the provinces exclusive authority to make laws in the area of education. University programs, diploma oversight, and proficiency tests in the field of health are all matters coming under provincial authority.[19] This authority also affords the provinces a role in the field of research.

Other Powers
A province's ability to intervene in the field of health is not limited to the specific jurisdictions already listed. In constitutional law, the exercise of its powers is also valid to the extent that such exercise can be tied in with any other area of jurisdiction explicitly set out in section 92 (Lajoie and Molinari 1978, 600). Accordingly, it was judged that under subsection 92(9), a province can impose a mandatory registration procedure for health professionals (*Ex Parte Fairbain*)[20] or assign professional associations the authority to impose fines and other penalties under subsection 92(15) (*Landers v. Dental Society (New Brunswick)*).[21] Its powers in the area of agriculture[22] (sec. 95), direct taxation (subs. 92(2)), or prisons and reformatories (subs. 92(15)) also afford it an incidental role in health (Beaudoin 1990, 510).

Constitutional Basis of the Federal Role

From a constitutional standpoint, we can see that health has been viewed by and large as a general envelope for which the provinces have primary responsibility. Today, however, the federal government is also very active in this area. It was when the Parliament of Canada became involved in social measures that the courts were called on to identify the constitutional basis for this intervention and to specify its limitations (Lajoie and Molinari 1978, 586). Except for an area of jurisdiction explicitly enumerated, federal authority over health matters generally derives from a triple source, namely, Parliament's authority to legislate in the area of criminal law, the federal government's spending power, and perhaps its authority to ensure peace, order, and good government (Canadian Bar Association 1994). For its part, the doctrine examines this question mainly to verify whether Parliament, from a constitutional standpoint and as the architect of a pan-Canadian public health-care scheme, can compel the provinces to comply with national standards that it, itself, sets.[23]

Relevant Provisions

Quarantine and Marine Hospitals
Subsection 91(11) assigns Parliament exclusive authority to make laws concerning 'quarantine and the establishment and maintenance of marine hospitals.' This explicit exception to provincial jurisdiction in this area is attributable to the fact that primary jurisdiction in marine matters was assigned to Parliament, particularly for navigation and the merchant marine (subs. 91(10)) and the naval service (subs. 91(7)).

Criminal Law
Subsection 91(27) assigns Parliament exclusive authority to legislate with regard to 'the criminal law, except the constitution of courts of criminal jurisdiction, but including the procedure in criminal matters.' This assignment must be viewed in its broadest sense.[24] The definition of criminal law is not rooted to a specific era or field; it evolves. The only characteristic common to all crimes is that they are prohibited and liable to sanction.[25] This jurisdictional assignment authorizes Parliament to prohibit, for either preventive or punitive purposes,[26] any act or behaviour and to impose sanctions for an offence; and it can proclaim new crimes.[27] But because a crime cannot be proclaimed in a void, it must be associated with situations deemed undesirable. In criminal law, federal statutes must not only decree a prohibition and sanctions, but they must also pursue an objective which is in the public realm and generally recognized in criminal law. In this regard, the

Supreme Court of Canada has already defined a public objective as being – and the list is not exhaustive – public peace, order, safety, *health*, and morality.[28] In addition, federal legislation must not constitute a specious encroachment upon provincial jurisdiction. Disguised legislation is not allowed under Canadian constitutional law (Brun and Tremblay 1997, 503).

From a constitutional standpoint, health occupies a grey area. Both Parliament and the provinces can intervene within their respective jurisdictions – hence the importance of highlighting the plenary nature of the jurisdiction that Parliament exercises in criminal law. It was determined that pursuant to this jurisdiction, Parliament may prohibit or control the manufacture, sale, and distribution of products posing a public health risk. Parliament may impose labelling and packaging requirements for hazardous products and warnings on cigarette packages.[29] Federal legislation on food and drugs is perfectly valid,[30] just as it is on narcotics.[31] Parliament is also authorized to criminalize abortion[32] and to ban the sale of furniture considered hazardous for children.[33] It can make it illegal to produce and sell hazardous products and therefore prohibit certain substances in food products.[34] But it may not impose standards on food composition, as this does not involve public health.[35] Similarly, the prohibition on the sale of margarine was not aimed at protecting public health; rather, this measure was aimed at protecting the dairy industry.[36] To sum up, if its jurisdiction in criminal law enables the federal government to play a significant role in public health protection, this single area of jurisdiction has little impact on the implementation and maintenance of a public health care scheme.

Spending Power
Generally, one level of government may spend in areas coming under the jurisdiction of the other. This can be likened to an owner exercising his or her power to dispose of property as he or she sees fit. But in so doing and from a constitutional standpoint, it must not attempt to control or regulate those areas that come under the other's jurisdiction (Brun and Tremblay 1997, 443–4; Hogg 2001, 163–73).[37] In the area of health, the federal government played a key role in implementing a public health care plan in all the provinces. To that end, it availed itself of its spending power. There is no explicit provision for this in the constitution. Rather, it derives from the manner in which these are interpreted, particularly the provisions of the Constitution Act, 1867, which deal with federal taxation power (subs. 91(3)), the authority to make

laws with regard to public property (subs. 91(1A)), and the power to appropriate federal funds (sec. 106) (Gibson 1996; Jackman 1977).[38]

Federal legislation, which provides for the allocation of funds in provincial areas through transfer or grant programs, sometimes contains conditions that must be observed by the provinces if they wish to receive this funding. To avoid regional disparities, lawmakers have often inserted into this legislation what is now called 'national standards.' In order to be constitutionally valid, the conditions must not alter the true substance of the statute or be tantamount to regulations governing a matter which comes under provincial jurisdiction. A province that enacts a law in order to conform to these standards is considered to be doing so of its own volition, since there is nothing obliging the province to do so from a legal standpoint.[39]

But can the contents of these conditions or 'national standards' alter the true nature of the federal statute in question and thus constitute a disguised attempt at regulating an area of provincial jurisdiction? As we know, the Canada Health Act contains conditions to which the provinces must adhere if they wish to remain eligible for federal funds. This legislation has never been challenged in the courts – one can understand why, from the provinces' viewpoint. But seen in a different light, the Supreme Court of Canada has already ruled that the simple withholding of funds by federal authorities in the event that a province fails to abide by the conditions prescribed in the federal statute does not in and of itself amount to regulating a provincial matter.[40] In *Winterhaven Stables Ltd. v. A.G. Canada*, the Alberta Court of Appeal ruled that pursuant to its spending power, Parliament may impose conditions while exercising this power, even if this creates pressure on the provinces to adapt their legislation accordingly. This does not amount to regulating a provincial matter. It was also stated that a distinction must be made in this field between the power to make laws and the power to enter into contracts. In the latter case, nothing would prevent the federal authorities from setting the conditions they want in an agreement or contract to which the provinces remain free to adhere (Hogg 2001, 166).[41]

In any case, federal activity in the field of health care is a clear affirmation of federal spending power. Obviously, the exercise of this power is generating enormous tension within the Canadian federal system. On the one hand, the Canadian government is acting on its commitment in section 36 of the Charter to provide all Canadians with reasonably comparable levels of public services at reasonably comparable levels of taxation. On the other hand, the provincial governments are demanding the right to fully exercise their sovereignty in this area. In this regard, a province does not really have the choice of accepting or refusing the conditions unilaterally put forth by the federal authorities. If a province refuses to participate in a federal initiative aimed at, say, implementing a new program, the taxpayers of that province would pay (through their federal taxes) for the program to be implemented in the participating provinces without being able to reap the benefits themselves. Thus the federal government's ability to use its spending power to influence provincial schemes and impose so-called national standards depends in large part on its financial wherewithal; this influence is likely to diminish in step with the decrease in federal transfers to the provinces, especially since a province may hesitate to implement a federal proposal, even a generously funded one, in the knowledge that a few years down the road the federal authorities may unilaterally decide to terminate their payments to the province. It should be pointed out that a disadvantage of such a system is that it creates some confusion in terms of accountability. Since maintaining existing programs and their quality depends on both provincial and federal funding, it becomes difficult to determine who is responsible for what, and when difficulties do arise, the two levels of government take turns passing the buck to one another.

Peace, Order, and Good Government
The introductory portion of section 91 of the Constitution Act, 1867, authorizes the Parliament of Canada 'to make laws for the peace, order, and good government of Canada.' Because the distribution of powers is comprehensive, this authority to make laws for peace, order, and good government is exercised in respect of all matters not coming within the classes of subjects assigned exclusively to the provinces or enumerated in section 91 (Brun and Tremblay 1997, 552–67; Hogg 2001, 421). This authority has been interpreted by case-law to comprise two elements. The first empowers Parliament to legislate in situations of emergency or national crisis. By its very nature, this authority can be exercised only on a temporary basis.[42] The second involves Parliament's ability to make laws on any matter that is in the interest of the federation as a whole. This is where the doctrine of national dimensions or national concern comes in.

In *R. v. Crown Zellerbach Canada Ltd.*,[43] the Supreme Court of Canada spelled out this theory of national interest.

1 The national concern doctrine ... is separate and distinct from the
   national emergency doctrine ...;
2 [The national concern doctrine] applies to both new matters which
   did not exist at Confederation and to matters which, although originally matters of a local or private nature in a province, have since,
   in the absence of national emergency, become matters of national
   concern;
3 For a matter to qualify as a matter of national concern in either sense
   it must have a singleness, distinctiveness and indivisibility that
   clearly distinguishes it from matters of provincial concern and a
   scale of impact on provincial jurisdiction that is reconcilable with the
   fundamental distribution of legislative power under the Constitution;
4 In determining whether a matter has the requisite singleness, distinctiveness and indivisibility, it is relevant to consider what would
   be the effect on extra-provincial interests of a provincial failure to
   deal effectively with the control or regulation of the intra-provincial
   aspects of the matter. (431–2, Le Dain J.)

The mere fact that a matter is of importance to the Canadian population as a whole does not necessarily mean that it has a national dimension nor makes it a national concern. The mere fact that health
insurance is perceived as a Canadian value does not alter its nature,
from a constitutional standpoint. In *A.G. Canada v. A.G. Ontario*, the
federal authorities' argument that unemployment insurance had
attained a national dimension was not upheld.[44] The merely local or
private nature of health constitutes an important basis for provincial
intervention in this area. But health also comprises aspects that come
under federal authority. Do certain aspects of the public health care
system – in particular national standards governing public administration, comprehensiveness, universality, portability, and accessibility –
constitute a matter possessing a singleness, distinctiveness, and indivisibility that make it distinct from provincial powers in this area?
More important, can a province's failure or inability to deal effectively
with these aspects inside its territory have an adverse effect on extra-
provincial interests? Some say that by virtue of this authority, the Parliament of Canada could indeed intervene in such areas as AIDS,
abortion, smoking, or foreigners' access to the medical profession (Gibson 1996, 19–24; Jackman 1996, 8–11). But all these aspects have no
bearing on the actual nature of today's health care system. The useful-

ness of the discussion lies, of course, in providing a basis for federal intervention without federal authorities necessarily having to use their spending power.

Other Powers
As in the case of a province, the federal government's ability to intervene in health matters also remains possible to the extent that such intervention can be associated with another area of jurisdiction expressly assigned to the Parliament of Canada by the Constitution Act, 1867. It is by virtue of their authority with regard to the militia, military and naval service, and defence (subs. 91(7)) that the federal authorities established and maintain veterans' hospitals. Parliament's exclusive jurisdiction over patents of invention and discovery (subs. 91(22)) and copyrights (subs. 91(23)) enables federal authorities to intervene in the area of scientific research and, more specifically, bio-medical, genetic, and pharmaceutical research. Parliament's jurisdiction over interprovincial and international trade enables the federal government to oversee exchanges of medical technology and of hospital equipment.

In the area of agriculture and immigration-related health matters, federal legislation prevails (sec. 95). In businesses that come under its jurisdiction, Parliament can regulate health and safety matters as well as labour relations (subs. 92(10)) (*Bell Canada v. Quebec*). The Constitution Act, 1871, enables it to exercise provincial health powers in federal territories (Beaudoin 1990, 501). Last, Parliament's authority with respect to Aboriginals, and lands reserved for them (subs. 91(24)), certainly enables federal authorities to deal with Aboriginal health matters (*R. v. Swimmer*). Curiously, federal authorities consider Aboriginal health matters to fall under provincial responsibility.[46]

Health in Other Federations

Contrary to unitary systems, a federal system distributes the exercise of internal sovereignty between a central State and member States. This model is adopted by a State because it constitutes a form of government adapted to its specific needs and characteristics. How have other federations gone about the task of distributing powers in the area of health? In this regard, the Canadian system is but one model among others, and all variations remain possible. Our purpose here is not to systematically review the manner in which other federal systems operate in this field. Rather, and for purposes of comparison, we would like to touch on and summarize a few experiences in other countries that might be of interest to Canada, in view of their level of economic development, their population and territory, and their proximity and influence.

Australia

At the time of Confederation in 1867, and influenced by the United States where the same thinking prevailed, Canada's population looked on health care as a private matter. During the same period, Australia took the opposite position. It was very receptive to European ideas in this field, which held that health care was a personal right; thus, public access to health care and hospitals seemed to go without saying. At a time when most Canadian hospitals were private and many were managed by religious communities, Australia already had a public hospital network (see Gray 1991, 26–49).

In the beginning, it was the federated States rather than the federal State which dispensed health services to the public. Responsibility for health stemmed from the residual jurisdiction vested in the federated States under the Australian Constitution, which assigned the federal State only the authority for quarantine. But the federal State's interest in promoting social measures led it to create a federal ministry of health in 1921 and to become more involved in setting health policy. It seems that the relationship between the two levels of government had been a collaborative one, all the more so since, unlike the Canadian provinces, the federated States were far more dependent on the central State for funding. Similarly, while Canada's politicians were concerned about removing financial barriers to access to health care, Australia was firmly committed to developing the actual provision of health services (Gray 1991, 50–2).

An amendment to the Constitution in 1943 specifically authorizes the federal State to adopt measures relating to pharmaceuticals, disease, and hospital, medical and dental services. Today both levels of government are concurrently and actively involved in the field of health, often in concert with local communities. Australia has a universal system of health benefits (Medicare) guaranteeing residents access to medical care and drugs at a reasonable cost, as well as free access to hospital care. Three-quarters of hospitals are public and their services are complemented by a network of private clinics. It is the federal State, with its exclusive authority to levy taxes, which funds the bulk of the system through a general tax and an income-related deduction for health insurance (Organization for Economic Cooperation and Development 1994, 59–61).

United States

The health care system in this country is relatively complex. It involves both the public sector, comprising the federal State, member States, and local communities, and the private sector, comprising insurance carriers and individual plans. Health care is dispensed locally within a loosely structured system. There is a free market when it comes to hospital services. There is no health planning at the federal level, although several reforms have been put forth with a view to controlling rising costs and improving accessibility to care. At the member States level, the role of the public authorities appears modest and is often limited to overseeing projects to create hospitals or health care centres. Most hospitals are managed by private, not-for-profit institutions, but some are owned by private, for-profit corporations or public authorities (OECD 1994, 343–7).

The United States does not have a general health insurance system. The public sector offers Medicare, a universal, national health insurance plan for seniors and persons with disabilities. The federal government manages this scheme, which serves about 13 per cent of the population. It is financed through a formula combining pay deductions, federal funds, and premiums. The public sector also operates Medicaid. This health insurance program is aimed at the disadvantaged and serves about 10 per cent of the population. Funding comes from the federal government and the federated States. Federal funding varies according to the federated State's wealth (between 50 and 83 per cent of the total). Medicaid is managed by the federated States, but this is done in accordance with federal guidelines on categories of recipients and the range of services covered. The federal authorities, the federated States, and the local communities also subsidize health care centres or hospitals for those most in need, or reimburse the institutions dispensing the care. But the vast majority of the public has recourse to the programs run by the private sector (OECD 1994).

Belgium

At the time of its founding in 1831, Belgium was a unitary State, but has become, following recent constitutional reforms, a highly decentralized federal State. It comprises, in addition to the federal government, three cultural communities (French, Flemish, and German), and three regions (Flemish, Walloon, and Brussels-Capital). The Constitution assigns the regions mainly economic powers; the regions are also involved in health and safety policies. The communities have exclusive jurisdiction over cultural matters, including education and 'personal matters' – the latter being matters closely linked with an individual's life within his or her community (Patenaude 1991, 21–39).

'Personal matters' encompass hospital and social services, which are organized and managed by the communities. The communities apply health policy, which comprises care delivery measures, health education, and preventive medicine activities and services. Individuals are required to join a mutual company, which reimburses the cost of services. But the federal government plays a very important role in the field of health through its financial support, public health initiatives, and, above all, regulation of access to and exercise of health professions (ibid.).

Conclusion

From a constitutional standpoint, primary responsibility for health services and care belongs to the provinces. The main reason for this is that the current public system is modelled after the insurance sector, a matter of ownership and civil rights in the provinces, and also because from very early on health was seen as a local or private matter. The creation and structuring of hospitals and health care centres, education, health professions, coverage of insured services, allocation and distribution of financial and medical resources are all sectors for provincial intervention. And it would appear that this is how it should be, to the extent that a province, because of its proximity to the population, is well acquainted with their real needs and seems to be the level of government most able to meet these needs.

But health, in view of the realities involved, definitely has elements that come under federal authority. The Canadian government intervenes in this field by means of specific powers. Its criminal law authority and, in particular, its spending power enable it to play an important role. While this spending power has not been challenged in the courts, it is nevertheless a source of tension. And although the Canadian Charter does not confer any right of access to health care, the fact remains that as things stand today, the Canadian public believes it has this right. In our opinion, the fact that access to health care constitutes a value in the eyes of Canadian society does not necessarily make it a matter of national concern, thereby opening the door to federal intervention in the interest of peace, order, and good government. Clearly, however, the federal authorities – if only because of their commitments – have an important role to play in this field.

The public health-care system is in the midst of a crisis. Increasingly, the decisions that must be taken in this regard involve governments' social policies and their financial situation. The rules of law can be used to identify who does what. They cannot, however, solve the problems currently plaguing the health care system. As in other federations, it is through a process of consultation and negotiations, rather than unilateralism, that the federal and provincial governments make their decisions. Is this not the true spirit of federalism? It is through political action that any development concerning the role played by each level of government in this field must take shape. When all is said and done, the law is simply a reflection of the agreements reached in this field, and any proposal in this regard oversteps the strictly legal boundaries of the present study.

NOTES

1 According to the terms of our mandate.
2 As early as 1919, the Liberal Party of Canada included this element in its political program. See also Taylor 1987.
3 It should be pointed out that at the instigation of their New Democratic governments, certain provinces, notably Saskatchewan, played a major role in implementing a public health system. Hospital insurance was introduced in Saskatchewan in 1947. British Columbia followed suit in 1949.
4 See the *Report of the Royal Commission on Health Services* (Ottawa: Queen's Printer, 1964–5), chairman: E. Hall.
5 See the Federal-Provincial Fiscal Arrangements and Established Programs Financing Act, S.C. 1977, c. 10. This legislation was later amended in step with the decline in federal contributions.
6 Certain matters, like immigration and agriculture, were assigned to both

levels of government, which have 'concurrent' jurisdiction over these areas. If there is a conflict between a federal statute and a provincial one, the federal statute prevails. See section 95 of the Constitution Act, 1867.

7 It should be pointed out that federal or provincial lawmakers are autho-rized to delegate jurisdiction to an organization subordinate to the other level of government. This form of cooperation conforms to the spirit of fed-eralism and was found to be constitutionally valid by the courts. See *P.E.I. Potato Marketing Board v. H.B. Willis Inc.; Coughlin v. Ontario Highway Trans-port Board.*

8 Section 33 of the Charter provides for an express declaration mechanism for exceptions to fundamental freedoms (sec. 2) or to legal and equality rights (ss. 7 to 15). Under section 1, the rights and freedoms set out in the Charter are subject only to such reasonable limits prescribed by law as can be demonstrably justified in a free and democratic society.

9 Including the territories, according to sec. 32 of the Canadian Charter. See *R. v. S.(S).*

10 Contrary to provincial charters of rights and freedoms, the Charter gener-ally does not apply to private matters. See *Douglas/Kwantlen Faculty Associa-tion v. Douglas College.*

11 Section 41 states: 'The Government of Canada is committed to (a) enhanc-ing the vitality of the English and French linguistic minority communities in Canada and supporting and assisting their development; and (b) foster-ing the full recognition and use of both English and French in Canadian society.'

12 See also *La municipalité du village de Saint-Louis du Mile-End v. Cité de Montréal; Re George Bowack; Canadian Pacific Navigation v. City of Vancouver.*

13 Section 91 *in fine* states: 'And any matter coming within any of the classes of subjects enumerated in this section shall not be deemed to come within the class of matters of a local or private nature comprised in the enumeration of the classes of subjects by this Act assigned exclusively to the legislatures of the provinces.'

14 See also *Reference re: Intoxicated Persons Detention Act (Manitoba).*

15 See, e.g., *In the Matter of a Reference as to Whether the Parliament of Canada Had Legislative Jurisdiction to Enact the Employment and Social Insurance Act; A.G. Canada v. A.G. Ontario.* In 1940, the Constitution was amended by the addi-tion of subsection 91(2A) on unemployment insurance. See the Constitution Act, 1940.

16 See *Reference: Validity of Section 5(A) of the Dairy Industry Act.* See also *Labatt Breweries v. A.G. of Canada.*

17 Pursuant to the federal authority over regulation of trade and commerce, see subsection 91(2) of the Constitution Act, 1867. See also Hogg 2001, 489–502.

18 See *Ex Parte Fairbain; Metherwell v. The Medical Council of British Columbia; Stinson v. College of Physicians & Surgeons (Ont.); Hunt v. College of Physicians & Surgeons (Sask.); R. v. Sirkis; Re Hayward; Landers v. Dental Society (New Brunswick)*; and, in general, *Re Underwool McLellan Associated Ltd. & Ass. of Professional Engineers.*

19 See *Metherwell v. The Medical Council of British Columbia.*

20 Subsection 92(9) assigns the province authority over 'shop, saloon, tavern, auctioneer, and other licences in order to the raising of a revenue for provincial, local, or municipal purposes.'

21 Subsection 92(15) assigns the province authority over 'the imposition of punishment by fine, penalty, or imprisonment for enforcing any law of the province made in relation to any matter coming within any of the classes of subjects enumerated in this section.'

22 In the event of conflict, however, the provincial statute must yield to the federal statute.

23 *In Re Shelley*; see also Hogg 2001, 163–8.

24 See, e.g., *RJR-Macdonald Inc. v. Canada (A.G.); Scowby v. Glendinning; A.G. for Ontario v. Hamilton Street Railway Co.*

25. See, e.g., *RJR-Macdonald Inc. v. Canada (A.G.); R. v. Zelensky; Proprietary Articles Trade Association v. A.G. of Canada.*

26 See, e.g., *R. v. Swain; Morgentaler v. R.; R. v. Furtney.*

27 See *Goodyear Tire & Rubber Co. v. The Queen.*

28 *Reference: Validity of Section 5(A) of the Dairy Industry Act; R. v. Vaillancourt; R. v. Morgentaler.*

29 See *RJR-MacDonald Inc. v. Canada (A.G.).*

30 See *R. v. Wetmore; Standard Sausage Co. v. Lee; R. v. Perfection Creameries Ltd.* See the Food and Drugs Act, now R.S.C., 1985, c. F-27.

31 *Ex Parte Wakaboyaski; Belleau v. Minister of National Health and Welfare.* Contra: *R. v. Hauser* in which the validity of the federal legislation was upheld on the basis of Parliament's authority to make laws for peace, order, and good government. Now see the Controlled Drugs and Substances Act.

32 *Morgentaler v. R.; R. v. Morgentaler.*

33 *R. v. Cossman's Furniture (1992) Ltd.*

34 *R. v. Wetmore; Standard Sausage Co. v. Lee, supra,* note 30; *Berryland Canning Co. v. The Queen.*

35 *Labatt Breweries v. A.G. Canada, supra,* note 16.

36 *Reference: Validity of Section 5(A) of the Dairy Industry Act, supra,* note 16.
37 For example, in *Dunbar v. A.G. Saskatchewan* provincial legislative authorization for payment of $1 million in international assistance was found to be valid.
38 See also, in general, Lederman 1967; Driedger 1981; Magnet 1978. For an opposing viewpoint, see Petter 1989.
39 *Mercer v. A.G. for Canada; Central Mortgage & Housing Corp. v. Cooperative College Residence Inc.; YMHA Jewish Community Centre v. Brown; Finlay v. Canada; Re Canada Assistance Plan.*
40 In *Re Canada Assistance Plan* British Columbia contested the reduction in federal funds for the wealthiest provinces in the fields of public assistance and social policy.
41 See also Scott 1977, 297, where the author states: 'Generosity in Canada is not unconstitutional, making a gift is not the same as making a law.'
42 For an explanation of this authority and its exercise, see *Reference Re Anti Inflation Act.*
43 At question was whether the Parliament of Canada could regulate the dumping of waste in provincial waters when it had not been proven that the said waste had a polluting effect on extra-provincial waters.
44 Unemployment insurance was found to be first and foremost a contractual matter coming under provincial authority in the area of property and civil rights.
45 See also Canadian Bar Association 1994, 18–20. For an opposing viewpoint, see Lajoie and Molinari 1978, 600–1.
46 Indian and Northern Affairs Canada, 'Indian Affairs in Canada and the United States.' http://www.ainc-inac.gc.ca/pr/info/info122_e.html (1 May 2001).

CASE LAW

A.G. Canada v. A.G. Ontario, [1937] A.C. 355.
A.G. for Ontario v. Hamilton Street Railway Co., [1930] A.C. 524.
Alltrans Express Ltd. v. Worker's Compensation Board, [1988] 1 S.C.R. 897.
Bell Canada v. Québec (C.S.S.T.), [1988] 1 S.C.R. 749.
Belleau v. Minister of National Health and Welfare, (1948) R.C.E. 288.
Berryland Canning Co. v. The Queen, [1974] F.C. 91.
Canadian Indemnity Co. v. A.G. British Columbia, [1977] 2 S.C.R. 504.
Canadian Pacific Navigation v. City of Vancouver, (1892) 2 B.C.R. 193.
Carruthers v. Therapeutic Abortion Committee, (1983) 6 D.L.R. (4) 57.

C.E. Jamieson and Co. v. A.G. Canada, [1988] 1 F.C. 590.

Central Mortgage & Housing Corp. v. Cooperative College Residence Inc. (1977), 71 D.L.R. (3) 183.

Citizens Insurance Co. v. Parsons (1881), 7 A.C. 96.

C.N. v. Courtois, [1988] 1 S.C.R. 868.

Coughlin v. Ontario Highway Transport Board, [1968] S.C.R. 569.

Douglas/Kwantlen Faculty Association v. Douglas College, [1990] 3 S.C.R. 570.

Dunbar v. A.G. Saskatchewan (1984), 11 D.L.R. (4) 374.

Eldridge v. British Columbia (A.G.) (1997), 151 D.L.R. (4) 577.

Ex Parte Fairbain (1877), 18 N.B.R. 4.

Ex Parte Wakaboyaski (1928), 49 C.C.C. 392.

Fawcett v. A.G. of Ontario & A.G. of Canada, [1964] S.C.R. 625.

Finlay v. Canada, [1986] 2 S.C.R. 607.

Goodyear Tire & Rubber Co. v. The Queen, [1956] S.C.R. 303.

Hunt v. College of Physicians & Surgeons (Sask.), [1925] 3 W.W.R. 758.

In re Shelly, [1913] 4 W.W.R. 741.

Labatt Breweries v. A.G. of Canada, [1980] 1 S.C.R. 914.

Landers v. Dental Society (New Brunswick) (1957), 7 D.L.R. (2) 583.

Mercer v. A.G. for Canada, (1971) 3 W.W.R. 375.

Metherwell v. The Medical Council of British Columbia, [1892] 2 B.C.R. 186.

Morgentaler v. R., [1976] 1 S.C.R. 616.

La municipalité du village de Saint-Louis du Mile-End v. Cité de Montréal, [1886] 2 M.L.R. S.C. 218.

P.E.I. Potato Marketing Board v. H.B. Willis Inc., [1952] 2 S.C.R. 392.

Proprietary Articles Trade Association v. A.G. of Canada, [1931] A.C. 310.

R. v. Cossman's Furniture (1992) Ltd. (1976), 73 D.L.R. (3) 312.

R. v. Crown Zellerbach Canada Ltd., [1988] 1 S.C.R. 401.

R. v. Furtney, [1991] 3 S.C.R. 89.

R. v. Hauser, [1979] 1 S.C.R. 984.

R. v. Hydro-Québec, [1997] 3 S.C.R. 213.

R. v. Morgentaler, [1988] 1 S.C.R. 30.

R. v. Morgentaler, [1993] 3 S.C.R. 463.

R. v. Perfection Creameries Ltd., [1939] 3 D.L.R. 185.

R. v. Sirkis, [1930] 2 W.W.R. 93.

R. v. Swain, [1991] 1 S.C.R. 933.

R. v. Swimmer, [1971] 1 W.W.R. 756.

R. v. Vaillancourt, [1987] 2 S.C.R. 636.

R. v. Wetmore, [1983] 2 S.C.R. 284.

R. v. Zelensky, [1978] 2 S.C.R. 940.

Re Canada Assistance Plan, [1991] 2 S.C.R. 525.

Re George Bowack, [1892] 2 B.C.R. 216.
Re Hayward, [1934] O.R. 133.
Re Underwool McLellan Associated Ltd. & Ass. of Professional Engineers (1980), 103 D.L.R. (3) 268.
Reference Re Anti Inflation Act, [1976] 2 S.C.R. 373.
Reference re: Intoxicated Persons Detention Act (Manitoba), [1981] 1 W.W.R. 333.
Reference: Validity of Section 5(A) of the Dairy Industry Act, [1950] 4 D.L.R. 689.
Rinfret v. Pope, [1886] 12 Q.L.R. 303, p. 315.
Schneider v. The Queen, [1982] 2 S.C.R. 112.
Scowby v. Glendinning, [1986] 2 S.C.R. 226.
Standard Sausage Co. v. Lee, [1934] 1 D.L.R. 706.
Stinson v. College of Physicians & Surgeons (Ont.) (1911), 22 O.L.R. 627.
Winterhaven Stables Ltd. v. A.G. Canada, [1988] 53 D.L.R. (4) 413.
YMHA Jewish Community Centre v. Brown, [1989] 1 S.C.R. 1532.

REFERENCES

Beaudoin, G.A. 1990. *La constitution du Canada*. Montreal: Wilson and Lafleur.
Brun, H., and G. Tremblay. 1997. *Droit constitutionnel*. 3rd ed. Montreal: Édition Yvon Blais.
Canadian Bar Association. 1994. *What's Law Got to Do with It?* Report of the Task Force on Health Care. Ottawa.
Driedger, E. 1981. 'The Spending Power.' *Queen's Law Journal* 7: 124.
Dupéré, T. 1987. *La perspective fédérale/provinciale dans le système de santé et de services sociaux du Québec*. Commission d'enquête sur les services de santé et les services sociaux. Quebec City, August.
Gibson, D. 1996. 'The Canadian Health Act and the Constitution.' *Health Law Journal* 4: 1–5.
Gray, G. 1991. *Federalism and Health Policy: The Development of Health Systems in Canada and Australia*. Toronto: University of Toronto Press.
Hogg, P.W. 2001. *Constitutional Law in Canada*. Student ed. Toronto: Carswell.
Jackman, M. 1996. 'The Constitutional Basis for Federal Regulation of Health.' *Health Law Journal* 5: 3–10.
Lajoie A., and P.A. Molinari. 1978. 'Le partage constitutionnel des compétences en matière de santé.' *Canadian Bar Review* 56: 579.
Lederman, W. 1967. 'Some Forms and Limitations of Cooperative Federalism.' *Canadian Bar Review* 45: 409.
McKall, R.T. 1975. 'Constitutional Jurisdiction over Public Health.' *Manitoba Law Journal* 6: 317–26.

Magnet, J.E. 1978. 'The Constitutional Distribution of Taxation Powers in Canada.' *Ottawa Law Review* 10: 473.

Organisation for Economic Co-operation and Development. 1994. *The Reform of Health Care Systems: A Review of Seventeen OECD Countries*. Paris: OECD.

Paternaude, P., dir., *Québec–Communauté française de Belgique: autonomie et spécificité dans le cadre d'un système fédéral*. Sherbrooke: Wilson and Lafleur, 1991.

Petter, A. 1989. 'Federalism and the Myth of the Federal Spending Power.' *Canadian Bar Review* 68: 448.

Scott, F.R. 1997. 'The Constitutional Background of Taxation Agreements.' In *Essays on the Constitution*. Toronto: University of Toronto Press.

Swartz, D. 1993. 'The Politics of Reform: Public Health Insurance in Canada.' *International Journal of Health Services* 23 (2): 219–30.

Taylor, M.G. 1987. *Health Insurance and Canadian Public Policy*, 2nd ed. Montreal: McGill-Queen's University Press.

2 Constitutional Jurisdiction over Health and Health Care Services in Canada

HOWARD LEESON

This chapter examines the various questions related to the origin and exercise of constitutional jurisdiction over health care in Canada. In particular, it examines four questions that are of importance for the future of publicly funded health care. These questions are:

1 What are the constitutional bases for the federal and provincial roles in the provision of health care in Canada?
2 What is the constitutional basis for the exercise of the federal spending power as it relates to health?
3 Does the Charter of Rights and Freedoms affect the distribution of jurisdiction with respect to health care and the delivery of health care?
4 Insofar as Canadian health policy increasingly involves broader definitions of 'health' each year, how might the interrelationship of broader parameters and overlapping jurisdictions affect health care policy and the discharge of responsibilities for the delivery of health care in the future? In particular, how do various jurisdictional responsibilities for economic matters affect health policy?

This chapter is divided into four sections that parallel these questions. The first section outlines the historical development of constitutional jurisdiction over health care in Canada. This development has been characterized by two long-term trends. First, important heads of power that might have been relevant to health care have taken on different meanings from those anticipated in 1867. This has occurred largely as a result of judicial interpretation. Second, during the period

1867–2002, the exercise of federal and provincial jurisdiction has changed profoundly in response to changing conceptions of the role of the state. Despite this complexity, there is a discernible body of case-law and convention to guide us in examining the present situation.

The second section looks specifically at the federal spending power and its impact on the development of health care policy and the delivery of health care services in Canada. The federal spending power provides the basis for much of federal involvement in the policy areas of the social safety net. The ability to give or withhold funding for specific programs has been a potent force in shaping all areas of social policy. In health care, it forms the basis for the Canada Health Act, which seeks to provide 'national standards' for medicare.

The third section deals with one of the most interesting points that has emerged in this debate, the impact, if any, of the Canadian Charter of Rights and Freedoms (the Charter) on the matter of the provision of health care services. Discussion in this area has usually revolved around the right to equality in the provision of care. Specifically, do people have some form of 'charter right' to health care? To date, the courts have resisted interpretations of equality rights that guarantee equality of condition as a public right, but they have not tolerated discriminatory treatment of individuals or groups in the provision of care. As well, the courts have resisted using place of residence as a basis for insisting on equality of condition or service. However, the law in this regard is evolving. This chapter deals with a more precise question, however. That is, Does the Charter affect jurisdiction over health care in Canada? The answer to this question is easier to determine.

Finally, and most interestingly, the definition of what constitutes a 'health' matter continues to expand. Thirty years ago a health matter was generally thought of in curative terms, which involved a doctor and a hospital, but that definition has broadened considerably. Determinants of health now include such things as genetic factors, lifestyle, social and economic status, occupational and environmental conditions, and even race or gender. This fourth section explores the constitutional implications that flow from this kind of broad definition. While it may be useful to aggregate policy into clusters, it becomes problematic when constitutional powers are not distributed in a way that facilitates these kinds of aggregations.

The chapter concludes with a summary of its descriptive and analytical findings. As well, some suggestions on constitutional interpretations and directions that might be useful in shaping future policy in this area are provided.

Health Care and the Constitution

Any examination of constitutional powers with regard to health care in Canada must be based upon the recognition of two important considerations. First, 'health care' is not a head of power in the Canadian Constitution in the same way that banking, buoys, or Sable Island is. The common perception is that health care is a matter of provincial jurisdiction. Such a statement is at best misleading. As Peter Hogg, one of Canada's pre-eminent constitutional experts, says:

> Health is not a single matter assigned by the Canadian constitution exclusively to one level of government. Like inflation, and the environment, health is an 'amorphous topic' which is distributed to the federal parliament or the provincial legislatures depending on the purpose and effect of the particular health measure at issue. (Hogg 1998, 445)

Why, then, is there a perception that the provinces have exclusive jurisdiction in this important social area? Part of the misunderstanding arises from the fact that section 92(7) assigns exclusive provincial control over hospitals and psychiatric institutions. In 1867, health care was thought of in terms of disease and hospitals. More will be said about this later.

The second important consideration has to do with the evolution of the federal system in Canada. More precisely, the exercise of various constitutional powers by the federal and provincial governments in Canada has been altered profoundly by two important events: the growth of the involvement of the state in the lives of all Canadians, and the way that judicial interpretation and conventional usage have altered the original intentions of those who drafted the British North America Act.

Let's first look at the second event. It is important for our discussion to understand that exclusive provincial power over what has become such an important matter as health care could not have been anticipated by the 'Fathers of Confederation.' As Smiley points out: 'The Confederation settlement contemplated a centralized federal system. Most of what were then regarded as the major functions of government were vested in the Dominion (Smiley 1980, 19). Insofar as this distribution of power is concerned, many federal heads of power that were thought to be important in 1867 have come to be restricted by judicial interpretation. These include, most importantly, the general power (Peace, Order and Good Government [POGG]) and the trade and commerce power. In contrast, specific heads of provincial power were interpreted more broadly to enhance the provincial role and jurisdiction. In particular, this was the case with the interpretation of section 92(13), Property and Civil Rights. The Judicial Committee of the Privy Council in Great Britain, through its disposition of appeal cases primarily during the period 1892–1930, effectively turned 92(13) into a broad provincial residual clause.[1] It is not possible to review the role of judicial interpretation in constitutional development in Canada in this chapter. It is important to point out, however, that such a process of interpretation could be expected where constitutional sections are either ambiguous or potentially susceptible to broad interpretation. Whyte and Lederman put this dilemma very well in their landmark book, *Canadian Constitutional Law*:

> The danger is this, that some of the categories of federal power and those of provincial power are capable of very broadly extended ranges of meaning. If one of these concepts of federal power should be given a broadly extended meaning, and also priority over any competing provincial concept, then federal power would come close to eliminating provincial power. The converse could happen just as easily, with the federal power suffering virtual eclipse. (Whyte and Lederman 1977, 4–10)

Thus, it is important to understand the actual heads of power with regard to health care and understand how they interrelate with other heads of power, how they have changed, and why.

This brings us to the second important event. The roles of the federal and provincial governments, and the exercise of their jurisdiction, have changed in response to changing conceptions about the role of government in society. In 1867, matters like education, health care, family care and control, and most of what we now consider social services were all considered private, charitable, or religious matters. These services, insofar as they existed, were not generally thought to be included in the responsibilities of the State, except in a very limited and regulatory way. The conceptions and expectations about the role of government in this area changed profoundly during the twentieth century, especially after the Great Depression. Canadians demanded that the State ensure that many basic social services in society be guaranteed by entrusting them to government. This raised the question of which government – federal or provincial – ought to be responsible for these services, and concomitantly, what the relationship between the governments was to be. As Bakvis and Skogstad point out in their recent book on federalism, it has made for interesting times:

> Despite occasionally turbulent relations between governments, and despite the high degree of centralization, the Canadian federation has successfully faced several major policy challenges. These challenges include those related to the construction of the post-war social safety net, including Medicare. (Bakvis and Skogstad 2001, 4)

The most crucial questions involved capacity and power. The lesson of the Depression was that the provinces had the constitutional power in matters relating to unemployment, pensions, and social services, but lacked the fiscal capacity to cope with the problems. By contrast, the federal government had the plenary taxing power and the fiscal capacity but no constitutional jurisdiction in relation to these costly areas of social welfare. This led to intense pressure from Canadians on the federal government to become involved in areas of provincial responsibility. Some provinces resisted this pressure, but fought a losing battle, as Russell points out: 'A rising tide of political sentiment ran in the opposite direction. From the 1930's through the end of the 1950's the centralist perspective was the dynamic initiating force in Canadian constitutional politics. Centralism was never stronger than during this quarter century' (Russell 1993, 62).

For the most part, this centralization did not involve specific constitutional amendment. Instead, the federal government found new ways to become involved, and, as we will see, it did so primarily through the use of its spending power. The desire of Canadians for social services legitimated the federal government's involvement in areas that were previously considered to be provincial responsibility. This is an important point. No federal government could resist the chance to secure political credit by ensuring that Canada would not return to the deprivation of the 1930s. The small matter of jurisdiction could be overlooked in the circumstances. Thus, together with the increasing complexity and expansion of health care delivery, crucial political imperatives dictated that both orders of government become involved in a profound way in this area.

With this background in mind, we can now examine the explicit heads of constitutional power involved in health care.

Provincial Powers

Below are the major provincial constitutional powers over health care. They are supplemented by the general power over provincial public lands and assets, as well as by provincial taxation power.

92(7): *The Establishment, Maintenance, and Management of Hospitals, Asylums, Charities, and Eleemosynary Institutions In and For the Province, Other Than Marine Hospitals*
This section constitutes one of the central sources of provincial jurisdiction in the area of health care. By natural implication, the regulation of personnel and the functions associated with these institutions broadens the ambit of jurisdiction. Originally, these institutions were under the control of private and religious groups. The fact that most are now owned by the government makes their control a matter of government proprietorship also. It should be noted that there are major exceptions to the above. The first is marine hospitals, which are explicitly mentioned in 91(11), as well as hospitals and care in federal territories and defence establishments.

92(10): *Local Works and Undertakings ...*
This section could be used to bolster provincial control since most hospitals are not part of interprovincial enterprises. However, many health care delivery organizations, such as nursing homes, are now both private and national in scope, and might be susceptible to federal regulation through competition legislation, or by virtue of the fact that they are economic enterprises that are covered by treaties such as the North American Free Trade Agreement (NAFTA).

92(13): *Property and Civil Rights in the Province*
This section, aside from the fact that it has received wide ambit in judicial interpretation, is the basis by which the provinces regulate labour relations and the professions involved in the health care field.

92(16): *Generally All Matters of a Merely Local or Private Nature in the Province*
This section is similar to section 92(10) but involves private matters as well. This would bolster the provincial power to regulate religious health care delivery agencies.

93: *In and for each province the Legislature may exclusively make laws in relation to education.*
This section allows the provinces to regulate the education and training of all health care delivery personnel. It also allows them, in conjunction with section 92(13), to establish self-regulating professions and registration procedures in the field.

95: *In each Province the legislature may make laws in relation to ... immigration*
This is a concurrent power with the federal government and provincial laws may not be 'repugnant' to federal laws. Immigration has been important in those provinces attempting to cope with a lack of domestic health care personnel by bringing immigrants into the province.

Federal Powers

Section 91: Powers of Parliament
The most important powers in this section have been the enumerated heads, which we will examine below. It is worth noting, however, that the residual or general power remains. Despite the fact that it was restricted by judicial interpretation in the period up to 1930, some think it possible that it could be important in the future. Indeed, the Supreme Court has indicated several times that it remains a possible potent source of federal power.[2] The most often cited examples of 'national concern' usually involve health matters:

> There are, however, cases where uniformity of law throughout the country is not merely desirable but essential, in the sense that the problem 'is beyond the power of the provinces to deal with' ... The often-cited case of an epidemic of pestilence is a good example. The failure by one province to take preventative measures would probably lead to the spreading of disease into those provinces, which had taken preventative measures. (Hogg 1998, 415)

The events following the attacks in the United States on 11 September 2001 have led the federal government to look at health measures designed to combat the release of deadly diseases such as smallpox. As well, the federal government has stockpiled drugs needed to cope with the deadly anthrax bacteria. No one would dispute that these are health measures, but they are generated from security and national defence concerns.

91(2): The Regulation of Trade and Commerce
This head of power was thought in 1867 to be one of the most important. Given the economic expectations associated with Confederation, and the anticipated role of the federal government in this area, it was a reasonable expectation. However, judicial review of this section in relation to section 92(13) led to the diminution of the federal power over trade and commerce. There is too little time in this chapter to fully explore the constitutional changes and debates involved in this matter. However, one crucial aspect is the regulation of international trade and commerce.

How is this related to health care – and the delivery of health care services? For the most part it relates to the production and trade in health care–related goods and services. Most of the products relevant to the delivery of health care – machines, drugs, tools, and construction of facilities – are produced in the private sector. Quite often they are imported from another country. They are treated no differently than other products that are produced or traded. As well, many of the services related to health care delivery, such as training programs, are also undertaken by the private sector, often with manuals or procedures developed in other countries and sold in Canada. In short, the economic aspect of health care is both international and subject to regulation by the federal government.

This is especially true when it comes to comprehensive international agreements. In agreements like NAFTA, general regulations about trade and trade practices are put in place, even though the implementation of those regulations may encroach on an area of provincial jurisdiction. Thus, obligations in the field of health care may result from general trade agreements, despite the fact that health care delivery is largely a provincial responsibility.[3] We will explore this more fully later on.

91(9): Beacons, Buoys, Lighthouses, and Sable Island
The federal government was given exclusive jurisdiction over all matters on Sable Island.

91(11): *Quarantine and the Establishment and Maintenance of Marine Hospitals*
The federal government has exclusive jurisdiction over marine hospitals in Canada. As well, it has the health-related power of quarantine.

91(22): *Patents of Invention and Discovery*

This power has had a major impact on health care in Canada. Patents allow the individual or corporation to claim the exclusive right to manufacture and profit from 'inventions.' This is particularly important with regard to drugs that are now used extensively in the prevention and treatment of illness. The cost of these drugs has risen dramatically over the past two decades, in part because Canada, along with other governments in the developed world, has extended the time of patent protection. In Canada, it was lengthened from seven years to twenty-one years. The effect of this has been to prevent generic manufactures from providing cheaper copies of the patented products until after their effectiveness has been superceded by newer patented drugs.

91(24): *Indians and Land Reserved for Indians*

Initially, this power included all health matters for 'Indian' people (excluding Metis in most cases). This is no longer the case. The matter of health care and the delivery of health care services for 'Indians' is a matter of ongoing negotiations between federal, provincial, and First Nations governments. First Nations want to deliver their own services wherever possible. However, they believe that the federal government is responsible for the cost of this care under treaty obligation. For its part, the federal government has now restricted its fiscal role to First Nations people on reserves. Provincial governments have now unwillingly assumed the cost of health care for all Aboriginal peoples off reserves.[4]

91(27): *The Criminal Law ...*

The criminal law power is intimately associated with matters of health care. By using its power to declare something a crime, the federal government has the power to restrict or expand many health activities. Current examples that illustrate this are the criminalization or decriminalization of sperm banks and of such procedures as abortion, cloning, or genetic research on embryos. As well, the use of certain foods and drugs can be made illegal or restricted. For example, marijuana can be used for medicinal or recreational purposes. By classifying it as illegal, the use of this substance is restricted to health purposes only.

92(10c): *The Power to Declare Works ...*

Federal power in this area results from its declaration of a 'work.' As a result, for example in the uranium area, the federal government becomes responsible for labour relations, work safety, and health issues, all of which would normally be under provincial jurisdiction. Thus, if the political will were present, any hospital or group of hospitals could be declared to be a 'work' for the general advantage of Canada by Parliament.

Federal Territories

The territories of Yukon, Northwest Territories, and Nunavut are ultimately under federal jurisdiction, since their own jurisdiction is delegated from Parliament. Although the three jurisdictions have various legislative bodies and treaty arrangements that govern the delivery of health care services, constitutional power in these areas remains with the federal government.

International Treaties

It is possible for the federal government to intrude on or frustrate provincial jurisdiction through the power to sign international treaties. In other federal countries, this power is virtually unchecked.[5] In Canada the situation is somewhat more complex. The constitutional power to implement treaties originally resided in section 132 of the Constitution Act. It allowed the federal Parliament to implement treaties signed on behalf of the empire.[6] However, in a landmark decision rendered in 1937, the Judicial Committee of the Privy Council declared this section to be exhausted as a result of the fact that treaties had ceased to be treaties of the empire. It rejected the idea that the federal Parliament would automatically have the right under section 91 to intrude on areas of provincial jurisdiction in order to implement the provisions of international treaties. This has left Canada with a 'bifurcated treaty power.' Simply put, if the federal government signs a treaty in an area of provincial jurisdiction, it means that the provincial legislature must implement the provisions of the treaty in its area of jurisdiction. It may or may not do so. Since 1937, the Supreme Court of Canada has 'nibbled' around the edges of this decision, but never reversed it.[7]

This has meant that economic treaties such as the FTA (Free Trade Agreement) and NAFTA, which obviously have implications for health care, have yet to be tested. It could be that the Supreme Court may find that the power exercised over international trade by the federal government can incidentally encroach on the provincial power over the delivery of health care. This would be especially relevant in the matter of private sector hospitals, and so on.

These sections do not represent an exhaustive list of specific powers, nor are the discussions about them as fully developed as they could be. However, they do touch on most of the relevant major heads of power. Of equal interest are those areas that are either ambiguous or that overlap.

Unassigned or Ambiguous Jurisdiction

As with any constitutional document, powers assigned to governments at one time often become redundant or inapplicable in another time. This has been especially true in Canada in the last century as the political and social roles of the federal and provincial governments have changed dramatically. Sometimes these ambiguities have been directly remedied through judicial decision or constitutional amendment. For example, neither the radio nor the airplane was contemplated in 1867. The question of regulation of these devices and activities associated with them became a question in the early twentieth century. The courts resolved both matters in 1930, assigning jurisdiction for both to the federal government.[8] No one contemplated the need for a national unemployment insurance scheme in 1867, but the savage Depression of the 1930s made it a social necessity. The problem was solved by assigning the matter to the federal government by amending the British North America Act in 1940. The same was true for pensions in 1951, although the provincial governments retained paramountcy in that case.[9]

Not all matters have been so easy to categorize, however. In some cases both federal and provincial legislatures have legitimate and pressing concerns. The question of the environment is an example. Both the Parliament of Canada and the provincial legislatures have dealt with 'environmental' matters when they thought it necessary. In part this is because the 'environmental matters' are not easily classifiable. They may involve a number of jurisdictional heads. For example, air pollution can be thought to be a matter involving natural resources if it comes from the operation of a mine, or water pollution can be a fisheries matter if it involves the rivers emptying into the ocean. It can be a local matter if it involves a lake; a federal matter if it affects inland streams; an international matter if it involves the Great Lakes. The type, extent, and time of the matter all affect the exercise of jurisdiction. Finally, the matter of politics also enters into the equation. It may be politically desirable for one order or the other to be seen to be doing something about a particular issue or problem at any given time. The environment is only one example – communications, intellectual property, and other matters could be said to fit into this category.

Of greater concern, perhaps, are matters that require federal and provincial governments to coordinate their areas of jurisdiction to deal with a particular issue. For example, in the matter of inflation, the primary powers are federal, but the exercise of provincial jurisdiction with regard to spending and borrowing is very important. In a modern interconnected and complex society, it is almost impossible to have watertight jurisdictional compartments. This is certainly true in the case of health care and the delivery of health care services. Even without the exercise of the spending power by the federal government, health care is an area where constitutional coordination is required. Thus, while it is useful to know the specific areas of jurisdiction, such knowledge alone gives you no sense of how the two orders of government actually exercise their power. Other matters, such as spending, become equally important.

Health and the Federal Spending Power

For the purposes of this chapter, we will assume that much of the history and detail involved with this issue is already known to the reader. The crucial elements revolve around the matter of the federal use (or non-use) of its ability to raise and spend revenue in Canada, and its impact on provincial legislatures and governments when it does so.

The term 'spending power' requires some definition in order to ensure that we deal with it in a precise manner. There are many ways that a government can use its power to 'spend.' The first and most obvious use of the federal spending power involves the expenditure of monies on projects and services within the federal jurisdiction. These can include direct payments to individuals or corporations for goods or services. As well, the federal government expends monies on various programs that are within the federal jurisdiction, which can include the expense of the public service in managing these programs.

The federal government also makes direct payments to individuals for a variety of purposes. There is nothing to restrict the federal government in these payments, although restrictions may revolve around the purpose involved or the qualifications required to receive the payment. The purpose may be something that is offered or regulated by the provinces. For example, there is nothing to prevent the federal government from giving cash bursaries to students attending educational institutions, or from providing research grants to university faculty engaged in research at a provincial university.

The federal government may also use its taxing power as part of the spending power. We have all heard of the term 'tax expenditures.' This usually means revenue forfeited by not exercising or transferring certain taxes, most often to the provinces. These are considered to be real expenditures, and their transfer is often referred to by federal ministers when talking about their 'share' of the cost of programs like medicare.

Another way to use the spending power is to transfer monies to other governments. In the case of the federal government, this application has a long and honourable history. Many of the crucial arrangements and debates in 1867 involved the level of Dominion payments to the new provinces, division of property, and assumption of debts. Several parts of the original British North America Act refer specifically to such arrangements.[10] This has continued to be the case, and has often been the subject of federal-provincial conferences. Transfer payments, as they are now called, are intimately bound up with shared-cost programs, the spending power, and federal/provincial questions about jurisdiction.[11]

Debate about the use of the spending power usually revolves around questions about its use in areas of provincial jurisdiction. The general arguments in this case are also well known. In the post–Second World War era, the Liberal federal government sought to establish a number of social programs in Canada. The motivation for this move has been a matter of some discussion. Some argue that it was simply the product of electoral concerns, a move to the left by the Liberals to blunt the rise of the Co-operative Commonwealth Federation (CCF). Others have argued that it resulted from the need to legitimate the capitalist economic system, to prevent a move towards socialism. For example, Garth Stevenson has argued this point of view in his work on Canadian federalism:

> Generally speaking, however, conditional grants [by the federal government] have been mainly devoted to legitimization, precisely because the provinces cannot be relied upon to spend money in this field of policy without substantial incentives, and in some cases actual coercion.
>
> It would be wrong, however, to overestimate the federal enthusiasm for

spending on legitimization ... By accepting only partial financial responsibility and leaving provinces to assume the rest, the federal government purchases the political benefits (or avoids the political cost of inaction), at minimum expense to its treasury. (Stevenson 1982, 157, 158)

Others explain the rise of shared-cost programs as a reaction by the state to the unreformed federal system, as a way to circumvent an unusable constitutional system. Barker, for example, writes:

Historically the fiscal arrangements for social policy have served various purposes, all of which can be related to the handling of social policy in the Constitution. At times, the purpose has been to bridge the vertical 'fiscal gap' caused by the constitutional allocation or mismatch of revenues and expenditures, while at other times the desire has been to assist the poorer provinces in such a way that all parts of the country are able to offer comparable levels of public services. Sometimes the intent is to convince provinces to establish programs that might otherwise not have been developed sufficiently or even introduced ... Lastly, national unity has been the object of the arrangements. In this form, the arrangements amount to 'bonds of nationhood' forged out of a sense among Canadians that they share common services with each other. (Barker 1998, 145)

Whatever the motivation, the outcome was that over one hundred shared-cost programs were established after the war, the best known of which were in the health care field. The constitutionality of this use of the spending power has caused considerable debate.

Generally, arguments against federal involvement in shared-cost programs involve two matters. The first is that by its use of the spending power, the federal government skews provincial priorities. By offering federal dollars for certain programs in the area of provincial jurisdiction, it ensures that other programs, not funded by the federal government, will be relegated to a lower priority. Insofar as the area of health care is concerned, this was an initial argument when the federal government first attempted to induce the provinces to establish a national medicare system. No province now seriously argues against a medicare system, but there is considerable debate about the lack of adequate federal financing, and, consequently, its role in determining the shape and priorities of the system.

The centre of debate over the past two decades, however, has concerned the use of the federal spending power in order to 'enforce' certain health care principles outlined in the Canada Health Act (CHA). These 'principles' are public administration, comprehensiveness, universality, portability, and accessibility. If a provincial system does not meet these criteria, it is liable to lose some or all of the federal funding designated for health care delivery.

There are, therefore, two important questions involved. Is it constitutional for the federal government to use its spending power in the area of health care? Is it constitutional for the federal government to impose conditions upon provinces like those in the CHA?

While there are still many who argue against a positive answer to the first question, the majority of scholars support the kind of interpretation outlined by Peter Hogg:

> It seems to me that the better view of the law is that the federal parliament may spend or lend its funds to any government or institution or individual it chooses, for any purpose it chooses; and that it may attach to any grant or loan any conditions it chooses, including conditions it could not directly legislate. There is a distinction in my view, between compulsory regulation, which can obviously only be accomplished by legislation enacted within the limits of legislative power, and spending or loaning or contracting, which either imposes no obligations on the recipient (as in the case of family allowances) or obligations which are voluntarily assumed. (Hogg 1998, 157)

He supports this view in two ways. First he refers to Parliament's power under sections 91(3), the power to levy taxes, 91(1A), the power to legislate in regard to public property, and 106, the right to appropriate federal funds. Second, he refers to the judgment of the Supreme Court in *Re Canada Assistance Plan*, in which Mr Justice Sopinka wrote the following for the unanimous decision:

> The written argument for the Attorney General of Manitoba was that the legislation 'amounts to' regulation of a matter outside of federal authority. I disagree. The Agreement under the Plan set up an open-ended cost-sharing scheme which left it to British Columbia to decide what programmes it would establish and fund. The simple withholding of federal money which had previously been granted to fund a matter within provincial jurisdiction does not amount to regulation of the matter. (Hogg 1998, 158)[12]

Hogg is supported in his view by many other scholars. Martha Jackman, writing in the *Health Law Journal*, outlines exhaustively the arguments and cases supporting the legitimacy of the federal government's role in health care. For example, she reviews the criminal law power involving environmental cases:

> Following its decision in *RJR-MacDonald*, the Supreme Court confirmed Parliament's ability to rely on its criminal law power to justify broader forms of health regulation in *R. v. Hydro-Québec*. (f.#55) The case involved a challenge by Hydro-Québec to the regulation of PCBs under the Canadian Environmental Protection Act. In rejecting Hydro-Québec's claim that the environmental controls contained in the Act touched upon matters of provincial jurisdiction, Justice La Forest asserted that the goal of protecting human health supported federal regulation of toxic substances under the criminal law power. The Supreme Court's reasoning in *RJR-MacDonald* and in Hydro-Québec provides considerable scope for future federal legislation aimed at controlling activities which put human health at risk, including those which have historically been perceived as entirely legitimate in nature. As Justice La Forest's decision makes clear, the federal government may not only exercise its criminal law power in emerging areas of public health concern, it may also invoke section 91(27) in support of regulatory schemes which, like the Tobacco Products Control Act, are relatively detailed and complex in their structure, penalties and scope. In this regard, the *RJR-MacDonald* decision represents an important departure from the earlier view (f.#56) that legislation of a regulatory rather than more strictly prohibitive form could not be justified under section 91(27). By allowing for a regulatory approach to public health issues under section 91(27), the decision significantly expands the potential for federal reliance on the criminal law power in the area of health. (Jackman 2000, f55 and 56)

She concludes that 'The need for cooperation between the federal government and the provinces in the area of health is therefore as much a matter of constitutional law as it is of sound health policy' (Jackman 2000, f142).

If Hogg and Jackman are categorical in this matter, some others are not. In an excellent article on this issue, Dale Gibson, Belzburg Fellow at the University of Alberta Law School, worries that the justifications put forward by Hogg and others are not sufficient. He writes:

Two important cautions should be noted, however. First the power may not be quite as sweeping as some of the pronouncements [like those of Hogg] seem to suggest. Although some of those statements quoted above seem to indicate that the federal spending power provides limitless justification for conditional federal fiscal initiatives in provincial fields, the historical pattern of Canadian constitutional interpretation, which has maintained a rough balance between federal and provincial powers, strongly suggests that if such initiatives threatened to alter that balance the courts would interfere. The second (and related) caution is that the customary theoretical legal basis for exercising the federal spending power in provincial fields is open to considerable question when scrutinized in terms of long-standing general principles of Canadian constitutional law. These two matters are related since, as will be seen, the customary rationale for the federal spending power offers very limited scope for federal involvement ... Leaving these legal doubts unresolved may not be wise. (Gibson 1996, 7)

Gibson outlines his concerns in some detail. He concentrates in particular on legal justifications that rely on section 91(1A), the Public Debt and Property clause. He reviews the argument used by most in favour of this broad power, which concludes that monies raised by the federal government are really property, and that the federal government is allowed to dispose of its property in any way that it desires. In the case of the Canada Health Act, therefore, it is really an act about federal property, and not health care.

Gibson goes on to argue that this approach has two 'Achilles' heels.' First, there is doubt as to the ability of the federal authority to raise money for provincial purposes, and second, there is a legal requirement that legislation authorizing spending be, in 'pith and substance,' about the disposal of federal property and not some other purpose. The second is potentially more telling. In examining the Canada Health Act, no reasonable person would conclude that it is only about the distribution of federal property. Several parts of the act make specific reference to health objectives and requirements. However, the act could still survive if it was deemed to have a dual aspect. Again, Gibson notes that such a conclusion is by no means guaranteed. In particular, he cites the Supreme Court decision on the Canada Assistance Plan, and concludes by saying:

In light of this uncertainty, those who support federal health care initiatives under the Canada Health Act and other uses of the federal 'spend-ing power' would be well advised, as a safeguard against the possibility that the 'property' rationale will eventually succumb to siege, to explore alternative rationales. (Gibson 1996, 16)

In the remainder of his article, Gibson provides a cogent and well-argued case that suggest the Canada Health Act can be justified under section 91, the Peace Order and Good Government clause (POGG). In particular, he stresses the 'national dimension' aspect of several judi-cial decisions involving POGG:

While the applicability of the POGG power to federal legislation relating to health has never been determined conclusively, the Supreme Court of Canada has suggested that the power has a role to play in that field, [Mar-garine Reference, 1985] and in 1993 the Quebec court of Appeal held that federal legislation restricting tobacco advertising could be justified by POGG. (Gibson 1996, 17, 18)

Gibson's arguments are compelling, if not conclusive, especially as they relate to some elements of the CHA such as portability, one of the five principles in the act.

Gibson wrote his article before nine provinces and the federal gov-ernment negotiated and signed the Social Union Framework Agree-ment (SUFA), which obligates all governments to respect the principles in the CHA. It is possible that this agreement could bolster the legal case that the requirements of the CHA are justifiable.[13]

We are left, therefore, with the uneasy feeling that the present consti-tutional justifications of the Canada Health Act are assailable, while other justifications, such as those proposed by Gibson, are not yet accepted.

Recent initiatives by the government of Alberta in response to the provincial study on the health care system, headed up by former deputy prime minister Don Mazankowski, may serve as the catalyst for some judicial activity in this regard. The provincial government appears poised to privatize parts of the hospital system and to delist some services. It is possible that this could be construed as a violation of the principles of the CHA. Preliminary reaction by the federal gov-ernment is cautious, with no indication that the federal government might penalize the province of Alberta for these proposed actions. This approach is not shared by many in the province itself, or by some of the opposition parties in Parliament. The lack of federal response raises a corollary question, however. Should the federal cabinet not penalize the province of Alberta, is that the end of the matter? The answer by at least one scholar is that this is not the case. Choudhry argues in a lengthy article that the courts could be asked to force the federal government to enforce the legislation and penalize the province. In particular, this action could be taken by individuals seeking to enforce the principle of the act. Should such a court decision be forthcoming, the federal government would be forced to act or change the legislation (Choudhry 1996, 462–509).

In the final analysis, at least in the near future, the constitutional status of the CHA may not be of great consequence. All governments have shown a distinct lack of appetite for a judicial challenge to its requirements. This is true even of the PQ government in Quebec. However, the continuing reduction of the federal fiscal role in health care may yet prove to be the catalyst for legal action. The outcome of that action would not, as Gibson has indicated, be a foregone conclusion.

The Charter of Rights and Freedoms and Health Care Jurisdiction

This section deals with the effect, if any, the Charter of Rights and Freedoms on the provision of health care services. Discussion about the Charter and health care usually addresses the question of whether or not there is a justifiable right to equality of health care or to a minimum standard of publicly provided health care in Canada. Specifically, do people have some form of 'charter right' to health care?[14] As always, the law in this regard is evolving, and a Charter challenge is not out of the question. However, this chapter deals with a more precise question: Does the Charter affect jurisdiction over health care in Canada?

There are several ways to conceptualize this question. One would be to ask, Has the Charter transferred jurisdiction over health care in any meaningful way between the two orders of government? The short answer to this question is no. Insofar as provincial or federal jurisdiction over health care is concerned, the courts have not used the Charter to reallocate power or powers as a result of interpretation of the Charter. It is difficult to conceive of this happening, except in the instance where one order of government refused to exercise its jurisdiction, causing a breach of a Charter right. For example, if the federal government refused to use the power to quarantine in specific regions of the country, section 15 might be invoked to ensure 'equality' of treatment. We are on slippery ground here, however.

If the Charter has not been used to do this, is there the potential for the Charter to be used to alter jurisdiction, or to enhance the jurisdiction of one order or the other? The answer is less than clear, but it is not difficult to conceive of how this might occur. For example, Dr Marcia Rioux, in a book by Margaret E.A. Sommerville, outlines the basis for such an occurrence:

> As an absolute minimum, any health policy must conform not only to the five recognized principles of the Canada Health Act, but also to meet the standards of the constitutional guarantee of equality rights ... the acceptable bases for determining access to scarce resources must now be viewed in terms of the legal standards found in the Constitution and the Charter of Rights and Freedoms. (Rioux 1999, 144, 145)

She goes on to cite cases where provincial governments were required to amend treatment or practices to conform to the equality guarantee of the Charter, under section 15. That is, equal access to treatment was not being afforded to a recognizable group, in the most recent case, to those who are deaf in British Columbia. She concludes by emphasizing that the equality section must be used to ensure that no discrimination is allowed as between individuals or groups. She implicitly accepts the notion that equal health care access is a right of citizenship (Rioux 1999, 144, 145).[15]

Superficially this has little to do with jurisdiction. She does not speak to the question of equality being between provinces or the need for the power over health care to be transferred to the federal government in order to ensure equality. However, when wedded to some of the notions presented in the Gibson article cited above, it is easy to see how this could be the case. Gibson argued that the CHA could be supported by the POGG power in section 91. In particular, he noted that the portability section of the CHA could be justified as a 'national concern' and therefore supported by 91:

> The goal of the portability criterion is obviously to ensure (to the extent that federal and provincial contributions are capable of doing so) that everyone who resides somewhere in Canada is free to exercise his or her right ... to move about the country at will, without jeopardizing his or her access to satisfactory public health care benefits. The contention that legis-

lation in support of such a goal has a national dimension is rooted, again, in the fact that no single province could achieve it. ... Only the Parliament of Canada has the constitutional authority to ensure the portability of health care benefits for all Canadians. (Gibson 1996, 22)

The argument is clearly about equality of access. Curiously, however, Gibson supports this argument only with reference to section 6 of the Charter, the Mobility Rights section, and not by reference to section 15, Equality Rights. It seems that this argument could also be made.

The combination of sections 6 and 15 in the Gibson argument gives us a scenario where the jurisdiction of the provinces could be altered and/or reduced by the application of the Charter in order to ensure equality of access between the provinces. In this case, the federal government would legislate portability under POGG, using the argument of national dimension and sections 6 and 15. Gibson goes on to speculate that universality and comprehensiveness could also be supported, albeit with less guarantee of success in case of a legal challenge (Gibson 1996, 23). Such an enhancement of federal jurisdiction in this scenario would profoundly affect the jurisdictional balance in health care.

The possibility of using section 6, Mobility Rights, to enhance the right of the federal government to legislate in the area of health care has already been noted above. Again, the existence of intergovernmental agreements like SUFA and the Agreement on Internal Trade (AIT) might be used to bolster the case.

The need for brevity in this article means that we have only scratched the surface of this subject. We can conclude by saying that it is likely that the Charter will be used to ensure equality of access in the area of health care in the future. Indeed, it may even be used to guarantee the system itself.

The Interrelationship of Definitions of Health and Constitutional Jurisdiction

This section attempts to answer the questions that surround definitions of health, health care and health care services, and jurisdictional responsibilities. More specifically, since definitions of what constitutes 'health' have become more encompassing as we move away from the acute and chronic care model and towards the 'wellness' or 'preventative' model, does this have implications for the interrelationship of constitutional jurisdiction and jurisdictions that will come into play in the regulation and delivery of these increasingly broad services? Even more specifically, what future role will economic powers play in the area of health?

One way to reduce the scope and complexity of these questions is to focus on one or two major issues. Another way is to look at what has shaped broad trends in federal-provincial relationships during the past several decades and attempt to extrapolate future trends in the area of health care, in particular from those broad trends. The first approach might select, for example, the issue of privatization and examine how major moves in this area might affect jurisdiction. The second approach might look at the role of the federal government in health care as an indicator of its commitment to the equity goals that have characterized federal government involvement in programs that are largely in areas of provincial jurisdiction. In this section we take the second approach, and blend in issues such as privatization where relevant.

We looked briefly above at the conditions involved in the creation of a social program like medicare after the Second World War. There was a broad social consensus that such a program was needed, and the fiscal capacity of the federal government to initiate and sustain such a program. Both consensus and capacity remained until the latter part of the twentieth century. Harvey Lazar describes this interrelationship very well:

> Until the late 1970's or early 1980's, Canadian fiscal federalism had a 'mission statement.' Its sense of purpose mirrored the broader postwar consensus about the role the state could play, through programs of redistribution and macroeconomic stabilization, in building a fair and compassionate society and a prosperous and stable economy. In turn this consensus was predicated on the idea that there was a latent sense of Canadian political nationhood, which could be mobilized in pursuit of these noble goals. (Lazar 2000, 4)[16]

For the most part, this 'mission' was accomplished without formal jurisdictional change. It was undertaken and installed through various informal federal-provincial mechanisms of accommodation. These have at different times been called cooperative federalism, collaborative federalism, executive federalism, accommodative federalism, and, recently, flexible federalism. Results were achieved largely through negotiation and federal-provincial agreement. In other words, conventional practice altered formal jurisdictional capacity.

That process began to break down in the last two decades. Under fiscal and other pressures, both orders of government began to make unilateral decisions that had serious implications for the other order. The consensus on process was the first casualty of fiscal pressure, especially after the Liberal party took over government in 1993. As a result, the system lost some of its sense of purpose and some of its sense of process. This, coupled with other factors, produced a crisis of funding and services in health care, which led to a crisis of confidence and disagreement about the principles of medicare.

This process was compounded by the emergence of genuine ideological differences between the governing parties of the provinces, and, in some cases, the federal government. In Alberta and Ontario, Progressive Conservative governments were not only committed to fiscal integrity, they were committed to reducing the role of government, including its role in health care. This brought them into conflict with some other provinces, like Saskatchewan, and with the federal government. The result was more pressure yet on the post-war consensus about social programs, with the expected fragmentation of program and purpose.

At the same time, there have been broad pressures in the other direction. Lazar, in the same article noted above, outlines these pressures:

> If the federal and provincial governments were operating in watertight compartments, this [trends towards unilateralism and loss of a sense of mission] might not matter much. But the forces of global and continental integration are increasing interdependence among economies and politics. For functional reasons, therefore, they are making intergovernmental collaboration a growing necessity for an ever-broadening range of issues not only across international borders, but also for governments within Canada. For that collaboration to be effective, however, the various governments have to have a minimum level of trust for one another. The 'rules of the game' must entail a measure of predictability about the behaviour of the partners. (Lazar 2000, 5)

Where, then, are these countervailing trends headed? Part of the answer lies in assessing how ever-broadening definitions of health, together with increasing economic globalization and integration, will integrate with the now re-emerging fiscal pressures that have fragmented the sense of national purpose described by Lazar.

Definitions of Health

As noted earlier in this chapter, conceptions of what constitutes health and health care services have changed dramatically since the time of Confederation. Indeed, they have changed more dramatically over the past three decades than at any time in between. We now conceive of 'health' in broader social terms, indicating that we understand that disease and its implications arise in a more holistic sense from everyday life and being. Many of the recent commissions studying health in the past two years have taken pains to point this out. Saskatchewan's Commission on Medicare, for example, referred to this in its report:

> High tech medicine and emergency room dramas may get all of the media attention, but a quiet revolution has been taking place at the other end of the health system that is just as important. The evidence from around the world is clear. When it comes to improving health, high tech care takes a back seat to primary health services. The 'miracles of modern medicine' are not limited to drugs and surgery. Research on heart disease and diabetes, for example, demonstrates that years can be added to people's lives by healthy lifestyles, early intervention, monitoring and health management-simple everyday health measures. (Saskatchewan 2001, 9)

The Commission goes further to say that the 'health effects of poverty and inequality are becoming more evident, particularly in the case of aboriginal people' (ibid., 12).

Lifestyles, poverty, inequality, drugs, high tech equipment, and the equity goals of accessibility, and comprehensiveness, all make for a complex multi-faceted system that does not fit neatly into the constitutional categories of 1867. It is clear, however, that as the definitions of health change and expand, they bring with them new ideas on what to do, and in many cases, how to do it more efficiently. Thus, promotion of health prevention measures is justified not only on the grounds that it will keep people healthier but also because it will be cheaper. The old maxim 'an ounce of prevention is worth a pound of cure' is at the heart of much of the reform of medicare and health care in general in Canada. Yet, despite cost savings, there is still the need to deal with rapidly expanding and costly health care measures in the existing system, while investing in new approaches that will ultimately save money. In other words, we need to invest now to save later. The first part of this equation is what has caused so much consternation over the past ten years.

It is obvious that how health, health care services, and even medical necessity are defined has profound implications on federal-provincial relations. If, as suggested in the Mazankowski Report in Alberta, certain medical services are removed from the list of covered services, it will undoubtedly cause discussion if not confrontation with the federal government. But will it affect constitutional jurisdiction? The answer is probably that it could, although this answer is hardly satisfactory. The most obvious way that this could happen would be through a court challenge involving the Canada Health Act, or even a Charter challenge, as discussed earlier. If such a challenge were successful, it could alter the jurisdiction of the provinces or the federal government. The more likely outcome, however, is that such definitional changes will alter federal provincial discussion and agreement.

Cost Containment, Federalism, and Jurisdiction

Given the widening definitions of health, it is inevitable that there will be increasing overlap with the federal government as the economic decisions of that government impact on health care. We saw this happen in the period after 1993. The federal government made massive cuts to transfer payments in all programs, including health. According to studies, when adjusted for inflation, public spending on health care declined by 1.1 per cent from 1992 to 1997. This brought the national share of the GDP spent on health care down from 10.2 to 9.2 per cent. As one study said, 'This absolute decline is unprecedented' (Rachlis et al. 2001, 6). The immediate impact of this was, as noted above, to increase unilateralism. The consensus on both role and process virtually collapsed. The now conventional ability of the federal government to shape the health care system by using its spending power was challenged and remains in question.

Another ramification of fiscal retrenchment was an increase in the amount of private spending in the system. In the same time period of 1992 to 1997, private spending, principally on drugs, dentistry, and related private-sector institutional care, rose by 16.4 per cent (Rachlis et al. 2001, 6). This has had an impact on jurisdiction as well. Take drugs as an example. We noted above that the power over patents has meant that the federal government has enormous influence on health care development and expenditures. These are largely private commercial enterprises whose product is tested, patented, and regulated by the federal government. The period of patent protection is a direct result of international agreements on patent protection. As individuals increasingly pay for their own drugs, these become significant private transactions, unregulated by provincial governments. The same is true of private home care services, such as those provided by corporations like the Extendicare Company, an international corporation that provides institutional care to the elderly. The federal government has considerable jurisdictional control over these services through taxation, and control of interprovincial economic activities. Should the privatization of direct health care delivery continue, the federal government would undoubtedly acquire more jurisdictional influence because of the increasing control it will attain through its economic jurisdiction over international treaties, patents, and so on.

Globalization and Health Care

At its simplest, we know that globalization will affect health as it has affected other economic and social areas. It will bring with it access to greater and more complex systems of knowledge, the production of the goods and services for health-related activities will probably become global in origin, and the ability for smaller national and subnational governments to control these international organizations will become increasingly problematic. How, if at all, might this influence jurisdiction in health care? There are many who put forward the 'end of territory' thesis, which proposes that through the process of international integration, territorial governments will lose real and legal sovereignty to international organizations. In this process, the nation-state will become increasingly irrelevant as social and economic activities are organized on an international basis. By implication, so will subnational governments.

Most believe that this approach is overly simplistic. The complexity of the interrelationship of social economic and political actions is not as deterministic as this thesis would have us believe. In an excellent article on this subject, Keating points out some of the problems with the 'end of territory' approach:

> We need to be careful about the 'end of territory' thesis. One cannot reason directly from functional re-structuring or economic processes to political power and governing institutions, without giving an independent

role to politics, a role which varies from one case to another ... Yet today, in the face of all of the forces apparently undermining the territorial basis for politics and government, the territorial principle for organizing government is not only surviving but extending. So, as in the past, we are seeing not the end of territory but its transformation and reinvention in new forms. (Keating 1999, 15)

Keating goes on to note that the new territorial politics will be characterized by four features: competition, context, complexity, and asymmetry. For our discussion of jurisdiction, the most important of these are complexity and asymmetry. Complexity means that the link between territory and function, identity, and institutions becomes complicated and variable. In particular, political accountability becomes blurred and innovation is less likely to occur. Asymmetry may also be one of the results of complexity, as the interrelationship of politics and complexity means that 'one size' is unlikely to fit all. If we accept the argument of Keating and others, politics and territory will still matter in the future, but in a different and more complex way. Thus, Lazar's argument that globalization will increase interdependence and blur jurisdictional lines even further in the future is probably correct.

How will governments respond to this blurring and asymmetry and what might be the form of their response? We can quite likely rule out formal constitutional change. Given the history of constitutional amendment in Canada during the past twenty years, and the continuing strong role of the PQ in Quebec, the possibility of some comprehensive new arrangements is 'just not on,' as they say.

More probably, we will see two contradictory directions, especially in the health care field. First, given the current fiscal arrangements and the expectation that governments are again going to cut spending, we can expect to see more unilateral moves. What has happened in Alberta and British Columbia in the past few months will probably be replicated in other provinces. This will lead to the possibility that some of these changes might be challenged by the federal government as violations of the CHA. While this is not a certainty, the actions of some provinces make it more of a possibility. Second, if provincial governments proceed with major privatization initiatives, the federal government's role through its economic powers over international trade might be enhanced. For example, private hospitals and other institutions might be covered by provisions of NAFTA. Unilateral moves by the federal government could lead to friction, as control over these institutions in different provinces becomes a matter of economic as well as health interest.

Another response, given globalization and the increasing importance of economic powers to the health field, may be that the federal and provincial governments will seek to extend the model of SUFA specifically to the field of health care. A comprehensive federal provincial accord in the field of health, akin to AIT or SUFA, would certainly be preferable to formal amendment or continued confrontation. This might allow for some more specific matters to be included in the agreement. Whether or not Quebec could be brought into such an arrangement is problematic, to say the least.

Finally, given the economic role of the federal government, there is the possibility that the courts might be used by individuals, companies, or governments to 'smooth out' complex jurisdictional overlap. Such challenges might arise from particular interest groups or private companies seeking to attain specific goals.

Much depends on how the federal government perceives its role in the field of health in the future. Recent initiatives stemming from September 11 seem to indicate that there is little chance that the federal government will enhance its fiscal role in the field in the near future. If it remains determined to put security, fiscal, and economic objectives ahead of matters like health care, it is likely that there will be further decentralization of control in the field of health. This could raise questions of equity and concern about national standards. Conversely, as noted above, the federal government's economic role, and the increasing complexity stemming from the influence of globalization, might force the federal government to re-evaluate its role and the tools it might use to ensure that it has a role in the future.

We can conclude that the increasingly comprehensive definitions of what constitutes a health matter, together with globalization, privatization, and the reduction of the fiscal role of the federal government will probably cause friction and disorder in health care matters. The result may not be a diminished role for the federal government but a changed one. The shape of that role is not entirely clear, but international agreements will ensure that the role remains important.

Conclusions

This chapter set out to answer these four questions:

1 What are the constitutional bases for the federal and provincial roles in the provision of health care in Canada?

2 What is the constitutional basis for the exercise of the federal spending power as it relates to health?

3 Does the Charter of Rights and Freedoms affect the distribution of
jurisdiction with respect to health care and the delivery of health
care?

4 Insofar as Canadian health policy increasingly involves broader
definitions of 'health' each year, how might the interrelationship of
broader parameters and overlapping jurisdictions affect health care
policy and the discharge of responsibilities for the delivery of health
care in the future? In particular, how do various jurisdictional
responsibilities for economic matters affect health policy?

The answer to the first question has raised some interesting issues.
Actual heads of power have changed little since the original British
North America Act was adopted. However, judicial interpretation of
some of those provisions has altered their ambit significantly. During
the same period, both orders of government have increased their overall involvement in general social matters, including health care. As a
result, although provincial governments have a firm jurisdictional
basis for the delivery of health care services, the increasing overlap and
expanding scope of services means that the federal government has
become a major player in the area.

Given the recent history of constitutional amendment in Canada,
there is little likelihood of amendments that would either clarify the
current heads of power or add new jurisdiction to the federal or provincial governments. It may be that the courts might reinterpret some
existing powers in an effort to remedy a specific problem, but they
would be loath to cast a broad net into such a sea of overlapping jurisdiction. As a result, we can anticipate that changes will occur, if at all,
by way of practice or agreement.

The answer to our second question has also provided some interesting insights. As noted above, the common conception is that health
care is a matter of provincial jurisdiction. We have demonstrated that
the actual situation is more complex than that simple understanding.
The second common conception is that the federal government is on
firm ground using its spending power in the area of health care. Put
differently, most agree that health is a matter of provincial jurisdiction,
but also agree that the federal government can make transfer payments
to provinces for health care purposes and attach conditions to those
transfers, even if they appear to invade provincial jurisdiction. Prov-

inces agree to this only because they want to keep federal funding. Although most constitutional experts agree that the federal government can dispose of its property in any way it sees fit, some, like Dale Gibson, think that this power may be on shaky ground.

Since the Canada Health Act is the main instrument of federal involvement, it is interesting that Gibson thinks that this Act may be assailable if it is defended solely as an exercise in the disposition of property. He believes that it can be defended under POGG on the 'national aspect' dimension. He may or may not be right, but it would be far better if the two orders of government could jointly agree on the principles involved and enshrine it in an agreement that carried with it a mutually agreeable dispute-settlement mechanism. Unfortunately, this is unlikely to happen without some agreement on long-term funding.

Question three dealt with the impact of the Charter on jurisdiction in the area of health care. Specifically, does the Charter affect the distribution of jurisdiction with respect to health care in Canada? We interpreted this to mean, Can the Charter be used to alter jurisdiction in health care? In a formal sense the answer is no. However, the potential to influence or enhance the exercise of jurisdiction is another matter. It is conceivable that the Charter, primarily through section 6, Mobility Rights, and section 15, Equality rights, might influence the role of the federal government. The kind of arguments made by Gibson that portability, for example, might be justified under POGG, could certainly be applied to sections 6 and 15 as well.

Finally, question four asked us to speculate on broadening definitions of health and how that might relate to the economic powers of the federal government. These were broad questions that were only partially addressed in this chapter. We concluded that economic powers would play an increasingly important role in health care because of globalization, economic powers like the power over patents, possible privatization, and finally, the important fiscal role that the federal government maintains in the funding of health care.

It is unlikely that there will be formal constitutional change in the area of health care. It is also probable that the courts will tread carefully in this area as well. If there is change needed in the exercise of jurisdiction, it will have to be brought about by political agreement, enshrined in some form of semi-permanent contract or arrangement. However, as one famous baseball person noted, making predictions is difficult, especially about the future.

NOTES

1 There are many good texts that discuss this matter. In particular, Smiley (1980), Stevenson (1982), and Meekison (1968).

2 In particular see Hogg (1988), 407–33, for a discussion of the 'branch,' 'gap,' and 'emergency' explanations of POGG. It would be worth noting, as well, that the Supreme Court has had an expanding view of federal legislative power under POGG (see *R. v. Crown Zellerbach Canada Ltd.*, [1988 1 SCR 401]) and has stressed the incapacity of the provinces to regulate effectively in some areas.

3 This is not as clear a federal power as this discussion might indicate.

4 For a good discussion of this, see the *Report of the Royal Commission on Aboriginal Peoples*, Volume 3, especially 107–77.

5 In the United States, the Supreme Court has given Congress virtually unfettered power to implement international treaties in areas of state jurisdiction.

6 Section 132 reads: 'The Parliament and Government of Canada shall have all Powers necessary or proper for performing the Obligations of Canada or of any Province thereof, as part of the British Empire, towards Foreign Countries, arising under Treaties between the Empire and such Foreign Countries.'

7 For a discussion of this decision and other related documents, see Howard Leeson and Wilfred Vanderelst (1973). Since 1937, as a result of the Labour Conventions Case, the federal parliament has lacked the ability to legislate obligations under international treaties that fall into areas of provincial jurisdiction. However, recent decisions by the Supreme Court of Canada, such as *Vapour Canada Ltd.*, [1977] 2 SCR 134 in 1974, *R. v. Crown Zellerbach Canada Ltd.* in 1988, and *General Motors v. National City Leasing* in 1989 have indicated that the federal government may be given more latitude under POGG to implement treaties in the future.

8 See the Radio and Aeronautics cases, [1932] A.C. 304 and [1932] A.C. 54, respectively.

9 There are a number of good articles on the events of the 1930s and how they affected Canadian federalism. The most eloquent portrayals are found in the Royal Commission on Dominion-Provincial Relations (Rowell-Sirois Commission) itself, especially the Saskatchewan submission. Other articles include Martha Fletcher, 'Judicial Review and the Division of Powers' and Bora Laskin, 'Reflections on the Canadian Constitution,' both in Peter Meekison, *Canadian Federalism: Myth or Reality* (1968); and the more recent article by Gerald Baier, 'Judicial Review and Canadian Federalism,' in Bakvis and Skogstad, *Canadian Federalism* (2001).

10 See sections 112, 118, 119, 142, and the Third and Fourth Schedules.
11 Once again there are several good sources for this discussion. In particular, Banting (1987, 1998) and Lazar (2000) have done considerable work on the evolution of the spending power in Canada.
12 Hogg reveals that he was counsel for the federal government in this matter.
13 In fact, the federal government and nine provinces agreed to a dispute-settlement procedure in the spring of 2002.
14 Interestingly, a corollary question is also being asked: Can the Charter be used to ensure the right to choose private care?
15 We may know more about this when the Supreme Court of Canada decides the *Lavigne* case from Quebec.
16 Professor Lazar's statement, while broadly true, fails to capture the regional commitment to this state of condition and the role of the federal government. In some provinces like Quebec, or in some regions like Western Canada, there was more or less a commitment at different times.

REFERENCES

Bakvis, Herman, and Grace Skogstad, eds. 2001. *Canadian Federalism: Performance, Effectiveness, and Legitimacy.* Don Mills, ON: Oxford University Press.
Banting, K.G. 1987. *The Welfare State and Canadian Federalism.* 2d ed. Montreal: McGill-Queen's University Press.
– 1998. 'The Past Speaks to the Future: Lessons from the Postwar Social Union.' In *The State of the Federation 1997: Non-Constitutional Renewal*, ed. H. Lazar, 44–69. Kingston: Institute of Intergovernmental Relations, Queen's University.
Barker, Paul. 1998. 'Disentangling the Federation: Social Policy and Fiscal Federalism.' In *Challenges to Canadian Federalism*, ed. Martin Westmacotte and Hugh Mellon, 144–56. Scarborough, ON: Prentice-Hall.
Choudhry, Sujit. 1996. 'The Enforcement of the Canada Health Act.' *McGill Law Journal* 41: 462–509.
Fierlbeck, K. 2001. 'Cost Containment in Health Care: The Federalism Context.' In *Federalism, Democracy and Health Care*, ed. D. Adams, 131–78. Montreal: McGill-Queen's University Press.
Gibson, Dale. 1996. 'The Canada Health Act and the Constitution.' *Health Law Journal* 4: 1–33.
Hogg, Peter. 1998. *Constitutional Law in Canada.* Scarborough, ON: Carswell Publishing.

Jackman, Martha. 2000. 'Constitutional Jurisdiction over Health in Canada.' *Health Law Journal* 95: 95–117.

Keating, Michael. 1999. 'Challenges to Federalism: Territory, Function, and Power in a Globalizing World.' In *Stretching the Federation*, ed. Robert Young, 8–28. Kingston: Institute of Intergovernmental Relations, Queen's University.

Lazar, Harvey. 2000. 'In Search of a New Mission Statement.' In *Canada: The State of the Federation 1999/2000*, ed. Harvey Lazar. Kingston: McGill-Queen's University Press.

Leeson, Howard, and Wilfred Vanderelst. 1973. *External Affairs and Canadian Federalism: The History of a Dilemma*. Toronto: Holt Rinehart and Winston.

Meekison, Peter, ed. 1968. *Canadian Federalism: Myth or Reality*. Toronto: Methuen.

Rachlis, Michael, Robert G. Evans, Patrick Lewis, and Morris L. Barer. 2001. *Revitalizing Medicare*. Vancouver: Tommy Douglas Research Institute.

Rioux, Dr. Marcia. 1999. 'An Appeal to the Charter of Rights and Freedoms.' In *Do We Care*, ed. Margaret Sommerville, 144–7. Montreal: McGill-Queen's University Press.

Russell, Peter H. 1993. *Constitutional Odyssey*. 2nd ed. Toronto: University of Toronto Press.

Saskatchewan. 2001. *Caring for Medicare*. Report of the Commission on Medicare. Ken Fyke, Commissioner.

Smiley, D.V. 1980. *Canada in Question: Federalism in the Eighties*. Toronto: McGraw-Hill Ryerson.

Stevenson, Garth. 1982. *Unfulfilled Union*. Rev. ed. Toronto: Gage Publishing.

Whyte, J.D., and W.R. Lederman. 1977. *Canadian Constitutional Law*. 2nd ed. Toronto: Butterworths.

3 How Will the Charter of Rights and Freedoms and Evolving Jurisprudence Affect Health Care Costs?

DONNA GRESCHNER

The Charter of Rights and Freedoms, as part of the Canadian Constitution, regulates governments' decisions about health care services. The Charter does not expressly guarantee either a right to health or a right of access to health care. However, its general rights provisions, such as equality rights, cover many aspects of the health care system. Since the Charter's enactment in 1982, persons have brought court actions that use Charter rights to challenge health care policies.

To date, the number of Charter challenges to facets of the health care system is not large, and the majority of them have been unsuccessful. Their impact has been uneven. The most successful litigants have been doctors, who have used Charter rights to prevent governmental policies that affected their remuneration and mobility. The least successful plaintiffs have been groups and individuals opposing hospital restructuring, with no victories grounded directly in the Charter. Patients have been only slightly more successful at using the Charter in their efforts to obtain particular health services at public expense. However, notwithstanding the small number of successful challenges since 1982, Charter litigation has the potential to affect significantly the allocation of health care resources – both the distribution of public money within the current Medicare system and the boundaries between the public and private components of health care. Consequently, health care reform needs to take into account the imperatives of Charter rights.

The first section of this chapter describes the Charter's application in the health care field. It focuses on the Charter rights with most relevance for health care decisions, summarizing briefly the jurisprudence under sections 7, 15, and, to a lesser extent, section 6. The second section examines in closer detail the jurisprudence under section 1 of the Charter; the third section discusses the relevance of international jurisprudence; and the fourth section looks at future developments in Charter litigation. (The relevant sections of the Charter can be found in Appendix I.)

The Charter and Health Care Policies

Because the Charter is an entrenched legal document, people may launch legal actions to change governmental decisions that they believe interfere with their rights. Indeed, people do not bring Charter actions for any reason other than to change governmental decisions. Every time a plaintiff succeeds with a Charter action, governmental decisions are modified or reversed. Since almost all governmental decisions involve expenditures, a successful court action means that money will be spent in ways different from those that governments had first wanted. Governments faced with a court order that requires expenditures have a number of options they can use to cover the cost, which includes diverting the money from other components of the health care system; managing the existing system more efficiently and using the savings to cover the costs of the court order; diverting more money into the general health care budget from other areas of spending; offloading some costs to users; decreasing the money paid to providers; raising taxes; or a combination of these. Regardless of the method it chooses, the government's spending decisions are affected. Indeed, the only way that the Charter could not affect government spending in some way is if plaintiffs never won their lawsuits.

The Charter's application to health care policies brings into play several other general features of Charter litigation. First, as with other areas of public policy, the Charter shifts a measure of power over health care reform to judges. They assess the merits of Charter claims and determine whether an aspect of the health care system complies with Charter rights. If it does not, they order governments to change the particular rule or practice. When governments first introduced medicare, beginning with Saskatchewan's legislation in 1962, judicial involvement in the program's design and implementation was minimal. The Canada Health Act, sometimes considered the bedrock of medicare, did not need to consider Charter litigation when it was enacted in 1984, as the Charter had come into force a mere two years earlier. Now, however, reform initiatives must take into account judicial interpretations of Charter rights and be defensible in a courtroom, not only an operating theatre. Generally, the availability of judicial review based on entrenched rights narrows the range of policy options available to governments (Manfredi and Maioni 2002, 217–19).

Second, the Charter has a homogenizing effect. Since constitutional rights apply across the country, an interpretation by one court will influence other judges and policymakers. Decisions from the Supreme Court of Canada are binding on lower courts, and decisions from provincial appellate courts have persuasive authority. This inescapable feature of Charter adjudication has consequences for health care costs. For instance, a ruling by a court in one province that the province must pay for a particular service means that other provinces will likely have to pay, too. A ruling that a specific reform, such as changing methods of paying doctors, is off limits to one province likely means that no province can introduce it. This tendency towards uniformity reduces sensitivity to local conditions (Manfredi and Maioni 2002, 219–21) and could dampen the increasing diversity in provincial reform initiatives (Gray 1998, 928).

Third, the Charter offers people additional arguments in political debates about health care policies. Because of the Charter, the discourse of rights is an increasingly important component of public policy formation. Even if people do not intend to launch legal actions to vindicate rights, they may resist controversial changes to health care services as encroachments upon their rights. Or, they may use rights language not as a shield to protect the existing system but as a sword to pressure governments into facilitating changes that they prefer, such as permitting private health insurance or adding particular treatments to the list of insured services. In the same way, governments may be able to justify reforms, or the status quo, as enhancing Charter rights. To the extent that deployment of rights language in political debates succeeds in influencing policy outcomes, the Charter has an impact upon costs, although in a more intangible and non-quantifiable way than with court actions.

There are many features of the health care system that are subject to Charter claims, such as those listed here.

1 The Charter may restrict a government's options for payment and supply of medical services. For instance, doctors in British Columbia successfully argued that their rights under section 7, Liberty Rights, and section 6, Mobility Rights, were infringed by policies allocating billing numbers (*Re Mia* 1985; *Wilson* 1988; *Waldman* 1999). However,

the Supreme Court has rejected the interpretations that succeeded in *Re Mia* and *Wilson*, and the New Brunswick Court of Appeal recently rejected a section 6 challenge to a similar billing number policy in that province (*Rombaut* 2001).

2 People have used Charter arguments to challenge integral aspects of the Medicare system, such as the prohibition on private health insurance, but thus far unsuccessfully (*Chaoulli* 2002).

3 The Charter affects governments' decisions about particular services to include within publicly funded medicare systems. These decisions may violate section 15, Equality Rights (*Eldridge* 1997; *Auton* 2000). If courts order governments to pay for these previously uninsured services, they expand the scope of publicly funded services, shifting the balance between public and private funding.

4 The right of parents to choose or refuse medical treatment for their children may be an aspect of their right to liberty in section 7, and, if they decide on religious grounds, their freedom of religion in section 2(a) (*R.B. v. Children's Aid Society* 1995).

5 The involuntary treatment of persons with mental illnesses is subject to section 7, Rights of Liberty and Security of the Person (*Carver* 2002).

6 The Charter is implicated in the 'right to die with dignity' cases, in which patients assert constitutional rights to choose the manner and time of their deaths (*Rodriquez* 1993).

7 The Charter affects the governments' prohibition of particular health services. In *R. v. Morgentaler* (1988), the Supreme Court's first involvement with the Charter and health care, the Court struck down the Criminal Code restrictions on abortion services as a violation of a woman's right to security of the person.

8 The Charter covers the employment relationship between governments and health care workers. However, not every work relationship in a health care facility falls within the Charter's purview (*Stoffman* 1990).

9 The Charter affects the legal power of professional organizations in the health care sector to regulate the activities of their members. The courts have struck down bans on advertising by dentists as a violation of freedom of expression (*Rocket* 1990) and a by-law preventing optometrists from having business associations with other optometrists (*Costco Wholesale* 1998).

Each type of litigation has an impact on costs. For instance, even

those decisions that reduce procedural complexities of accessing services, such as *Morgentaler*, will affect costs in several ways. For one
thing, complying with procedures always has direct and indirect costs,
and changing procedures will alter these costs. In addition, since procedural obstacles often have a deterrent effect, simplifying procedures
may increase total cost because more people will obtain the service.
However, the most important effects of the Charter on health care costs
result from cases in the first three areas. These areas comprise two
related categories: structure of payment and delivery of health care,
and scope of coverage with respect to publicly insured services
(Von Tigerstrom 2002).

The first category involves changes to the methods by which governments pay for health services and provide them. Generally, Canada has
a mixed system, with considerable public financing and mostly private
delivery. Whether and how to change the mix between the public and
private components of health care financing and delivery is one of the
key policy questions of our time. Charter rights may be invoked to
question the wisdom and constitutionality of proposals that alter the
mix or restructure in other ways the institutions of health care. This
category includes challenges by doctors to changes in physician management schemes (e.g., *Rombaut* 2001), attempts to enjoin hospital
closures (e.g., *Wellesley Central Hospital* 1997; *Ponteix* 1994), and actions
to permit private health insurance for services covered by medicare
(*Chaoulli* 2002). The last type of action, if successful, has the potential
for causing the most dramatic change to the health care system, since
removing the ban on private health insurance would create a two-tier
or multi-tiered system (Schrecker 1998, 143).

The second category involves challenges by patients who want the
government to pay for more services than those currently covered by
the medical insurance plan (e.g., *Cameron* 1999a; *Auton* 2000). Here,
again, successful court actions change the mix between public and
private funding. These lawsuits usually do not strike at the core of
medicare's principles. Rather, because they ask for public insurance to
include more services, they seek expansion of the principles of universality and accessibility. However, that does not reduce their potential
to affect significantly the distribution of health care costs.

Overall, Charter actions brought by patients and others have been
few in number. The table of cases in Appendix II lists Charter decisions
that involve, in some aspect or another, health care services, whether
provided in hospitals, clinics, nursing homes, or schools. (The table

excludes cases involving involuntary treatment of patients, fetal rights, and informed consent.) There are only thirty-three. Even if this number were doubled to compensate for any cases missed by the searches, the total number would not be large. This low number is surprising. Since health care affects everyone and is the largest single budget item for provinces, one would expect more litigation, especially in light of the state of flux in the health care system.

Of these thirty-three cases, claimants in eleven cases succeeded in obtaining remedies for a Charter violation. The rate of success, 33 per cent, is in line with the general success rate for Charter claims from 1982 to 1998, which most authors calculate at between 30 and 35 per cent (Kelly 1999). Moreover, in several cases in which plaintiffs have successfully proven a violation of a Charter right, the government has demonstrated that the violation is a reasonable limit under section 1 (*Cameron* 1999a). Courts have been cautious about judging governments' health care policies as unreasonable. Further, in several Charter actions where plaintiffs obtained remedies, governments did not attempt to raise section 1 arguments (*Re Mia* 1985; *Wilson* 1988). If they had, the results might have been different, and the number of successful challenges even lower.

The impact of these successful cases on health care costs is difficult to assess because no numbers are readily available. Nevertheless, it is possible to draw tentative conclusions. Overall, of the eleven cases in which courts gave a remedy, the ones with the greatest impact on health care costs were the doctors' mobility and liberty claims. The provinces' restricted ability to ration physician services likely had financial ramifications in the tens or hundreds of millions of dollars, not only in British Columbia, where the cases originated, but also in other provinces that were considering similar schemes in the late 1980s and early 1990s. At the other end of the cost spectrum, a few successful cases likely had a much smaller effect on overall costs: for example, *R. v. Morgentaler* (1988), which involved access to abortion services, and *R. v. Parker* (2000), which concerned access to marijuana for medical purposes. Somewhere in between are cases such as *Lalonde* (2001). *Lalonde* is similar to the doctors' mobility rights cases because it involves structural issues of health care delivery. On its face it involves a large sum of money because the Ontario government decided not to proceed immediately with restructuring services at the hospital in dispute. However, more precise information is needed to assess the monetary consequences of a failed attempt at hospital restructuring.

Whether closure of a particular hospital saves money in the long run depends on several factors, such as the inefficiency of the hospital in question, and whether services are managed efficiently among other hospitals in the area.

With respect to challenges about the scope of insured services, patients obtained remedies in only two cases. In *Eldridge* (1997), the Supreme Court accepted evidence that the cost of providing sign language interpreters was $150,000, which was approximately 0.0025 per cent of the provincial health care budget. Since all provinces now have to provide such a service, the nationwide cost is greater (assuming that some provinces did not provide the service before the Court decision), but still not significant. In *Auton,* the British Columbia court ordered specific treatment for autistic children, which was estimated to cost $40,000 to $60,000 a year per child, with treatment ranging from two to five years per child. Unfortunately, the court did not estimate the total cost of the service. Although several provinces already pay for this treatment when recommended by doctors, others do not. On a national basis, the cost implications of this ruling would not be negligible.

Overall, the direct effect of Charter litigation on health care costs has not been large, except with respect to restructuring physician services. However, the future may be quite different. One scholar's comment about the Supreme Court is apt: 'Offering predictions about the Court's future use of the Charter is a dangerous game' (Kelly 1999, 636). Kelly concludes that the Supreme Court's recent decisions indicate a trend towards minimizing conflict with the legislative branch (636), which would suggest that governments may not need fear too greatly an activist judiciary. However, studies also show that judges are more inclined to nullify recent policy choices by provincial legislatures (Manfredi and Maioni 2002, 221), which would mean that new provincial policy directions in the health care field are more susceptible to judicial reversal.

In grappling with the question of future judicial involvement, this chapter focuses on the courts' interpretation of the most important Charter rights. On the premise that courts rarely change jurisprudential direction overnight, the interpretations accepted to date for Charter rights would continue to structure arguments in the near future.

Appendix 1 reproduces the most relevant Charter provisions. Section 15, the Equality Rights provision, gives everyone the right to equality without discrimination on a number of grounds. Two of the enumerated grounds have direct relevance to the health care field –

physical and mental disability. Section 7 gives everyone the right not to be deprived of life, liberty, and security of the person, except in accordance with the principles of fundamental justice. Section 6 states that every citizen and permanent resident has the right to pursue the gaining of a livelihood in any province. If a court rules that a person's rights have been violated, governments may justify the limitation under section 1 as reasonable in a free and democratic society. However, justificatory arguments also come into play in interpreting the scope of rights.

Section 15

Claims under section 15 have focused on expanding the scope of insured services. Persons allege that a particular health care policy, which excludes them from coverage or reduces their share of resources, violates their rights to the equal protection and equal benefit of the law. The potential for claims is theoretically quite broad because one prohibited ground in section 15 is physical or mental disability. Although the courts have not issued an authoritative definition of this ground, it covers illnesses and a wide array of conditions. However, the total number of Charter claims under section 15 is very small, and only two, *Eldridge* and *Auton*, have been successful. Courts have been cautious about ordering governments to pay for particular health services.

This conclusion may seem surprising in light of the considerable media attention given to the Supreme Court's unanimous judgment in *Eldridge*. A group of deaf patients argued that the British Columbia government's decision not to fund sign-language interpreters for them when they received medical treatment violated their right to equality under section 15. Specifically, they argued that this failure constituted adverse effects discrimination on the basis of physical disability because their inability to communicate effectively with medical personnel denied them the equal benefit of the provincial medicare program. The Supreme Court agreed and directed the government to provide sign-language interpreters where necessary for effective communication.

The *Eldridge* ruling imposes a positive obligation on governments to provide a particular service for patients. However, it does not open the floodgates to constitutional challenges about the scope of 'insured medical services.' As the Court stressed in its reasons, the inequality was about access to insured health care services. The plaintiffs were not asking for a specific medical treatment that the government had decided not to fund, such as expensive fertility treatments. Rather, they wanted equal access to all the services, and no more than those services that were available to the hearing population. The problem was not the services offered by the government but the fact that the government provided the services in a manner that hearing people could readily access, but not deaf people. As in the earlier *J.C.* (1992) decision from a lower court about the exclusion of women from prisoners' treatment programs, the *Eldridge* claimants could not access equally services that were generally available to others because of an enumerated ground (disability in *Eldridge*; sex in *J.C.*).

The policy that distressed the patients in *Eldridge* is an example of 'rationing by characteristic' – a particular health care service is insured, but not everyone who can benefit from the service can access it. Governments also engage in 'rationing by service' – a specific medical treatment for a particular illness or condition is not funded for anyone. For example, in *Cameron* (1999, 1999a) the province funded some hospital services for infertility but not *in vitro* fertilization (IVF) or intra-cytomplasmic sperm injection (ICSI). In *Auton*, the province funded some treatment for autistic children, but not the Lovaas treatment preferred by the plaintiffs, who were parents of autistic children. These cases, which involve the scope of coverage, raise different questions. Governments assess a broad range of factors in making such decisions, including the cost of the treatment, its effectiveness in improving the patient's quality or length of life, and social and ethical concerns. Moreover, courts may hesitate to evaluate complex decisions about the clinical effectiveness and other medical standards for highly specialized treatments (Von Tigerstrom 2002, 171). Von Tigerstrom argues that cases involving 'rationing by services' are more difficult to resolve, but even if this is the case, one cannot underestimate the complexities of 'rationing by characteristics,' which may involve a multitude of interconnected assessments.

With respect to 'scope of coverage' cases, courts now assess claims in accordance with a general scheme that the Supreme Court articulated after its *Eldridge* decision. In *Law v. Canada* (1999), the Court held that a plaintiff must satisfy the following three steps in order to prove a violation of equality rights:

1 The impugned law or policy must draw a distinction between

groups of persons on the basis of a personal characteristic, or fail to draw such a distinction for a group already disadvantaged, in a manner that results in substantively differential treatment between the groups.

2 The differential treatment must be on a ground that is enumerated in section 15 (such as sex or age) or on a ground that is analogous to an enumerated ground (such as sexual orientation).

3 The differential treatment must constitute substantive discrimination, which means that it offends the plaintiff's essential human dignity.

The first two criteria are not too burdensome for plaintiffs who want an expansion of insured services. After all, the plaintiffs are patients who seek treatment for physical or mental health problems. The third criterion presents more problems, as it does generally for plaintiffs with section 15 claims. Not every distinction in health treatment between groups of patients is discriminatory; for instance, the mere fact that governments do not fund IVF or ICSI treatment for infertility is not automatically discriminatory. Patients must also convince a court that the distinction offends their dignity. The Supreme Court has said that such distinctions have 'the effect of perpetuating or promoting the view that the individual is less capable or worthy of recognition or value as a human being or as a member of Canadian society, equally deserving of concern, respect, and consideration' (*Law* 1999, para. 88).

The case-law to date does not provide clear guidelines to distinguish between exclusions from insured services that offend dignity and those that do not. In *Cameron* (1999a), the Nova Scotia Court of Appeal was split on whether the non-insurability of IVF and ICSI impinged upon the plaintiff's essential human dignity. A majority of the Court concluded that the exclusion did violate dignity because of historical stereotyping of infertile persons, especially women, and the stigma associated with infertility. By contrast, a minority opinion ruled that the exclusion of some infertility services did not offend dignity, stating that it was 'an inevitable consequence of the administration of health care' (682). However, the dissenting judge commented that if the government refused to fund any medical treatments for infertility, such a policy would likely offend essential human dignity (683–4).

Although the sparse case-law does not permit ready generalizations, it does seem that exclusions justified by cost, risk, safety, and low effectiveness will not violate human dignity. However, wholesale delisting of services might well do so. Governments will need to justify exclusions with evidence about the reasons for the exclusion; in short, they will need to prove that the exclusion is supported by sound medical evidence or other cogent reasons that are unrelated to any prejudice or stereotyping about the persons who wish to have the service. In this regard, the third criterion replicates the balancing that takes place in section 1.

In summary, section 15 does present possibilities for patients to challenge decisions about the scope of coverage. Perhaps one reason for the low number of cases in which persons seek more health services is the relative universality, accessibility, and comprehensiveness of Canada's existing Medicare system. Anyone in need of medical treatment to preserve life or health is usually entitled to receive it (Jackman 1995; Von Tigerstrom 2002). Thus, it is not surprising that Charter cases to date have involved expensive uninsured services, such as drug prescriptions (*Brown* 1990) and fertility treatments (*Cameron* 1999, 1999a). Consequently, if governments change significantly the current mix of public and privately funded health care services, section 15 will become more important as a shield to protect existing coverage. In addition, however, the Charter may be used as a sword to obtain more insured services, such as pharmaceutical products. With escalating drug costs and increasing reliance on life-saving drugs, it is surprising that major exclusions from medicare, such as most prescription drugs and home care, have not been subject to more Charter challenges.

If the courts do hold that a particular feature of the health care system violates equality rights, the government may justify the limit under section 1. For instance, in *Cameron* the majority of the Nova Scotia Court of Appeal held that the exclusion of IVF and ICSI treatments from insured services violated section 15, but was a reasonable limit under section 1 (which is discussed more fully below).

Section 7

Section 7 protects the right not to be deprived of life, liberty, or security of the person except in accordance with the principles of fundamental justice. Its power as a tool to challenge health care policies has been limited because plaintiffs must overcome significant obstacles in proving a violation of section 7.

First, plaintiffs must show that either 'liberty' or 'security' encompasses health or health care services. The courts have not interpreted the rights in section 7 in a manner sufficiently broad to encompass a general right to health, or, except in exceptional circumstances, a right to access health care services. With respect to liberty, a majority of Supreme Court judges has ruled that the phrase covers only freedom from physical restraint and not economic liberty, such as the right to engage in contractual relations (Hogg 2001, 920). With respect to security, the Court has held that it includes the right of access to health care (*R. v. Morgentaler* 1988), and the right to refuse medical treatment for oneself (*Rodriquez* 1993). Lower courts have ruled that security does not include the right to have health care of one's choice provided at public expense, such as public funding of drug prescriptions (*Brown* 1990) or enhanced public funding for nursing homes (*Ontario Nursing Home Assn.* 1990). In Nova Scotia, a claim under section 7 for public funding of fertility treatments was curtly dismissed by the trial court (*Cameron* 1999, para. 160), and not pursued on appeal (*Cameron* 1999a).

Second, even if plaintiffs can prove a deprivation of liberty or security, they must also show that the deprivation contravened the principles of fundamental justice. The Supreme Court has interpreted the phrase 'principles of fundamental justice' to mean basic tenets of the legal system, such as the presumption of innocence (*Reference Re Motor Vehicle Act* 1988). These basic tenets clearly include the rules of fair procedure, but whether they include substantive principles is more debatable. In a recent decision involving child protection hearings, the Court suggested that section 7 is restricted to situations where the infringements to liberty or security are 'a result of an individual's interaction with the justice system and its administration' (*New Brunswick* 1999, para. 65). With health care services, when plaintiffs challenge governmental decisions about 'medically necessary services' or other funding provisions, they will find proving a violation of these principles exceedingly difficult because generally the health care system is administrative, not criminal.

One example of criminal prohibitions was the therapeutic abortion committee provisions that the Supreme Court struck down as a violation of section 7 in *R. v. Morgentaler* (1988). These provisions made abortion a criminal offence unless the abortion was approved by a cumbersome hospital committee structure. The unusual feature of this legislative regime was that women seeking abortions and doctors performing them were guilty of a criminal offence unless they received prior approval from a committee. A woman's access to health services and a doctor's freedom to perform the service were severely constrained by the most onerous legal sanction – criminal punishment. In this context, the Supreme Court held that a woman's right to security of the person included the right to access health care services without threat of criminal sanction, and that the convoluted and often elusive committee structure violated the principles of fundamental justice. One judge, Justice Wilson, went further and held that the Criminal Code provisions also violated a woman's right to liberty.

The legal rule in *Morgentaler* was exceptional because it was situated on the overlap between the criminal law process and the health care system. A similar example is *R. v. Parker* (2000), where the Ontario Court of Appeal struck down the criminal prohibition against possession of marijuana for people who use the drug for medicinal purposes. However, cases in which a form of health care is subject to severe criminal penalty are rare. In an effort to overcome the stricture of criminal or quasi-criminal sanctions as a condition of section 7 claims, several commentators have argued recently that principles of fundamental justice should encompass administrative procedures, which would include a wide variety of health care policies (Karr 2000; Hartt and Monahan 2002).

Moreover, in cases where plaintiffs challenge basic tenets of the health care system, governments may be able to rely on the principles of fundamental justice to defend their decisions because these principles include other Charter values, such as equality and human dignity. In *Chaoulli* (2000), the trial judge ruled that the prohibition of private health insurance for services covered by medicare, while perhaps infringing section 7 rights if the public system did not provide sufficient access to health services, did not contravene the principles of fundamental justice. The prohibition was adopted because allowing a parallel private system would impair the viability of the public system, and adversely affect the rights of the rest of the population. The judge concluded as follows: '[The prohibition is] motivated by considerations of equality and human dignity ... it is clear that there is no conflict with the general values promoted by the Charter' (qtd. in Von Tigerstrom 2002, 166). The trial judge's decision was upheld by the Quebec Court of Appeal (*Chaoulli* 2002).

One underlying reason for the judicial hesitancy about broadly interpreting section 7 is the more general reluctance to include economic interests within section 7. The Supreme Court has ruled that economic rights in the corporate or commercial context do not come within section 7. The courts are afraid of opening section 7 to a host of economic claims. Indisputably, health services are bundles of economic interests, not manna – someone must provide them, and someone must pay for them. At the same time, however, the Supreme Court has left open the question of whether section 7 could protect economic interests that are integrally connected to material well-being (*Irwin Toy* 1989, 1003–4). Since health care qualifies as essential for well-being in the same manner as food and clothing, it remains possible to protect health care under section 7 notwithstanding its economic aspect. For instance, if people were denied access to emergency medical services because they could not pay for them, their claim of a section 7 violation could receive a sympathetic judicial hearing. Moreover, the medicare system is extremely popular, and many citizens view it as a fundamental plank of Canadian society. This popularity may assist judges in overcoming their usual reluctance to evaluate and supervise benefits programs. The Supreme Court recently heard an appeal from a Quebec case that raises the issue of whether inadequate social assistance payments violate security of the person (*Gosselin* 1999). Its decision may foreshadow the Court's direction on analogous cases in health care.

In the near future, one can reasonably expect more Charter claims that address the phenomenon of waiting lists. Recently, several lawyers have argued, as in the *Chaoulli* litigation, that waiting lists impair patients' psychological health and, in some cases, threaten their lives (Karr 2000; Hartt and Monahan 2002). Further, they argue that the appropriate remedy is private health insurance that covers services now paid for by medicare. This line of argument is attractive not only to wealthy patients who could afford private insurance but also to those doctors and other health care providers who wish to establish private medical facilities. If successful, these arguments would have a major impact on health care costs; parallel private systems reallocate existing resources and cause an increase in the total budget, as well as raise issues of equity and access (Gray 1998, 910–13). But success for these arguments is not assured. Besides the difficulty of showing a violation of principles of fundamental justice, patients and health care providers who argue for more private insurance face an additional obstacle. Even if waiting lists violate section 7, the appropriate remedy may be more public funding or better management of waiting lists, rather than creating a system of parallel private health care by removing the ban on private insurance. For instance, since waiting lists for a specific procedure may vary greatly among a group of specialists, it might be appropriate for a court to order publication of wait times for all specialists in the province. Such an order would give patients valuable information on how to choose a specialist. What is not obvious, however, is that the remedy for wait times is private insurance; this remedy would only fix the constitutional violation for wealthy people who could afford insurance, and may substantially worsen the constitutional violation of wait times for poor people, who would endure longer wait times because of a drain of medical resources to the privately funded system (Schrecker 1998, 143). As noted above, the government's egalitarian objective in prohibiting private insurance was recognized by the trial judge in *Chaoulli* (2000).

The debates about remedies for correcting wait times illustrate a major difficulty with Charter review of health care policies. The health care system is fiendishly complicated and simple answers to problems (such as allowing private insurance as a response to waiting lists) could wreak considerable damage to the system and cause constitutional violations for other groups of people. Judges are not well equipped to deal with the enormous ramifications of changing elements of the health care system. They may not obtain much help from counsel, who may have neither the expertise nor interest in assisting judges in understanding fully the variables and dynamics of health care policy. For instance, it is distressing that a major article arguing for the unconstitutionality of the prohibition on private health insurance (Karr 2000) does not cite a single study from health economists or policy analysts on the causes of, and remedies for, wait times. The more recent study by Hartt and Monahan (2002), arguing that wait times violate section 7 rights, refers briefly to several studies about wait times but fails to consider the wider consequences of judges creating a two-tier health system. The complexities of wait times and options for solving them (Lewis et al. 2000) illustrate that assessing health care policy is a quintessentially interdisciplinary undertaking. Yet judges will be wading into these thorny areas without expertise. For understandable reasons, they may adopt an attitude of extreme caution, if not deference, as they have generally done with health care cases to date (*Cameron* 1999a; *Chaoulli* 2000, 2002).

One last point must be made about section 7. In several cases, judges have said that violations of section 7 can only be justified under section 1 in exceptional circumstances (*Reference Re Motor Vehicle Act* 1988, 518). In practice this means that the justificatory arguments for limiting rights occur within the interpretation of the section itself (Hogg 2001,

916), defining the scope of 'liberty' and 'security' and the content of principles of fundamental justice. One example of this practice is the trial judgment in *Chaoulli* (2000).

Mobility Rights and Fundamental Principles

Of the other Charter provisions that affect the health care system, mobility rights deserve attention. Section 6 states that every citizen has a right to earn a livelihood in the province. Mobility rights have impaired the provinces' ability to reform their policies of physician management. British Columbia's efforts to rationalize physician services have been particularly hard hit in this regard (*Re Mia* 1985; *Wilson* 1988; *Waldman* 1999).

However, mobility rights may no longer protect doctors' freedom from regulation. The Supreme Court recently issued a major decision about section 6 in which it held that a violation of mobility rights required discrimination on the grounds of provincial residency (*Canadian Egg Marketing Agency (CEMA)* 1998). Consequently, policies that regulate doctors' practices within a particular province do not violate mobility rights, contrary to the holding in *Re Mia* and the trial judgment in *Waldman*, unless the particular scheme distinguishes between doctors on the basis of past or present residency. Most proposals for equitable distribution of doctors do not draw such distinctions, and therefore do not violate section 6. Accordingly, when the British Columbia Court of Appeal heard the appeal in *Waldman*, it applied the *CEMA* decision to hold that only one provision of the scheme violated section 6, although it refused to sever the offending provision and thus struck down the entire law (*Waldman* 1999, para. 51). Recently, when a group of doctors in New Brunswick challenged that province's rationing scheme for physician services, the New Brunswick court applied the *CEMA* decision to dismiss their claim (*Rombaut* 2001).

One recent case involving a hospital restructuring attracted considerable media attention, but on closer scrutiny it does not herald a new era in judicial regulation of health care policies. In *Lalonde* (2001), a group of francophone citizens challenged the decision of the Ontario Health Services Restructuring Commission to change the mandate of Hôpital Montfort, the only French-language hospital in Ontario. They argued that the decision adversely affected medical services to their official-language community. The Ontario Court of Appeal held that the Commission must respect the Constitution's fundamental organizing principles, which include the protection of minorities, in its restructuring decisions. The Court quashed the decision and remitted the matter to the minister for reconsideration in accordance with its reasons. The judgment's only novel feature was the ruling that administrative agencies must consider fundamental constitutional principles in addition to Charter values. It is a long established principle that governmental agencies, such as health services commissions, must respect Charter rights and exercise their discretion in a manner consistent with the Charter. The plaintiffs in Lalonde, however, could not rely on section 15 because of a line of cases holding that language was not an analogous ground under section 15. Hence, they relied on the fundamental constitutional principle of protection of minorities. Given section 15's broad scope with respect to enumerated and analogous grounds, cases such as *Lalonde* where plaintiffs must resort to deeper constitutional values in challenging administrative discretion may be quite rare.

Jurisprudence under Section 1

Section 1 serves a dual purpose. It guarantees rights and freedoms, but also permits governments to limit those rights if the limits are reasonably justified in a free and democratic society. In the classic case of *R. v. Oakes* (1986), Chief Justice Dickson established the basic criteria by which to assess whether violation was a reasonable limit. The *Oakes* test is twofold. First, the government must establish that the impugned law had an important objective. This criterion has proven easy for governments to satisfy. Indeed, there have been virtually no cases in which the test is not met (Hogg 2001, 743). In the context of health care, the government has invariably argued that its objective for a particular policy, such as not insuring particular services or rationing billing numbers, is to protect the viability of medicare and use its resources effectively. This objective satisfies the first branch of Oakes.

The second branch of the *Oakes* test assesses the government's means of achieving its objective. The test is one of proportionality, with three parts. First, the means must be rationally connected to the objective. Second, the means must impair as little as possible the right or freedom; there must not be a less drastic alternative by which to achieve the ends. Third, the means must not have a disproportionately severe effect on persons to whom it applies. Generally, in almost all section 1 cases, the disputes have turned on the second part of this three-pronged test – the least drastic means (Hogg 2001, 743). The language in *Oakes* was quite stringent: the law had to impair the right as little as possible. However, later cases have softened the language considerably. Quite soon after *Oakes*, the Supreme Court recognized that governments needed a margin of appreciation in designing laws, and that courts should give some degree of deference to legislators in crafting policies. Courts now look for reasonable efforts by governments to minimize legislative infringements of Charter rights, rather than the least minimal interference. In short, a range of governmental policies, not merely the least drastic, will satisfy section 1.

Generally, courts are more willing to give a margin of appreciation to governments when one of several considerations is present: if the law is intended to protect a vulnerable group, such as children or poor people; if the law reconciles the interests of competing groups; if the law allocates scarce resources; or if the law rests on complex, and often competing, social science evidence (Hogg 2001, 764). Laws regulating the health care system usually possess all four of these characteristics. Accordingly, in cases involving components of the health care system, all of these considerations should come into play, resulting in a wide margin of appreciation when governments justify restrictions under section 1.

The wide margin of appreciation for governments is demonstrated in the jurisprudence. Judges understand that health care budgets are complex and controversial, involving difficult trade-offs. They have been reluctant to second-guess governments about the best way to spend health care dollars. The majority opinion in *Cameron* (1999a), in ruling that a section 15 violation was justified under section 1, illustrates the general judicial attitude. After reviewing the government's evidence about increases to the health care budget and federal cut-backs to cost-sharing programs, which resulted in compelling pressures on the Department of Health, it expressed considerable reluctance to find that the government's policies were unreasonable under section 1: 'the evidence makes clear the complexity of the health care system and the extremely difficult task confronting those who must allocate the resources among a vast array of competing claims ... The policy makers require latitude in balancing competing interests in the constrained financial environment. We are simply not equipped to sort out the priorities. We should not second guess them, except in clear cases of failure on their part to properly balance the Charter rights of individuals against the overall pressing objective of the scheme' (*Cameron* 1999a, 667).

With respect to predicting when the government will fail in meeting its burden under section 1, the two 'scope of coverage' cases in which courts rejected the section 1 arguments are not especially helpful for drawing generalizations. In *Eldridge*, where the Supreme Court ordered the government to pay for sign-language interpreters for deaf patients, it stressed that the cost was minimal. Unfortunately, it did not consider the impact of its ruling on other provinces, who might have different financial circumstances. Nor did it assess the cogency of the evidence about cost, accepting without question an intervenor's somewhat dubious estimate (Manfredi and Maoini 2002, 229). In *Auton*, the rather skimpy discussion of section 1 is unsatisfactory. The Court seems to duck the issue of money, noting the cost per child, but not the total amount of the treatment. It apparently regarded the situation as identical to that in *Eldridge*, which was erroneous since the Supreme Court stressed that *Eldridge* involved access to existing services, not adding new ones. In *Auton* it seems that the most important consideration was the Court's assessment that the savings created in the long run by assisting autistic children would likely offset the cost of the controversial treatment.

The exception to this general deference is the doctors' claims that physician management schemes violated their Charter rights. Overall, courts have been unusually insensitive to the enormous cost ramifications of invalidating provincial rationing schemes for physician services. Although, as noted previously, the jurisprudential foundations of the doctors' victories are now shaky, the general judicial fondness for doctors' claims may carry over into new challenges brought by doctors to preserve their dominant position within the health care system. For instance, it is not unrealistic to expect challenges if a regional health authority required all doctors in its area to be paid by capitation or employment contracts, rather than permitting 'fee for service' arrangements. Although section 7 does not cover the right to exercise a profession (*Reference Re Criminal Code* 1990, 527), past Charter victories by doctors would give their challenges more chance of success than analogous claims by other professions. Nevertheless, the odds of victory in challenging contractual requirements with health authorities would still be low (Flood 1999, 193).

Two clear points emerge from the case-law. First, cost is indeed a consideration in section 1 balancing. In its early Charter jurisprudence, the Supreme Court stated rather categorically that cost could not justify infringements of rights; in other words, governments could not use money as a reason to violate Charter rights (*Singh* 1985, 469). If fair hearings for refugee claimants would cost hundreds of millions of dollars, as did the remedy in the *Singh* case, then the government must pay the bill. However, this rigid view about the role of costs has considerably loosened. With many rights, providing the right to one group without regard to costs may result in another group being denied its rights. Arguably, health care decision-making is a paradigmatic example of these trade-offs. The courts may ignore the cost of providing a service if it is small (*Eldridge*) but not when it is relatively large (*Cameron*).

Second, there is a great need for cogent evidence. Even with a margin of appreciation and judicial sensitivity to the complexities of health budgeting, section 1 justifications will require evidence that the government considered alternatives to the impugned policy. This evidence could involve the cost-benefit analysis engaged in by policymakers, the medical studies that were examined, and any other relevant factors that were taken into account. If governments do not adduce evidence, their likelihood of success under section 1 is greatly diminished. In *Eldridge*, for example, the Court emphasized several times the government's failure to adduce evidence of undue strain on the health care system if the service was provided (*Eldridge* 1997, paras. 92, 94).

The obligation to produce evidence in an open court about the merits, expense, and risks of different health care options may have positive benefits for health policy. For one thing, it may deter policymakers from making decisions based on the decibel level of the group asking for a particular service at a particularly sensitive time, such as immediately before an election. Overall, it may hasten the incorporation of what has been called 'evidence-based medicine' into public policy about health care.

However, there remain significant problems with judicial assessments under section 1. One major problem inheres in the very nature of adjudication: telescopic vision. As the litigation in *Eldridge* and *Auton* illustrates, in each case the court assesses only one tiny part of a very large puzzle. And, because it focuses on only one part, that part is magnified. What adjudication usually fails to consider is the opportunity cost of its orders – where else could the money be spent? Yet this is the question that necessarily preoccupies policymakers. Judicial recognition of the telescopic nature of adjudicatory methods ought to strengthen their caution about reviewing health care decisions.

International Law

Canada is a signatory to international conventions about human rights. The right to health is firmly embedded in many conventions, albeit with slightly different language in each one (Toebes 1999). These conventions are binding at international law. Canada is obliged to act in accordance with these conventions, but convention rights are not directly enforceable in Canadian courts (Hogg 2001, 689). Nevertheless, they are important to a study about the Charter because of the long-standing principle that domestic law should be interpreted in a manner consistent with international obligations. In a recent decision, the Supreme Court emphasized that this principle includes Charter interpretation: '[I]nternational human rights law ... is also a critical influence on the interpretation of the rights included in the Charter' (*Baker* 1999, para. 70).

This section briefly discusses one important convention, the *International Covenant on Economic, Social and Cultural Rights (ICESCR)*, as an example of the right to health in international law. Article 12 recognizes 'the right of everyone to the enjoyment of the highest attainable standard of physical and mental health.' It provides further that State Parties shall take steps necessary to achieve the full realization of this right, including reducing infant mortality, improving environmental and industrial hygiene, preventing and treating disease, and creating 'conditions which would assure to all medical service and medical attention in the event of sickness' (*ICESCR* 1966, Art. 12[2]). This right clearly includes the right to health care, such as immunization services, essential drugs, and emergency medical treatment. But it also includes health-related issues, such as safe water, adequate sanitation, and environmental health (Toebes 1999).

International conventions require State Parties to file periodic reports describing their efforts to comply with the convention's obligations. The *ICESCR* reports are filed with the Committee on Economic, Social and Cultural Rights. With each report, the Committee publishes concluding remarks that indicate the direction of international law developments.

Canada filed its third periodic report to the Committee in 1998. In its concluding observations, the Committee did not comment negatively on health care services, except with respect to the 'significant cuts to services on which people with disabilities rely' and programs for people discharged from psychiatric institutions (Committee on Economic, Social and Cultural Rights 1998, para. 36). However, it expressed concern about many aspects of Canada's social programs, including the cuts to social assistance, the restrictions on unemployment insurance, the growing problem of homelessness, and the inadequate protection of women's rights. It drew attention to the adverse consequences for poor people that flowed from the replacement of the Canada Assistance Plan with the Canada Health and Social Transfer (CHST), including the absence of national standards for social assistance programs. Furthermore, it found inexplicable the double standards in the CHST: '[The CHST] did, however, retain national standards in relation to health, thus denying provincial flexibility in one area, while insisting upon it in others [social assistance]. The delegation provided no explanation for this inconsistency' (para. 19). Overall, one can conclude that Canada's medicare program fulfills its international obligations, but its social programs need improvement. Insofar as a right to health includes basic necessities, such as income and shelter, Canada is failing to meet its obligations.

International obligations may influence proposals to reform the existing health care system. In a number of reports, the Committee asked State Parties to report on whether disparities exist between the public and private sectors in their health care systems. Furthermore, it has noted that plans to decentralize and privatize health care services do not relieve a State Party from its obligations to promote access to health care services, especially for poor people (Toebes 1999, 105–6). Thus, if Canadian governments were to privatize health care services to a significant degree, they may run more afoul of their international obligations.

One issue in international law debates is whether social and economic rights, such as the right to health in Article 12 of the *ICESCR*, should be given the same priority as civil and political rights, such as freedom of expression. Many scholars have argued that international law should be governed by a principle of indivisibility: social and economic rights are indivisible from civil and political rights, and should have the same priority in terms of enforcement (Schabas 1999). Critics of this approach argue that social and economic rights involve different considerations, such as imposing positive obligations on governments, and should not be lumped in with civil and political rights (Richards 1999).

This debate has relevance to the question about the future impact of the Charter on the health care system. If the principle of indivisibility becomes more widely accepted, courts will be more willing to interpret Charter rights broadly to include a general right to health and to issue Charter remedies for the enforcement of social rights. Insofar as judicial deference is grounded, at least in part, on acceptance of a distinction between political rights and social rights, a removal of the distinction weakens that particular argument for deference.

The Charter and Future Developments

This chapter addresses the question of the impact of the Charter on health care costs. The case study shows that the number of successful Charter challenges since 1982 is not large, and the impact of these decisions, except for the doctors' challenges, has not yet been significant. Most claims have played around the edges of the current health care system, rather than attacked its foundations, and many court decisions have been sensitive to the dynamics of health care reform.

One reason that the Charter's impact has not been revolutionary is the relative comprehensiveness and accessibility of the medicare system. A number of basic principles informed the Hall Commission in the 1960s and are currently articulated in the Canada Health Act. In particular, the three principles of universality, accessibility, and comprehensiveness can be cast as manifestations of the Charter values of equality and protection of human dignity. In this respect, Charter rights augment the existing health care system; to state the obvious, section 15 claims about the scope of coverage do not introduce equality as a foreign concept to the health care system. However, apparent compatibility between medicare's principles and Charter values does not forestall continued litigation. Since general principles do not mechanically translate into a single set of practical policies (Okma 2002, 46), agreement in principle does not erase sharp disagreement about implementation. Moreover, more litigation can be expected if governments engage in reform measures that are perceived to depart from Charter values, or if courts change their views about what are Charter values.

Two structural factors will also influence the extent of future Charter litigation. First, litigation is expensive. Individuals rarely have sufficient personal resources to initiate a major constitutional challenge. If individuals with complaints about inadequate health services do have money, they are more likely to use it to buy the medical services they need rather than go to court. Moreover, public funding for litigation is not available. The Court Challenges program, which provides limited funding for individuals and groups to launch legal actions, only has power to fund cases that challenge federal laws. Since health care is a matter of provincial responsibility, and provinces make most health policy decisions, most challenges to health care policies are outside the program's purview. Second, time is an important consideration. Legal actions take a long time to proceed through the judicial system, and the very nature of some health decisions means that many patients cannot effectively use the courts.

These factors, however, have less salience for providers, such as doctors, or for private providers, such as dentists and pharmaceutical companies. With less cost constraints, they may initiate Charter litigation as a sword to obtain favourable policy changes, or as a shield to maintain their position. For instance, litigation to strike down the ban on private health insurance uses the Charter as a sword to increase private health care. The hypothetical doctors' challenge to employment or capitation contracts would use the Charter as a shield to prevent structural changes in physician remuneration. Moreover, Charter actions may be initiated as a tactic to pressure governments and influence public debate, even if the likelihood of success in court is low.

Governments could forestall some litigation by using the section 33 override. For those Charter cases involving sections 2, and sections 7 to 15, Parliament and provincial legislatures may declare that a law operates notwithstanding those Charter rights and freedoms. However, the override is not often used because of the fear of negative political repercussions. Moreover, some Charter rights (such as section 6's mobility rights) and the Constitution's fundamental principles fall outside the override's ambit, and governments are unable to immunize themselves from constitutional challenges on these grounds. Governments will have no recourse other than section 1 to justify interference with rights, as they have done successfully with some challenges to date.

One important question involves deciding what constitutes governmental action in the health care area. Section 32 states that the Charter applies to Parliament, the federal government, and the legislatures and governments of each province and territory. Hypothetically, if a government decided to privatize health care entirely – whatever that might mean (Gray 1998, 908) – the Charter would no longer govern the health care system. However, even if this most unlikely scenario were to unfold, the Charter will likely not be avoided. The question of what is government action under section 32 is notoriously complex, and it may be quite possible to find sufficient government action to ground Charter claims, especially since wholesale privatization does not avoid Canada's obligations under international law. The very point of positive governmental obligations is to require governments to provide particular services. Insofar as Charter jurisprudence develops more positive obligations (and *Gosselin* may be a harbinger), privatization options might become more difficult. In any event, the private sector is regulated by statute and the common law. The Charter directly regulates the former, and its values regulate the latter.

In considering reforms to the health care system, governments should take Charter values into account. This can be done in a number of ways that not only show respect for constitutional values but may also diminish the risk of courts striking down health care policies. These ways are not startling, but are integral to good governance in any policy area. Specifically, policies should be justified with evidence, such as economic studies about the merits and drawbacks of particular changes. In addition, reforms should be publicly justified as furthering important Charter values, such as equality, and decision-making within the health care system should be transparent and include procedural safeguards, such as appeals from funding decisions. Space does not permit fuller consideration of implementing these methods, but they are worthy of further study. For instance, a statutory Patients' Bill of Rights may assist courts in elucidating the core requirements of rights in the health care context. More judicial education about the economics of health care systems would do no harm. The health care system is one that every Canadian uses but few know much about, including members of the legal community. If judicial review in a democracy is a dialogue between judges and legislatures, more and better information about the content of the dialogue – in this instance, health care policy – would only enrich the debate.

Conclusion

There will always be Charter litigation seeking to enforce and expand upon constitutional rights as a means of effecting health policy. The dynamic between the Charter and the health care system, or to put the matter more precisely, between judges and health care officials, is an inescapable component of Canada's health care system. To date, there have only been a few successful Charter challenges to the health care system, and, with the exception of the British Columbia doctors' cases, their financial impact on the system has not been great. Several fundamental Charter values, such as equality and non-discrimination, animate the existing medicare system. The principles in the Canada Health Act fulfill Canada's international obligations with respect to health services, and go a long way towards satisfying the requirements of sections 7 and 15. Courts have shown considerable sensitivity to the dynamics of Canada's health care system, recognizing the importance of accessible health care for everyone, the unbelievably complex system in place for its delivery, and the need to give governments a wide margin of appreciation. However, the number, type, and likely success of challenges depend on many factors, including the nature of reforms introduced by governments. If governments delist more services or significantly change the mix of public and private sector delivery, they can expect more Charter claims from individuals using the Charter as a shield to preserve the current system. Alternatively, if governments do not change the system, or if they change in a controversial direction, they will face challenges from people using the Charter as a sword to force changes in a different direction. To lessen the impact on health care costs of the inevitable Charter challenges, governments can explicitly take Charter values into account in their health care policies, and justify their decisions with the best available evidence.

Appendix 1: Canadian Charter of Rights and Freedoms

Guarantee of Rights and Freedoms

Rights and freedoms in Canada
1. The Canadian Charter of Rights and Freedoms guarantees the rights and freedoms set out in it subject only to such reasonable limits prescribed by law as can be demonstrably justified in a free and democratic society.

...

Mobility Rights

Mobility of citizens

6.(1) Every citizen of Canada has the right to enter, remain in and leave Canada.

(2) Every citizen of Canada and every person who has the status of a permanent resident of Canada has the right
   a) to move to and take up residence in any province; and
   b) to pursue the gaining of a livelihood in any province.

(3) The rights specified in subsection (2) are subject to
   a) any laws or practices of general application in force in a province other than those that discriminate among persons primarily on the basis of province of present or previous residence; and
   b) any laws providing for reasonable residency requirements as a qualification for the receipt of publicly provided social services.

(4) Subsections (2) and (3) do not preclude any law, program or activity that has as its object the amelioration in a province of conditions of individuals in that province who are socially or economically disadvantaged if the rate of employment in that province is below the rate of employment in Canada.

Legal Rights

Life, liberty and security of person

7. Everyone has the right to life, liberty and security of the person and the right not to be deprived thereof except in accordance with the principles of fundamental justice.

...

Equality Rights

Equality before and under law and equal protection and benefit of law

15.(1) Every individual is equal before and under the law and has the right to the equal protection and equal benefit of the law without discrimination and, in particular, without discrimination based on race, national or ethnic origin, colour, religion, sex, age or mental or physical disability.

(2) Subsection (1) does not preclude any law, program or activity that has as its object the amelioration of conditions of disadvantaged individuals or groups including those that are disadvantaged because of race, national or ethnic origin, colour, religion, sex, age or mental or physical disability.

...

Application of Charter

Application of Charter
32.(1) This Charter applies
　　　a) to the Parliament and government of Canada in respect of all matters within the authority of Parliament including all matters relating to the Yukon Territory and Northwest Territories; and
　　　b) to the legislature and government of each province in respect of all matters within the authority of the legislature of each province.
　(2) Notwithstanding subsection (1), section 15 shall not have effect until three years after this section comes into force.

Exception where express declaration
33.(1) Parliament or the legislature of a province may expressly declare in an Act of Parliament or of the legislature, as the case may be, that the Act or a provision thereof shall operate notwithstanding a provision included in section 2 or sections 7 to 15 of this Charter.
　(2) An Act or a provision of an Act in respect of which a declaration made under this section is in effect shall have such operation as it would have but for the provision of this Charter referred to in the declaration.
　(3) A declaration made under subsection (1) shall cease to have effect five years after it comes into force or on such earlier date as may be specified in the declaration.
　(4) Parliament or the legislature of a province may re-enact a declaration made under subsection (1).
　(5) Subsection (3) applies in respect of a re-enactment made under subsection (4).

Appendix 2: Cases on Health Care Costs (as of June 2002)

Case name and citation	Facts	Argument, right claimed	Analysis	Disposition
Patients – specific treatment				
Brown v. British Columbia (Minister of Health), [1990] BCJ 151 (BC SC)	AIDS patients, drug AZT was placed on Pharma-care plan, which meant that all AIDS patients except those on social assistance or in long-term facilities had to pay for part of the drug's cost.	S.15: discrimination against AIDS patients as compared with other patients, such as cancer patients.	No violation: the reason for AIDS drugs being on a different plan than cancer drugs has to do with a difference between the drugs, not inequality as contemplated by s.15.	Plaintiffs lost
		S.7: deprivation of right to life, liberty, and security of the person.	No violation: s.7 does not contemplate economic deprivation.	
Ontario Nursing Home Assn. v. Ontario, [1990] OJ 1280 (Ont. HCJ)	Plaintiffs challenge the provision of more funding to homes for the aged than for other nursing homes.	S.7: deprivation of right to life, liberty, and security of the person because better care was available at homes for the aged than at other nursing homes.	No violation: no evidence that plaintiffs were not adequately cared for; s.7 does not entitle person to additional benefits that might enhance a plaintiff's life, liberty, or security of the person.	Plaintiffs lost
		S.15: discrimination.	No violation: type of residence (aged/nursing) not an enumerated or analogous ground.	

Appendix 2: (Continued)

Case name and citation	Facts	Argument, right claimed	Analysis	Disposition
Fernandes v. Manitoba, [1992] MJ 279 (Man. CA)	F was in hospital but wanted to live in an apartment; if he did, he would need an attendant for 16h/day; Director of Income Security refused F's request for additional allowance.	S.7: life, liberty, security of the person. S.15: discrimination on the basis of disability.	No violation: desire to live someplace in particular is not a right protected by s.7. No violation: no discrimination on the basis of personal characteristics or disability.	Plaintiff lost
Cameron v. Nova Scotia (Attorney General), [1999] NSJ 297 (NS CA)	Infertile couple, wanted government to pay for fertility treatments.	S.15: infertile people have a disability, denial of payment was substantially different treatment on the basis of disability; found to be discrimination.	Violation, but justified under s.1. Best possible health care with limited financial resources requires flexibility in apportioning social benefits; the violation minimally impaired s.15 right because it denied funding for only two procedures.	Plaintiffs lost
Irshad v. Ontario (Minister of Health), [2001] OJ No. 648 (Ont. CA)	Immigrants to Ontario not eligible for medicare; upon reaching a certain immigration status, had to wait 3 months.	S.15: denial of medical coverage on the basis of residency in Ontario.	No violation: residency requirement did not offend dignity; there were alternatives to provincial medical coverage.	Plaintiffs lost
N (DJ) [Niznik] v. Alberta (Child Welfare Appeal Panel), [1999] AJ 798 (Alta. QB)	N's son is autistic; N received some funding for family support, and wanted funding for further therapy and training; Director, Appeal Panel refused.	S.15: discrimination.	No violation: no evidence that N was treated differently than other similarly-situated children, N received some therapy at school; special needs were of the type that School Act provided for.	Plaintiff lost [overruled by *Auton*?]

Appendix 2: (Continued)

Case name and citation	Argument, facts	Argument, right claimed	Analysis	Disposition
Auton v. British Columbia (Minister of Health), [2000] BCSC 1142 (BC SC)	Parents of autistic children want government to pay for Lovaas behavioural therapy for pre-school children; government would not fund until school age be-cause treatment was consid-ered 'education,' and it was very expensive treatment.	S.15: discrimination: pri-mary health care need of children with autism is early behavioural intervention, a necessary treatment.	Violation: Lovaas was medical treatment; gov-ernment failed to give children the treatment they needed. Violation not justified under s.1.	Plaintiffs won; court ordered government to pay for Lovaas treat-ment when doctor rec-ommended it.
Martin v. NS WCB, [2000] NSJ 353 (NS CA)	Workplace injury caused chronic pain that caused disability; WCB did not compensate except in lim-ited circumstances; at trial plaintiffs won.	S.15: discrimination against people who suffer chronic pain.	No violation: no evi-dence that sufferers of chronic pain experi-enced historical disad-vantage or stereotyping; overall purpose of com-pensation scheme was compensatory.	Plaintiffs lost
Eldridge v. British Colum-bia (Attorney General), [1997] 3 SCR 624	Deaf patients wanted gov-ernment to provide sign-language interpretation [SLI] when they communi-cated with health care providers.	S.15: failure to provide SLI, where necessary for effec-tive communication, is dis-crimination on the basis of disability.	Violation: discrimination because deaf patients denied equal access to health services available to everyone. Failure to provide SLI was adverse effects discrimination; decision not to fund SLI was not justified under s.1.	Plaintiffs won; Court directed government to administer medicare legislation in manner consistent with s.1; dec-laration suspended for 6 months.

Appendix 2: (Continued)

Case name and citation	Argument, facts	Argument, right claimed	Analysis	Disposition
RR v. Alberta (Child Welfare Appeal Panel), [2000] AJ 580 (Alta. QB)	Rs had 3 children: 2 with cerebral palsy, 1 with spastic hemiplegia; wanted funding for conductive education during school year and at summer camp; Director, Appeal Panel refused; parents knew other children with CP who got funding.	S.15: these children (denied funding) with CP were treated differently from other children with CP (received funding).	No violation: children were subjected to differential treatment, but not on listed or analogous ground; differential treatment was not on the fact of disability, but personal characteristics, specific medical needs and family situation.	Plaintiff lost
Patients – criminalized treatment				
R. v. Morgentaler, [1988] 1 SCR 30	Doctor violated Criminal Code by performing abortions on women who had not obtained certificate from therapeutic abortion committee at an approved hospital; women also guilty of Criminal Code offences.	S.7: breach of life, liberty, and security of the person, not in accordance with the principles of fundamental justice.	Violation: State interference with bodily integrity (forcing woman to carry to term; delay and subsequent risks) and state-induced psychological stress (at least in criminal law) is a breach of women's security of the person. Deprivation not in accordance with principles of fundamental justice: defence is illusory, not all hospitals qualify to have a committee; even if they do qualify, having the committee is not mandatory. 'Security of the person' includes a right of access to medical treatment for a condition representing a danger to life or health, without fear of criminal sanction.	Court declared the Criminal Code provisions invalid, and of no force and effect.

Appendix 2: (Continued)

Case name and citation	Argument, Facts	Argument, right claimed	Analysis	Disposition
Rodriquez v. British Columbia (1993), 107 DLR (4th) 342	Plaintiff, who suffered from terminal illness, sought declaration that Criminal Code prohibition on assisting suicide was unconstitutional.	S.7: prohibiting persons from helping plaintiff commit suicide violates plaintiff's security of the person. S.15: violation of equality rights on the ground of physical disability.	No violation: The security interest was infringed, but the deprivation did not infringe the principles of fundamental justice. S.15: assuming a violation, it was justified under s.1.	Plaintiff lost
R. v. Parker, [2000] OJ No. 2787 (Ont. CA)	P had severe epileptic seizures, conventional medicine did not control his condition, but marijuana did; he could not find a legal source so he grew his own; charged with criminal offences of possession and cultivation.	S.7: prohibiting P from using a necessary medication infringed right to security of the person; threat of jail engaged right to liberty.	Violation: depriving access (via criminal sanction) to medication reasonably required for a medical condition that threatens life or health violates security of the person. Liberty violated by threat of imprisonment; liberty also includes right to make decisions of fundamental importance, including choice of medication. Deprivations violated the principles of natural justice because blanket prohibition did little or nothing to enhance state interest.	Court declared the criminal prohibition of marijuana invalid, and of no force and effect. It suspended the declaration for 12 months, and gave a personal exemption to P.
Hospital Restructuring *Lachine General Hospital v. Quebec* (1997), 142 DLR (4th) 659 (Que. CA)	Pursuant to restructuring legislation, several hospitals in the Montreal region were ordered closed, including an English-language hospital.	S.15: closing hospital that primarily served anglophone patients violated equality rights of patients and personnel.	No violation: no discrimination proven; difference in bilingual hospitals before and after closure was minimal.	Plaintiffs lost

Appendix 2: (Continued)

Case name and citation	Argument, facts	Argument, right claimed	Analysis	Disposition
Ponteix (Town) v. Saskatchewan, [1995] 1WWR 400 (Sk. Q.B.)	Pursuant to restructuring legislation, many local hospitals converted to health centres, with reduced emergency/over-night service. Rural coalition reached agreement with government about such service, which plaintiff alleges was breached.	S.7 and s.15: reduced availability of emergency/over-night service violated security of the person and equality rights.	No violation: even if Charter applies, it does not require the same standard of health care for all residents, regardless of where they live.	Plaintiffs lost
Russell v. Ontario, [1998] OJ 4116 (Ont. Ct. of Justice)	Ontario Health Services Restructuring Commission ordered Hôtel Dieu, a hospital run by nuns, to shut down and transfer its operations to another hospital.	S. 2(a): freedom of religion – plaintiffs, the nuns who run Hôtel Dieu, cannot carry out their religious mission to minister to the sick poor.	No violation: freedom of religion does not entitle anyone to State support for one's religion. Nothing prevents nuns from ministering to the sick poor on that site.	Plaintiffs lost
Wellesley Central Hospital v. Ontario, [1997] OJ 3645 (Ont. Div. Ct.)	Ontario Health Services Restructuring Commission ordered Wellesley Hospital to transfer its services to another hospital, which was administered by a religious order; individual plaintiffs, who were HIV-positive gay men, objected.	S.2(a), s.15: compelling gay men to receive treatment at a hospital administered by a religious order violated freedom of religion and was discriminatory.	No violation: no evidence that gay men would be compelled to receive treatment at the hospital; no evidence of breach of other Charter rights.	Plaintiffs lost
SGEU v. Saskatchewan (1997), 145 D.L.R. (4th) 300 (Sask. QB); affirmed 149 DLR (4th) 190 (Sask. CA)	Hospital restructuring plan would move 20% of SGEU membership to other unions, who would be bargaining agents for these employees.	S.2(d): mandatory move of some employees to other unions violated freedom of association.	No violation: freedom of association does not include freedom to choose one's bargaining unit.	Plaintiffs lost

Appendix 2: (Continued)

Case name and citation	Argument, Facts	Argument, right claimed	Analysis	Disposition
Jewish Hospital of Hope v. Quebec (1997), 139 DLR (4th) 456 (Que. CA)	Pursuant to hospital restructuring legislation, hospital became subject to a regional board of directors.	S.2(d): freedom of association violated by imposing a regional board of directors.	No violation: freedom of association does not include a hospital's administrative autonomy.	Plaintiffs lost
Pembroke Civic Hospital v. Ontario, [1997] OJ 3142 (Ont. Ct. Gen. Div); dismissed [1997] OJ 3603 (Ont. CA)	Heath Services Restructuring Commission ordered Pembroke Civic Hospital to merge with another one, operated by the Roman Catholic Church.	Ss. 2(a), 7, and 15: the religious views of RC hospital would influence health care.	No violation: Charter challenge was premature. No evidence that Roman Catholic views were forced on patients or affected treatment.	Plaintiffs lost
Lalonde v. Ontario (Health Services Restructuring Commission), [2001] OJ 4767 (Ont. CA)	Bilingual hospital provided service in French 24 hours a day; government (HSRC) restructured hospital and limited its services.	S.15: discrimination against the francophone community. Fundamental constitutional principle of protecting minorities violated by HSRC.	No violation: language was not an enumerated or analogous ground. Violation: HSRC must respect fundamental constitutional principles. It failed to give serious weight and consideration to the hospital's importance to the francophone community.	Plaintiffs won. Court remitted matter back to minister (who replaced HSRC) for reconsideration taking into account fundamental constitutional principles.

Appendix 2: (Continued)

Case name and citation	Argument, Facts	Argument, right claimed	Analysis	Disposition
Doctors/Hospital Employees – Discrimination				
Sniders v. Nova Scotia (1988), 55 DLR (4th) 408 (NS CA)	Plaintiff, a member of a bargaining unit, challenged hospital's mandatory retirement policy.	S.15: age discrimination.	Violation: mandatory retirement is age discrimination, and cannot be justified under s.1.	Plaintiff won. Court ordered him reinstated as employee.
Stoffman v. Vancouver General Hospital (1990), 76 DLR (4th) 700 (SCC)	Plaintiffs had their admitting privileges terminated when they reached the age of 65, pursuant to the hospital's mandatory retirement policy.	S.15: age discrimination.	No violation: hospital was not covered by Charter. However, even if it was, the s.15 violation was justified under s.1.	Plaintiffs lost
Jamorski v. Ontario (AG), [1988] OJ 221 (Ont. CA)	Plaintiffs were graduates of Polish medical schools and had passed Canadian exam. They could not get internship because of differential treatment for foreigners; had to pass preinternship program, which only had 24 places.	S.15: discrimination on the basis of graduating from accredited or non-accredited schools.	No violation: was not differential treatment because grads of accredited vs. non-accredited schools are different, unreasonable to expect that grads of both would be the same; even if there was a violation, it would have been justified under s.1.	Plaintiffs lost. Appeal dismissed.
Doctors – Liberty and Mobility with Respect to Practice				
Jaeger v. Quebec (1998), 155 DLR (4th) 599 (Que. CA)	Foreign doctors could obtain license to practise in designated geographic regions, if they stayed in the region for 4 years. Penalty for moving earlier was $50,000/year. Plaintiff doctor, who obtained licence under the program, objected to the penalty.	S.7: requirement to stay in one place for 4 years violated liberty.	No violation: liberty does not include freedom to practise profession wherever one wishes, without financial penalty.	Plaintiff lost
		S.15: policy discriminated against foreign doctors.	No violation: equality rights not violated by special program that increased opportunities for foreign doctors.	

Appendix 2: (Continued)

Case name and citation	Argument, Facts	Argument, right claimed	Analysis	Disposition
Kirsten v. College of Physicians and Surgeons, [1996] SJ 462 (Sask. QB)	Plaintiff challenged agreement with College to practice in rural Saskatchewan for 5 years, in exchange for license.	S.6: mobility – 5-year agreement denied right to move to another province. S.7: liberty.	No violation: assuming that rights were violated, plaintiff waived his Charter rights.	Plaintiff lost
Mia v. British Columbia (Medical Services Commission) (1985), 17 DLR (4th) 385 (BC SC)	M studied and graduated in British Columbia, but interned, did post-graduate training, and practised outside province; British Columbia would not give M a billing number.	S.6: mobility; prima facie right to move to a province for work, and to work anywhere in province; S.7: liberty includes freedom to practise a profession.	Violation: s.6 protects right to practice on a viable economic basis anywhere in province. Liberty in s.7 protects freedom of movement within a province for purpose of pursuing professional practise; breach of principles be-cause policy was arbitrary.	Plaintiff won. Court declared that M entitled to billing number for services rendered anywhere in province.
Wilson v. British Columbia (Medical Services Commission), [1988] BCJ 1566 (BC CA)	Plaintiffs were 6 doctors: 4 graduated from UBC and practised outside British Columbia; 2 were educated outside British Columbia and now subject to British Columbia restrictions; legislation gave MSC power to not grant billing numbers, and, if granted, to restrict numbers to specific area or purpose (e.g., locums).	s.7: freedom to practice profession was so severely restricted that it violated liberty; 'liberty' should be interpreted generously to include right to choose an occupation and where to pursue it. S.6: mobility rights infringed by geographic restrictions within province.	Violation: liberty includes right to practise medicine in British Columbia without geographic restriction. Breach of principles of fundamental justice because of procedural unfairness (vague criteria; uncontrolled discretion of MSC) and the manifest unfairness of a scheme in which doctors with restricted numbers were at the mercy of doctors with unrestricted numbers, abuse of the system. Court did not address s.6 arguments.	Plaintiffs won. Court declared that legislation invalid, and of no force and effect.

Appendix 2: (Continued)

Case name and citation	Argument, Facts	Argument, right claimed	Analysis	Disposition
Waldman v. British Columbia (Medical Services Commission), [1999] BCJ 2014 (BC CA)	Plaintiffs challenged physician supply management. MSC created a new billing system: if new billers wanted to work in a place that already had enough doctors, they could only bill a maximum of 50% of the normal rate; after 5 years of practise in British Columbia the geographical restriction was lifted; preference was given to BC-educated new doctors.	S.6: mobility rights violated by geographic restrictions.	Violation: mobility rights violated by preference to doctors who were trained in British Columbia, or who started studies in British Columbia by a certain date; the remainder of the scheme did not violate s.6	Plaintiffs won. Court refused to sever invalid provision from valid provisions, and it declared entire scheme invalid.
		S.15: discrimination on the basis of province of training or residence.	Court of Appeal did not consider s.15; trial judge had held that s.15 not violated because billing system did not discriminate on enumerated or analogous ground.	
Rombaut v. New Brunswick (Minister of Health and Community Services), [2001] NBJ 243 (NB CA)	Plaintiffs challenged physician resource management plan. Doctors practising in New Brunswick before the plan came in were exempted or grandfathered; New Brunswick does not have a medical school, so there is no distinction between new doctors from here or new doctors from away.	S.6: grandfathering provisions are preferential for New Brunswick practitioners.	No violation: a purpose of s.6 is to protect dignity (human rights); there is a preference that would count as discrimination, but it is not on the basis of residency; even if there is a violation it is justifiable under s.1.	Plaintiffs lost
		S.15: gender discrimination because system perpetuates the gender imbalance of the status quo.	No violation: system is equally hard on men and women, it does not promote men over women.	
		S.7: right to practise with the partners they want and be paid for it.	No violation: s.7 is not concerned with economic deprivation.	

Appendix 2: (Concluded)

Case name and citation	Argument, Facts	Argument, right claimed	Analysis	Disposition
Practice Regulation				
Rocket v. Royal College of Dental Surgeons of Ontario (1990), 71 DLR (4th) 68 (SCC)	Several dentists challenged the rule of their professional association prohibiting advertising.	S.2(b): freedom of expression. Ban on advertising violated dentists' expressive freedom.	Violation: ban prohibits legitimate forms of expression, and cannot be justified under s.1.	Plaintiffs won
Costco Wholesale Canada Ltd. v. British Columbia (1998), 157 DLR 725 (BC SC)	Two optometrists challenged by-law of Board of Examiners in Optometry, which prohibited optometrists from having business associations with non-optometrists.	S.2(d): ban on business associations violated freedom of association.	Violation: freedom of association includes economic associations. Ban not justified under s.1. Absolute ban not proportionate to objective of maintaining high standards of professionalism.	Plaintiffs won
Medicare Structure				
Chaoulli c. Québec (Procureur Général), [2002] JQ 759 (Que. CA)	Plaintiffs challenged Quebec law that prohibited private health insurance for health services covered by medicare.	S.7: limits on access to the private insurance violates right of security; health care is an important personal decision, and therefore its curtailment infringes liberty right.	No violation: s.7 does not include economic rights. Even if s.7 applies, no violation of principles of fundamental justice. Prohibition aims to safeguard public system of protection of health.	Plaintiffs lost

REFERENCES

Auton (Guardian ad Litem of) v. British Columbia (Minister of Health). 2000. [2000] B.C.J. No. 1547 (BC SC).

Baker v. Canada (Minister of Citizenship and Immigration). 1999. (1999) 174 D.L.R. (4th) 193 (SCC).

Brown v. British Columbia (Minister of Health). 1990. [1990] B.C.J. No. 151 (BC SC).

Cameron v. Nova Scotia (Attorney General). 1999. (1999) N.S.J. No. 33 (NS SC).

Cameron v. Nova Scotia (Attorney General). 1999a. [1999] N.S.J. No. 297 (NS CA); leave to appeal to the Supreme Court of Canada denied, 29 June 2000.

Canada Health Act, R.S.C. 1985, c. C-6.

Canadian Egg Marketing Agency v. Richardson. 1998. [1998] 3 S.C.R. 157.

Carver, Peter. 2002. 'A New Director for Mental Health Law: Brian's Law and the Problematic Implications of Community Treatment Orders.' In *Health Care Reform and Law in Canada: Meeting the Challenge*, ed. Tim Caulfield and Barbara Von Tigerstrom, 187–222. Edmonton: University of Alberta Press.

Chaoulli c. Québec (Procureur général). 2002. [2002] J.Q. n° 759 (Cour d'appel du Québec).

Chaoulli c. Québec (Procureur général). 2000. [2000] J.Q. n° 479 (Cour supérieure du Québec – Chambre civile).

Committee on Economic, Social and Cultural Rights. 1998. *Concluding Observations on Canada*. UN Doc. E/C.12/1/Add.31.

Costco Wholesale Canada Ltd. v. British Columbia (Board of Examiners in Optometry). 1998. (1998) 157 D.L.R. (4th) 725 (BC SC).

Eldridge v. British Columbia (Attorney General). 1997. [1997] 3 S.C.R. 624.

Flood, Colleen. 1999. 'Contracting for Health Care Services in the Public Sector.' *Canadian Business Law Journal* 31: 175–208.

Gosselin c. Québec (Procureur général). 1999. [1999] J.Q. n° 1365 (Cour d'appel du Québec).

Gray, Gwen. 1998. 'Access to Medical Care Under Strain: New Pressures in Canada and Australia.' *Journal of Health Politics, Policy and Law* 23: 905–47.

Hartt, Stanley, and Patrick Monahan. 2002. *The Charter and Health Care: Guaranteeing Timely Access to Health Care for Canadians*. Toronto: C.D. Howe Institute.

Hogg, Peter. 2001. *Constitutional Law of Canada*. Student Edition. Carswell: Toronto.

International Covenant on Economic, Social, and Cultural Rights. 1966. Adopted 16 December 1966. UN Doc. A/6316.

Irshad (Litigation Guardian of) v. Ontario (Minister of Health). 2001. [2001] O.J. No. 648 (Ont. CA).

Irwin Toy v. Quebec (Attorney General). 1989. [1989] 1 S.C.R. 927.

Jackman, Martha. 1995. 'The Regulation of Private Health Care under the Canada Health Act and Canadian Charter.' *Constitutional Forum* 6:54.

J.C. v. Forensic Psychiatric Service Commissioner. 1992. (1992) 65 B.C.L.R. (2d) 386 (BC SC).

Karr, Andrea. 2000. 'Section 7 of the Charter: Remedy for Canada's Health Care Crisis?' *The Advocate* 58(3)(4): 363–74, 531–41.

Kelly, James. 1999. 'The Charter of Rights and Freedoms and the Rebalancing of Liberal Constitutionalism in Canada, 1982–1997.' *Osgoode Hall Law Journal* 37: 625–95.

Lalonde v. Ontario (Commission de restructuration des services de santé). 2001. [2001] O.J. No. 4767 (Ont. CA).

Law v. Canada (Minister of Employment and Immigration). 1999. [1999] 1 S.C.R. 497.

Lewis, Steven et al. 2000. 'Ending Waiting-List Mismanagement: Principles and Practice.' *CMAJ* 162(9): 1297–1300.

Manfredi, Christopher, and Antonia Maioni. 2002. 'Courts and Health Policy: Judicial Policy Making and Publicly Funded Health Care in Canada.' *Journal of Health Politics, Policy and Law* 27(2): 213–40.

New Brunswick (Minister of Health and Social Services) v. G.(J.). 1999. [1999] 3 S.C.R. 46.

Okma, Kieke. 2002. 'What Is the Best Public-Private Model for Canadian Health Care?' *Policy Matters* 3(6): 1–60.

Ontario Nursing Home Assn. v. Ontario. 1990. (1990) 72 D.L.R. (4th) 166 (Ont. High C. of Justice).

Ponteix (Town) v. Saskatchewan. 1994. [1995] 1 W.W.R. 400 (Sask. QB).

R.B. v. Children's Aid Society of Metropolitan Toronto. 1995. [1995] 1 S.C.R. 315.

R. v. Morgentaler. 1988. [1988] 1 S.C.R. 30.

R. v. Oakes. 1986. [1986] 1 S.C.R. 103.

R. v. Parker. 2000. [2000] O.J. No. 2787 (Ont. CA).

Reference Re Criminal Code, Ss. 193 & 195.1(1)(c). 1990. [1990] 4 W.W.R. 481.

Reference Re Motor Vehicle Act of British Columbia. 1988. [1988] 2 S.C.R. 486.

Re Mia and Medical Services Commission of British Columbia. 1985. (1985) 17 D.L.R. (4th) 385 (BC SC).

Richards, John. 1999. 'William Schabas v. Cordelia.' *National Journal of Constitutional Law* 11: 247–60.

Rocket v. Royal College of Dental Surgeons of Ontario. 1990. (1990) 71 D.L.R. (4th) 68 (SCC).

Rodriquez v. British Columbia (Attorney General). 1993. [1993] 3 S.C.R 519.

Rombaut v. New Brunswick (Minister of Health and Community Services). 2001. [2001] N.B.J. No. 243. (NB CA).

Schabas, William. 1999. 'Freedom from Want: How Can We Make Indivisibility More Than Just a Mere Slogan?' *National Journal of Constitutional Law* 11: 189–212.

Schrecker, Ted. 1998. 'Private Health Care for Canada: North of the Border, An Idea Whose Time Shouldn't Come?' *Journal of Law, Medicine and Ethics* 26: 138–48.

Singh and Minister of Employment and Immigration, Re. 1985. (1985) 17 D.L.R. (4th) 422 (SCC).

Stoffman v. Vancouver General Hospital. 1990. [1990] 3 S.C.R. 483.

Toebes, Brigit. 1999. *The Right to Health as a Human Right in International Law.* Antwerp: Intersentia.

Von Tigerstrom, Barbara. 2002. 'Human Rights and Health Care Reform: A Canadian Perspective,' in *Health Care Reform and Law in Canada: Meeting the Challenge,* ed. Tim Caulfield and Barbara Von Tigerstrom, 157–85. Edmonton: University of Alberta Press.

Waldman v. British Columbia (Medical Services Commission). 1999. [1999] B.C.J. No. 2014 (BC CA).

Wellesley Central Hospital v. Ontario (Health Services Restructuring Commission). 1997. [1997] O.J. No. 3645 (Ont. C. of Justice, Gen. Div.)

Wilson v. British Columbia (Medical Services Commission). 1988. [1988] B.C.J. No. 1566 (BC CA).

PART II

THE INTERGOVERNMENTAL CONTEXT

4 Intergovernmental Cooperation Mechanisms: Factors for Change?

RÉJEAN PELLETIER

Federalism is founded on the notion of shared sovereignty, in that none of the entities forming the federation – be it the central State or the provinces, Länder or cantons – can fully lay claim to sovereignty. To achieve shared sovereignty, the power to legislate is shared between the two orders of government. A written constitution sets out the distribution of jurisdictions defining the matters on which each may legislate or, in some cases, recognizing areas where each can intervene according to certain terms and conditions.

The famous formula devised by Daniel Elazar (1987, 12), known as self-rule plus shared-rule, translates well the reality of federalism and the main principles underlying it. On the one hand, federated entities (such as the Canadian provinces) as well as the central State must be autonomous in their jurisdictional sphere, thus precluding forms of subordination of one order of government by the other. This autonomy must translate into sufficient financial capacity with which to effectively exercise powers – otherwise, the autonomy becomes illusory.

On the other hand, the federated entities and the central State must share a few common rules: a constitution governing the federation; common institutions; and a political community characterized at once by the desire to live together and by the expression of the diversity present in the federation. Therefore, the central political institutions must reflect as best they can the country's unity and diversity. That is why, with rare exceptions, all federations have a second chamber (Watts 1999, 92), which is supposed to represent the diversity embodied by the federated entities. Participation by federated entities in the exercise of central power is essential in a federation. And yet not only must participation be effective, but the composition of the second chamber and the mechanism for appointing its members must also meet the objective of representation and real participation of federated entities in the exercise of central power.

Recently, the Supreme Court of Canada provided a good illustration of federalism, invoking the dual principles of autonomy and participation as well as the need to respect diversity.

> The principle of federalism recognizes the diversity of the component parts of Confederation, and the autonomy of provincial governments to develop their societies within their respective spheres of jurisdiction. The federal structure of our country also facilitates democratic participation by distributing power to the government thought to be most suited to achieving the particular societal objective having regard to this diversity. The scheme of the Constitution Act, 1867, ... was not to weld the Provinces into one, nor to subordinate Provincial Governments to a central authority, but to establish a central government in which these Provinces should be represented, entrusted with exclusive authority only in affairs in which they had a common interest. Subject to this, each Province was to retain its independence and autonomy and to be directly under the Crown as its head. (Supreme Court of Canada 1998, par.58.)

This kind of federalism is not static: it must evolve with time, and this includes the right of politicians to make amendments to the Constitution, the supreme law governing the country. Since 1867, there have been about forty constitutional amendments, some affecting the division of powers (such as unemployment insurance in 1940, and old age pensions in 1951), and others affecting institutions, the admission of new provinces, and political rules (such as the changes to representation in the House of Commons). However, since the failure of both the Meech Lake Accord in 1990 and the Charlottetown Accord in 1992, this avenue seems completely blocked, with the exception of bilateral amendments under section 43 of the Constitution Act, 1982. Unlike his predecessor, Prime Minister Jean Chrétien steadfastly refuses to go down the path of constitutional reform (Pelletier 2000, 73–7).

A federation engages only occasionally in reforming its constitution. Between these instances, courts are called upon to interpret the supreme law of the land. That is what the Judicial Committee of the Privy Council, based in London, did until 1949, and what the Supreme

Court of Canada has done since then. Both have acted as the final Court of Appeal in all matters, including constitutional disputes. In addition to the criticism that Supreme Court judges are appointed solely by the federal government, which is contrary to the spirit of federalism and the practice of most federations (Watts 1999, 100–1), many have noted the trend towards a 'judicialization of the political system' and a 'politicization of the judicial system,' especially since the Charter of Rights was adopted in 1982 (Monahan 1987; Knopff and Morton 1992; Mandel 1989). However, the courts have a say only if asked to settle a dispute between two parties, or if a government submits a question to the court through a reference proceeding (Tremblay 2000, 339–61).

Some federations, like Switzerland and Australia, modify their Constitution by referendum. They appeal directly to the sovereign people, considered the ultimate decision-maker on constitutional amendments. This avenue has rarely been taken in Canada, except for the Charlottetown Accord in 1992, and in some provinces such as Newfoundland and Quebec (in 1980, 1992, and 1995). Under the Constitution Act, 1982, the Constitution is primarily the responsibility of governments and provincial legislatures (Cairns 1991, 1992), not of citizens, as though representative democracy must always prevail over participatory democracy.

There is another avenue for making adjustments to the federal system without necessarily resorting to constitutional amendments. In a context of greater interdependence and with the aim of ensuring increased constitutional flexibility, the different orders of government have put in place intergovernmental cooperation mechanisms in order to engage in consultations and to develop better cooperation and coordination among themselves. This has allowed them to adapt to changes and to resolve disputes as they arise (Watts 1999, 57). These administrative agreements can affect the jurisdictional balance without the need for formal amendments or constitutional interpretation by the courts. These are the mechanisms of intergovernmental cooperation, involving first ministers, sectoral ministers, and senior officials – which have given rise to 'executive federalism' (Smiley 1980) – that are of particular interest here.

The idea of growing interdependence does not mean that one order of government is dependent on or subordinated to another, but that the actions of one order of government influence the other. This requires coordination and a certain amount of cooperation between governments. Nevertheless, this 'cooperative' federalism results just as often in competition and conflict as in cooperation and coordination.

In light of the above comments, this chapter looks more specifically at the question of whether the mechanisms for intergovernmental cooperation in the Canadian federation can contribute to or hinder change. In other words, to what extent have these mechanisms at the federal-provincial as well as the interprovincial level promoted or hampered desired changes?

By change, I mean any modification of a previous situation, whether it takes the form of a simple addition to an existing situation, a major reform or real innovation. At its inception, hospital insurance was a real innovation, while reforms enacted by Ministers Marc-Yvan Côté and Jean Rochon led to major changes to Quebec's health care network. However, expanding the range of health care covered by medicare is an addition to an existing program. In some cases, these changes are perceived in a positive light, while in others they are seen in a negative light (such as the major cuts made in health spending).

The Failure of Intrastate Federalism

Intergovernmental cooperation mechanisms, particularly federal-provincial mechanisms, should respond to the principle of *participation* mentioned in the above Introduction. I refer here to the central political institutions that should enable federated entities to participate in central decision-making. As Preston King (1982, 405) was already reminding us, the distinctive element of a federal system – that can contribute to the success of the whole – is the extent to which 'the central government incorporates regional units into its decision procedure on some constitutionally entrenched basis.'

What has been called *intrastate* federalism can be defined, according to Smiley and Watts (1986, 4), as the 'arrangements by which the interests of regional entities – either of the government or of the residents of these entities – are channelled through and protected by the structures and operations of the central government.' In Canada's case, we cannot help but note the shortcomings, if not the failure, of the mechanisms in expressing and conveying the interests of the federated entities to the 'structures and operations of the central government.'

Many analysts argue that the Canadian Senate, while it has adequately fulfilled its role of taking a sober second look at legislation and of investigating important issues, has failed to meet expectations concerning representation of regional interests. This is, after all, an essential, fundamental role that must be played by a second chamber in a federation.

Using the criteria of performance, effectiveness, and legitimacy developed by Bakvis and Skogstad (2002, 3–23), we can see that the Canadian Senate meets those very partially, if at all. Indeed, it enjoys only limited legitimacy by virtue of the fact that all members of the Senate are appointed by the federal Prime Minister alone, and remain in place until retirement. They cannot be expected to be accountable to the governments or population of the federated entity they are supposed to represent, or to uphold the interests of these entities. Moreover, their effectiveness, measured in terms of results obtained as representatives of the federated entities, is also very low because in the Senate, as in the House of Commons, party discipline rules. In this sense, the Senate is not a provincial Chamber, like the German Bundesrat, but a partisan one, like the House of Commons.

Accordingly, the Senate has an overall weak performance in terms of its ability to adequately represent the diversity of federated entities and to ensure their participation in the central decision-making process. On the one hand, appointing only Liberal or Conservative senators (the only two parties to hold power in Ottawa since 1867) fails to properly represent the wide diversity of Canadian politics, which is not limited to these two parties. On the other hand, given its limited legitimacy, the Senate cannot, in the end, oppose decisions taken by the House of Commons, which means that it will always capitulate when the House turns down an amendment coming from the Senate, unless a compromise satisfactory to both parties is found. It is interesting to note that the extensive powers of the United States Senate have not been altered by the fact that senators are now directly elected by the population of each state, whereas before (until 1913), they were elected indirectly by state legislatures.

The federalization of the federal cabinet is a custom dating back to the early days of Confederation. The first cabinet of John A. Macdonald included 'representatives' of the four provinces from which Canada originated. With few exceptions, this tradition has prevailed ever since. Next came the practice of mandating a minister to defend regional interests (Bakvis 1991), making up for the deficiencies of the Senate, which has not really risen to the task. But these ministers have never represented, nor wanted to represent, provincial governments.

The federalization of the cabinet comes up against two major obstacles. First, with the exception of the unionist government in power from 1917 to 1921, no Canadian government – not even a minority one – has ever included more than one political party. The problem stems precisely from the fact that the party in power does not always enjoy solid support in the various Canadian provinces. That was the case with, among others, the Liberal governments of Pierre Elliott Trudeau and Jean Chrétien during the last quarter century. Second, bound by party discipline and ministerial solidarity, which are 'the two sides of the same coin' (Pelletier 1999, 58), ministers must close ranks once a decision has been made and cabinet must display a show of unity behind the decision. This does not mean that there are no discussions about divergent regional interests around the cabinet table, but that these divergences must be kept quiet in the interest of ministerial solidarity once a decision has been taken.

Political parties have also been used both as a way to integrate a diverse population and as a means of representing an array of interests. At the federal level, parties have been required not only to carry out the traditional functions of political formations in democratic countries (e.g., running candidates in elections, formulating policy, and forming the government) but also to represent the regional, linguistic, or ethnic distinctions that characterize Canada. This process was to take place *within* each party rather than letting the parties divide among themselves the responsibility of representing and defending these various interests (Elkins 1991; Covell 1991; Carty, Cross, and Young 2000). The brokerage theory has been used to translate this reality and explain the Canadian party system (Clarke et al. 1991). If a party wants to capture and maintain power, it must cast the net wide and come to terms with Canada's diversity. This has been the key to the Liberal Party's success during the twentieth century, as it has succeeded more often than any other at building a coalition of these various interests.

Once again, two problems come to mind in analysing the representative role of Canada's political parties. First, Members of Parliament are bound by party discipline, which impedes the expression of regional interests in the House of Commons. Party discipline, as recognized by the Royal Commission on the Economic Union and Development Prospects for Canada in 1985, '(sharply limits) the ability of individual Members of Parliament to act as spokespersons for their province's interests' (3:79). Dissidence within a party is rare and often heavily sanctioned (exclusion from caucus). Second, the Canadian parliamentary system – inherited from Westminster – operates on a majority basis; hence, a single party finds itself in power, relegating other parties to play the role of opposition. The outcome of the last three federal elections (1993, 1997, and 2000) shows that the ruling Liberal Party received little support in the West, lukewarm support in Quebec, and a whopping majority in Ontario. At the same time, two 'regional' parties – the Bloc Québécois in Quebec and the Reform Party (now known as the Canadian Alliance) in the West – captured more than half the seats in their respective regions. The current fragmentation of Canadian politics certainly ensures better representation of regional interests in the House of Commons, but the parties defending these interests are relegated to opposition benches, while the party in power is muzzled by party discipline. With the exception of Ontario, which largely controls the Liberal caucus and exerts wide influence in cabinet, the other regions have felt, and still feel, excluded from power and from genuine participation in the decision-making process at the central level. This is especially true of the West.

In short, the current political situation reflects a crisis in representation marked by the failure of intrastate federalism in Canada. This crisis is apparent at four levels. First, there is the issue of electoral participation: in November 2000, only six out of ten voters (61.2 per cent) took time to cast their ballots, breaking a record that had stood since 1896. Second, one must consider the tepid support that the electorate has given the majority party: the Liberals managed to capture only 38.5 per cent of the vote in 1997 and 40.8 per cent in 2000. Third, the Senate has been unable to adequately play its role of representing regional interests, which should be the primary role of a second Chamber in a federation. Fourth, we must keep in mind the impact of party discipline, which impedes the expression, in Parliament, of the various interests found within parties, most notably the party in power – where this expression would be even more important since that party is the main source of policies that are eventually adopted and implemented.

In the long run, reforming central institutions would enhance the legitimacy of the federal authorities, which could then claim to represent not only Canada as a whole but also Canada's diversity and regional interests. For now, such is not the case, especially given the absence from the political agenda of any meaningful reform of Canada's central institutions.

Interstate Federalism Put to the Test

In response to the shortcomings of intrastate federalism, a form of interstate federalism characterized by ongoing relations between the two orders of government has emerged, especially after the Second World War (McRoberts 1985, 75). If cooperation and coordination cannot take place efficiently in central institutions, they can be achieved by other means. As in the Westminster model, where the government plays a dominant role, these mechanisms have taken the form of 'executive federalism,' characterized by the intervention of members of the executive branch, not only first ministers and sectoral ministers but also senior officials reporting to them. But these mechanisms of cooperation and coordination also give rise to competition and conflict between governments that do not pursue the same policies. That is why we must see the players in these intergovernmental cooperation structures as associates-rivals or *partners-adversaries*, reflecting the dual dimension of cooperation and conflict that marks many intergovernmental meetings.

At the same time, we need to examine whether intergovernmental cooperation mechanisms implemented long ago have brought real change to the Canadian federation. If the conflictual nature of certain issues can impede change, one must also ask whether the cooperative dimension can prevail in some areas, and under what conditions. To that end, I will review a number of agreements – or, on occasion, unilateral decisions by Ottawa – and from these, draw general conclusions after setting the basis for stakeholders' claims. I do so mainly (though not exclusively) from a Quebec perspective. Before looking at these case studies, it is important to provide an overall assessment of federal-provincial-territorial meetings held in recent years, and to depict the 'general mood' of intergovernmental relations over the past decade.

Early on, McRoberts wrote that 'federal-provincial liaison bodies, drawing together federal-provincial officials, primarily bureaucratic, in a wide range of areas grew from 64 in 1957 to, by one estimate, 400 in 1972' (1985, 75). That is a considerable increase, which is linked to the implementation of a large number of federal-provincial programs. Furthermore, the Secrétariat aux affaires intergouvernementales canadiennes of the Government of Quebec reports ninety-six meetings during the fiscal year from 1 April 1999 to 31 March 2000, and 103 meetings in 2000–2001. This includes federal-provincial-territorial meetings, federal-provincial meetings, provincial-territorial meetings, and interprovincial meetings in such diverse fields as agriculture, health, justice, the environment, transportation, social services, domestic trade, forestry, and the labour market. Two-thirds of these are administrative meetings involving deputy ministers or senior officials. However, there is also a large number of ministerial meetings – they make up almost one-third of the total.

Quebec has taken part in practically all of these meetings, the only exceptions being six in 1999–2000 and seven in 2000–2001, which it attended as an observer only. Most of these exceptions had to do with meetings on social policy that was linked to the implementation of the Social Union Framework Agreement, which Quebec refused to sign.

In the 1993 federal election, the Liberal government of Jean Chrétien was elected on the promise of putting aside Canada's constitutional problems and concentrating on other political priorities, particularly the economy. This commitment came in the wake of two resounding constitutional failures, namely the Meech Lake Accord in 1990 and the Charlottetown Accord in 1992. However, following the referendum held in Quebec in October 1995 on the sovereignty-partnership option, the federal government sought to regain the initiative both on the constitutional front (in reference to the Supreme Court and the Clarity Act) and in other sectors.

In the latter case, the main idea is to show that, while the constitutional path is practically blocked, it is nevertheless possible to resolve certain issues that concern the provinces. Using a pragmatic, case-by-case approach, the Chrétien government is trying to prove that agreements can be reached with the provinces, showing some flexibility as required. Appearing at times accommodating, at others more restrictive by using the carrot-and-stick approach, he is pursuing a dual objective: to show that federalism can evolve by concluding agreements with the provinces, thereby creating a heightened sense of belonging in Canada by emphasizing pan-Canadian mobility and a genuine national identity through shared values, especially in the social area.

With these notions in mind, let's now review certain agreements reached between Ottawa and the provinces in recent years.

Labour Force Training or Asymmetric Federalism

The Adult Occupational Training Act of 1967 brought an end to nearly fifty years of conditional grants in the field of vocational education. This legislation stemmed, in part, from the unilateral decision by federal authorities 'to transform the vocational training of adults into an adjunct of employment policy' (Dupré 1985, 9). From that point on, despite the transfer of this program from the vocational education sector to the employment sector, Quebec insisted on full control over this field, linked – in its view – to an integrated policy of training and re-entry into the labour force. In fact, according to Stefan Dupré, the federal manpower plan of the mid-1960s never got off the ground, because the ministries of education successfully intervened and forced federal officials to deal with them. In Dupré's opinion, this provincial victory sealed the fate of the federal plan in the months following its unveiling (1985, 10).

But the federal-provincial bickering did not end there. It finally ended thirty years later, in 1997, when Ottawa and the provinces concluded a labour force training agreement. The breaking of this deadlock was linked to the referendum of October 1995 in Quebec and to preparations for the federal election that took place later in 1998. In the wake of its referendum defeat, the government of Lucien Bouchard (who had just replaced Jacques Parizeau at the helm of the Parti Québécois) showed a willingness to strike agreements with Ottawa as long as they were in keeping with Quebec's interests, helped change situations deemed unacceptable, or helped increase Quebec's powers. For its part, the Liberal government of Jean Chrétien wanted to show Quebeckers – ahead of the upcoming federal election – that Canadian federalism was flexible and worked well. In short, conditions appeared very favourable on the heels of the Quebec referendum, since Ottawa needed to signal its openness to Quebec (Pelletier 1998, 302).

It is against this backdrop that the labour force training agreement (more precisely, the Canada/Quebec labour market agreement in principle) reached with the federal government should be analysed. From Quebec's standpoint, an agreement of this nature, first envisioned under the government of Jean Lesage in the 1960s, had become a major priority and enjoyed the support of all the province's socio-economic stakeholders. As for Ottawa, it did not want to sign such an agreement with Quebec alone, since it could be interpreted elsewhere in Canada as a concession to Quebec (following the 1995 referendum, that had been perceived as a threat) or as the granting of a special status (linked to the notion of distinct society, already rejected with the Meech Lake Accord in 1990) (Pelletier 1998, 302).

The agreement in principle reached with Quebec, combined with the related implementation agreement, provides an example of asymmetric federalism at work: an administrative agreement authorized by a very broad piece of federal legislation that allows the marked differences between the provinces' educational systems to be taken into account. Asymmetric in that five provinces, including Quebec and Alberta, obtained a complete transfer of labour market responsibilities, while three Atlantic provinces (with the exception of New Brunswick) settled for a joint management formula or participation in the federal program, and British Columbia concluded what was seen as a hybrid, temporary agreement.

The asymmetry can also be seen in the Quebec agreement, which stands apart from the others on a specific point (following an exchange of letters between the responsible ministers). Under Quebec's Bill 101, French is recognized as the official language of the public administration; hence, services to users are first offered in French, except if businesses wish to communicate in their language. On request also, services can be offered in English. However, the government's Web sites are bilingual. Such a policy contrasts with the bilingualism policy in effect at the federal level, which requires services to be offered to users in both official languages, but only in areas where the demand warrants it (Pelletier 1998 and 2002 interview). Implementation of these agreements is left to the provinces, which can select the formula best suited to their situation. Thus, Quebec and Alberta decided to amalgamate or integrate the various existing programs, but insisted on different methods of implementation (e.g., employment assistance in Quebec and loans/grants in Alberta).

All in all, this transfer of responsibilities and federal public servants has been favourably received in Quebec, even though Quebec authorities were initially confronted with major problems raised by a different classification system for federal employees, the status of Quebec's casual employees, and the need to adjust internal systems. Since then, the problems have been solved: the fact that these programs were amalgamated, it was stressed, helped a great deal.

Internal Trade Agreement or Federalism with the Provinces

Doern and MacDonald describe the Internal Trade Agreement (ITA) as the convergence and interaction of three policy spheres: industrial regional policy; trade policy; and federal-provincial policy. With respect to the latter point, which is of particular interest to us here, they indicate that the entire negotiating process provides an example of federalism at work (1999, 17–36).

This prompted Daniel Johnson, Quebec's premier at the time, to say that the agreement represented 'a perfect illustration of how federalism should work' (qtd. in Schwartz 1995, 214).

Already, the Free Trade Agreement with the United States, and then Mexico, had paved the way for a form of cooperation, if not participation, by the provinces in developing the central government's negotiating position for Canada. To be sure, this approach was modelled on 'executive federalism,' as described by Smiley (1980) and Cairns (1977). But opening up Canada's markets to the free flow of goods and services made it even more necessary to open up Canada's domestic market in the same way (Schwartz 1995).

As for the more traditional brand of executive federalism, the Internal Trade Agreement introduced two innovations: the first was the presence of a neutral presiding officer who acted as a mediator, seeking to reconcile thirteen different interests (the ten provinces, the federal government and the two territories) in fifteen policy areas and to reach compromises among the parties while taking into account their interests (Doern and MacDonald 1999, 32). The second innovation involved the creation of an Internal Trade Secretariat, ultimately responsible in part for the successful outcome of the negotiations. The Secretariat was charged not only with establishing common grounds for discussions on internal trade but also, and most importantly, during the intensive phase of the negotiations, with providing the necessary analyses to demonstrate the impact of a particular decision or the applicability of the framework rules (55–6). In particular, the actors were concerned with the agreement's effects on the distribution of powers defined in the Constitution. Thus, the Secretariat's role was to show that a negotiated agreement on internal trade would have no effect on the constitutional front.

Of course, each delegation had its own agenda and its own objectives. Generally speaking, there was a need to strike a balance between trade liberalization and the imperatives of regional economic development. That said, Alberta and Manitoba were wholeheartedly in favour of interprovincial free trade, while Quebec was rather favourably inclined, albeit with certain reservations in the energy and cultural sectors. But from Quebec's perspective, it was important to reach an agreement before the upcoming provincial election, scheduled for 1994. The provinces, then led by New Democratic governments (Ontario, British Columbia, and Saskatchewan), appeared fairly sceptical and criticized various aspects of free trade, seeking to maximize the exemptions and minimize the general rules. The Atlantic provinces and the Territories, while not opposed to the idea of opening markets, feared that regional development policies would fall by the wayside, with considerable fallout for them. Politically, they were negotiating from a position of weakness (Doern and MacDonald 1999, 59–81).

The agreement was signed in July 1994, following a First Ministers' meeting. What really got the negotiating process on track was an agreement by internal trade ministers, in December 1992, on three main principles, and on four main rules for applying these principles, to guide future negotiations. Soon after, in March 1993, that group – the Committee of Ministers on Internal Trade (CMIT) – reached agreement on a series of negotiating rules, and even set a firm date for the start of negotiations as well as a deadline (30 June 1994). The report prepared by the chief negotiators committee in January 1994 paved the way for more intensive talks; these, in turn, enabled the Internal Trade Secretariat to produce a draft text for discussion and further revisions. Following a second draft submitted in May, the CMIT reached an agreement on 28 June 1994, which was eventually signed by the first ministers in July 1994. The role played by First Ministers was more 'philosophical' than practical. But at the same time, they pressed for the negotiations to be completed within the required time frame (Doern and MacDonald 1999, 46–56). The agreement took effect on 1 July of the following year.

Implementation of the ITA partially lessened the need for bilateral agreements between any two provinces (e.g., between Quebec and New Brunswick and between Quebec and Ontario), particularly on procurement. This was by no means a panacea; problems still remained, especially in the area of labour mobility.

Indeed, implementation of the ITA has not resolved all the issues. The chapter on energy is still the subject of negotiations. The Internal Trade Secretariat, established under the agreement and based in Winnipeg, is examining what the parties to the agreement have achieved since its implementation and what remains to be done (Internal Trade Secretariat 2002b). Judging by the evidence, the achievements have been impressive and point for the most part to the creation of an internal common market. Which is not to say that everything has been settled, especially in light of a series of legitimate objectives, in all chapters, that give rise to numerous exceptions. In fact, during a conference held in Toronto on 31 May and 1 June 2001, participants said that progress had been slow and implementation even slower. They urged Ottawa to show leadership in this area (Internal Trade Secretariat 2001, 37). Opening up procurement to free trade, full labour mobility, and liberalizing the energy sector are the areas most often cited as not yet in line with the requirements of internal free trade.

We must bear in mind that the ITA is a *political* document, not a *legal* text, which might make it less restrictive for the actors involved. This non-legislative (and definitely non-constitutional) dimension is linked to the political backdrop against which the agreement was negotiated. After the Meech and Charlottetown failures, an agreement had to be reached at all costs (in the words of Mark MacDonald, 'federalism was in need of a victory – any victory ...' [2002, 143]) in order to show that federalism could work and that it was possible to agree on important questions, in this case questions pertaining to the economy. It should also be noted that the parties involved were fully aware of the costs of a failure to reach this agreement.

In sum, as one interviewee[1] noted, the ITA strikes a fragile balance between the desire for more liberalized trade and the desire to maintain regional distinctiveness. In this sense, the 'national' consciousness is not as developed as it could be. As the interviewee added, however, progress continues, albeit on a small scale (e.g., the gradual opening up of procurement). As for the dispute resolution mechanism provided for in the agreement, everything will depend on the willingness of politicians to negotiate in good faith and abide by the recommendations of the dispute settlement panel.

Social Union or Federalism without Quebec

To gain a proper understanding of the Social Union Framework Agreement (SUFA), one must consider two important issues that surfaced in the 1990s. First, a profound need was felt to reform social programs that had been in place for a quarter century. The question then arose as to which order of government should take on this controversial task, given the implications and the intervention of both orders of government in this area. Second, questions were raised as to the recurring deficits of governments in Canada since the mid-1970s, which worsened during the 1990–2 recession (Richards 2002, 1).

The governments of the prairie provinces were the first to act, cutting programs and eventually taxes. Ottawa was next, with across-the-board program cuts; only old age security and Aboriginal programs emerged unscathed. In 1995, the federal government created the Canada Health and Social Transfer (CHST) by merging the Established Programs Financing (EPF) and the Canada Assistance Plan (CAP). The new CHST featured block funding, as had been the case with EPF since 1977 but not with the CAP, the last major federal transfers program to the provinces where funding of social services and social assistance was split evenly between the two orders of government (except for the more well-off provinces). In addition, federal Finance Minister Paul Martin announced in his February 1995 budget that the provinces would see their transfers reduced by more than one-third, or $6 billion over a two-year period.

This major cut-back was the main focus of the meeting of provincial First Ministers in August 1995, which led to the creation of a provincial-territorial committee to look into the matter. The committee tabled a progress report in December 1995. In light of the unilateral approach taken by the federal government, it proposed an improved framework for Ottawa's spending power, a better definition of the exclusive jurisdiction of each order of government, efforts to reduce overlap as much as possible to enhance accountability, and adoption of joint decision-making mechanisms (Gagnon 2000, 12–13).

Subsequently, the Quebec government – concerned with maintaining its jurisdiction, as Premier Bouchard underscored in Jasper in August 1996 and reiterated a year later at the provincial First Ministers' meeting in St Andrews – decided to opt out of the talks. In the meantime, the federal government, at the behest of the provinces (except Quebec), engaged more actively in negotiating an agreement on the social union. In June 1998, all the provinces, without Quebec, agreed on an agenda for negotiating with Ottawa. However, the main agenda items were compatible with the key objectives pursued by Quebec (Richards 2002, 4).

The August 1998 Annual Premiers' Conference, in which Quebec participated, produced a consensus among all the provinces. Referred to as the Saskatoon consensus, it was founded on an essential, oft-reiterated demand by Quebec, namely, the ability of a province (or territory) to opt out of any new or modified Canada-wide social program in areas of provincial/territorial jurisdiction with full compensation, provided that the province/territory carries on a program or initiative that addresses the priority areas of the Canada-wide program (Noël 2000a, 24). This agreement allowed the provinces to maintain a common front, which held fast until the eve of the signing of the SUFA. Indeed, the final document that emerged from the January 1999 meeting of provincial ministers responsible for this area, in Victoria, set forth a common provincial position.

A few days later, however – on 4 February 1999, more precisely – the common front collapsed: the Social Union Framework Agreement was concluded between the federal government and nine provinces. Quebec did not sign the agreement, seeing it as legitimizing the federal government's spending power without Ottawa offering anything tangible in return (such as a guarantee of stable funding), beyond a requirement to consult the provinces. It entrenched the federal government's role in the social sector without recognizing the primacy of the provinces. Ottawa's flexibility and initiatives were preserved, while the constraints it would have to meet were fairly modest. Most important, the Agreement remained silent on a major demand by Quebec: 'the ability (of a province or territory) to opt out of any new or modified Canada-wide social program in areas of provincial/territorial jurisdiction with full compensation,' as stipulated by the news release issued in August 1998 at the Annual Premiers' Conference in Saskatoon.

As several analysts pointed out (Lazar 2000a, 28–9; Vaillancourt 2002, 38–9; Robson and Schwanen 1999, 3), it was the lure of money that swayed the nine provinces to sign the agreement and abandon their previous unanimous stance in favour of restraining Ottawa's spending power. Robson and Schwanen add that Ottawa and the provinces thereby forced Quebec to defend alone its constitutional rights (1999, 4). Beyond the lofty aims of the Saskatoon consensus, one thing is clear: most provinces wanted increased federal funding, something that Ottawa promised them in 1999 and which ended the common front, at least momentarily.

Ottawa's interest in SUFA stemmed from the fact that 'as the signing date approached, the fiscal circumstances of the federal government improved dramatically, and Ottawa was able to put cash on the table in exchange for looser constraints on its spending power' (Gibbins 2001, 7). At the same time it wanted to show that, in line with statements by Prime Minister Chrétien, federalism could be renewed without having to amend the Constitution.

According to federal officials interviewed for this chapter, SUFA is simply a 'code of conduct' for the various governments and a 'general framework' to guide the ministries involved. For the federal government, the deal has already led to significant progress, since it made it possible, among other things, to conclude an agreement on affordable housing based on the principles contained in the agreement.

However, it seems that the agreement has failed to live up to the expectations of most provinces. Quebec sees it as an unacceptable step backwards; indeed, even the Liberal Party headed by Jean Charest and Mario Dumont's Action démocratique du Québec refused to endorse the agreement. André Binette had this to say about the demise of the common front: 'The English-speaking provinces are trying to make the federation work, even if it means centralization. Quebec cannot bring itself to pay such a price, because it would pose a threat to its national identity' (2000, 50, my translation).

Three years have passed since the agreement was signed. Thus, governments have jointly undertaken, with the exception of Quebec (which has observer status), 'a full review of the agreement and its implementation' (article 7 of SUFA). The process is under way, but little progress has been made. All the provinces, but particularly Alberta and Ontario, want the dispute resolution mechanism issue resolved; they are even threatening to reopen the agreement. It is clear that if this issue were settled to the provinces' satisfaction, it would constrain the federal government and further restore a balance and a more level playing field between the 'partners.'

In any event, it is difficult at this point to assess the real effects of the Agreement, apart from increased federal funding on social programs – an increase that would have come about with or without the agreement. Given the magnitude of the federal surpluses, it would have been completely unacceptable for Ottawa to deny the provinces additional funding. But the way the provinces see it, federal funding remains inadequate, a position reiterated by the premiers at their annual conference in Winnipeg in August 2000 and again, with insistence, in Victoria in August 2001. There, they suggested that 'adequate and sustainable fiscal arrangements' might include not only restoration of federal funding through the CHST with an appropriate escalator, but also tax-point transfers as one possible alternative and fundamental changes to the equalization system (Canadian Intergovernmental Conference Secretariat 2001). They renewed this consensus at a special meeting held In Vancouver In January 2002.

In Addition, each First Ministers' meeting, along with each health ministers' meeting, is an opportunity to underline the magnitude of the task at hand: pharmaceuticals management, health human resources management, continuing care (primary care, home care, community care), clear accountability and reporting to citizens (the list goes on).

It should also be pointed out that in various news releases issued after these meetings, Quebec makes a point of reminding everyone of its position: while it declined to sign the Social Union Framework Agreement (and therefore does not feel bound by it), it usually adheres to the principles set out therein and is committed to cooperating with other provinces. But the point that truly emerges from the framework agreement process is the need for intergovernmental cooperation 'in full respect of each government's jurisdiction,' as stated in the news release issued at the conclusion of the federal-provincial-territorial First Ministers' meeting of September 2000 in Ottawa.

In sum, since SUFA is first and foremost a 'code of conduct' for the various governments, it is difficult to assess its concrete effects. In practical terms, the issue is as much about health care innovation as about mobility of persons; as much an issue about the fight against poverty (Osberg 2000) as about Millennium Scholarships; and as much about affordable housing as about the National Child Benefit. When all is said and done, SUFA will be assessed on the basis of the policies adopted and the programs implemented. Except for the first section dealing with principles, SUFA focuses on the processes (five sections) rather than on the substance (only one section, on mobility), notes Harvey Lazar (2000b, 101). Which is to say that in order to adequately assess SUFA, we cannot look solely at the substance of the Agreement (the programs put in place), but need to look also at the process (are these programs in line with the provisions of SUFA?).

Finally, it can be said that as of August 2002, SUFA had not delivered on its promises, neither in terms of federal-provincial cooperation and constraint on spending power – witness the ever-expanding unilateral actions by Ottawa in the form of ad hoc and targeted transfers (Millennium Scholarships, Canada Research Chairs, Canada Foundation for Innovation, the Medical Equipment Trust Fund) – nor in terms of dispute resolution, since the mechanism provided for in the agreement has yet to materialize, nor in terms of citizens engagement, since performance indicators, participation structures, and accountability procedures are still lacking. However, SUFA has led to Quebec's isolation, and has thus shown that Canadian federalism can be reformed without Quebec.

Health: The Dangers of Unilateralism

It is widely recognized that the federal government played a major role in implementing the hospital insurance program in 1957, followed by medicare in 1966; this is not to ignore the pioneering role played by the Government of Saskatchewan. As was the practice in that period of 'cooperative' federalism, these projects took the form of programs funded jointly and equally by the two orders of government (Lazar 2000a, 6–16). All the provinces, including Quebec, eventually came on board.

Painstaking negotiations between Ottawa and the provinces led to the creation, in 1977, of the Established Programs Financing (EPF) system, whereby the federal government pledged to provide, for health and postsecondary education, block funding in the form of tax-point transfers and cash. Thus, EPF gave the provinces greater leeway and in so doing, lessened Ottawa's control over sectors that, after all, were under provincial jurisdiction. By its very nature, block funding was not accompanied by any real control mechanisms for the federal government over funds given to the provinces, in contrast with the joint programs.

According to Monique Bégin (2002), former federal minister of Health and Welfare, the objective of the Canada Health Act of 1984 was precisely to restore federal control, lost with the introduction of EPF, over the implementation of health policies in the provinces. The 1984 Act's five fundamental principles – accessibility, universality, comprehensiveness, portability, public administration, which are still in effect – enabled the federal government to ensure that these principles were upheld; it could therefore exert once again some control over this sector. A recalcitrant province that accepted, say, user fees or physician overbilling would face a penalty.

After three years, penalties had been imposed on seven provinces, totalling $245 million – $134 million for overbilling and $111 million for user fees. All these fines were later reimbursed after the provinces banned these practices, which contravened the principles set out in the Act (Bégin 2002, 3). The key consideration isn't so much the penalties imposed – fairly minimal since 1984 – as the conditions or standards that continue to govern the payments made under the CHST. These conditions are currently at the heart of the debate surrounding the management of the health sector (Commission sur le déséquilibre fiscal 2002, 78–80).

This type of punitive federalism reduces the provinces' ability to make changes to health programs. To understand why the debates in this area have been so fierce, we should consider the principles of public administration, comprehensiveness, or accessibility. The Act of 1984 continues to play a major role in the field of health. Thus, it helps control the often conflictual relations between governments.

In this context, can we really talk about a collaborative federalism coming increasingly to the fore since the mid-1990s (Lazar 1998, 2000a)? This type of federalism would foster partnership and equality between orders of government rather than strong federal leadership. It would correspond to a period of belt-tightening and block funding that would hardly encourage federal activism. On the contrary, Ottawa would be obliged to accept a more egalitarian partnership on account of its inability to use cash transfers to shape the provinces' conduct (Lazar 2000a, 29).

Apart from the fact that reductions in federal spending have now given way to budget surpluses, we must bear in mind that on several occasions Ottawa has used trusts or foundations as new mechanisms for shaping the provinces' conduct, either by requiring them to invest in a particular sector (purchase of medical equipment), or bypassing them in dealing directly with citizens or organizations (Millennium Scholarships, Canada Research Chairs).

As for the notion of partnership and equal footing, Alain Noël – among others – argues that, on the contrary, the current 'collaborative' brand of federalism is hierarchical and must be viewed as 'hegemonic cooperation,' a label borrowed from Keohane. In this form of cooperation, one order of government wields dominant power, setting the rules and providing the necessary stimulus so that the other order conforms to these rules. It simply reflects a reality where cooperation emerges from conflict rather than harmony, but also where the conflicting parties are not necessarily on an equal footing (Noël 2000b, 6–14). In other words, cooperation is 'a regulated and institutionalized form of conflict' (Noël 2001, 17).

Some analysts blame the difficulties associated with collaborative federalism on the lack of a 'mission statement,' of clear objectives and of a long-term perspective to guide politicians, particularly about fiscal federalism (Lazar 2000a). Indeed, most political decisions taken by heads of government at federal-provincial conferences have implications for fiscal federalism. In turn, all the changes made over the years to federal transfers to the provinces have had a direct impact on provincial budgets. In this context, several policies announced in recent federal budgets – policies that had an impact on provinces – are not the product of federal-provincial negotiations. This mode of operation, which violates the principles set out in SUFA (e.g., the need to give advance notice), has led to increased uncertainty among provincial actors.

This observation, while shared by several analysts, is interpreted differently by others. According to Alain Noël, Ottawa's social and intergovernmental policies can seem improvised, inconsistent, or unpredictable; 'this approach, however, should not be taken as a sign of weakness or lack of purpose.' He adds, 'The cultivation of uncertainty is a prerogative of power' (Noël 2001, 3). The difficulties raised by collaborative federalism do not stem, according to Noël, from a lack of vision on Ottawa's part, but rather from an 'uneven relationship solidly rooted in a serious and growing vertical fiscal imbalance between the two orders of government' (ibid.).

This brings us to the heart of the debate on Canadian federalism. It is not a genuine partnership between equals, but an uneven relationship between politicians – one of whom exhibits his or her mastery of the situation by keeping the others in a climate of uncertainty through decisions that betray a lack of direction, especially when they negate an agreement signed a few years earlier (most notably, articles 3 and 4 of SUFA). Thus, there is no apparent transparency or accountability guiding federal budgetary policy, or even intergovernmental relations as a whole. This raises fears that collaborative federalism was linked to a particular set of conditions shaped by fiscal restraints, and that it has rapidly morphed into a form of unilateralism where the central government has reclaimed control over intergovernmental relations. In this context of inequality, it is harder to find evidence of transparency and accountability, unless what is meant by accountability is being answerable not to citizens but to the central government.

Health: A Dynamic Sector in Spite of It All

Beyond the Social Union Framework Agreement, which 'could turn out to be a major innovation in the workings of the federation, heralding a new era of collaboration (and) mutual respect among levels of government ... or could be ignored by its signatories and relegated to a footnote in the country's history' (Lazar 2000b, 100), the health sector remains of utmost importance in the lives of all Canadians.

Reading through the agendas for meetings of health ministers or deputy ministers over a period of four years, one notes that most of the (numerous) items deal with current issues of concern to the public or specific groups. From tainted blood and hepatitis C to health human resources (physicians, nurses, and so on), from anti-smoking initiatives to primary health care, from home care to medical equipment, from organ donations to pharmaceuticals management, from reproductive technologies to information on health and communications technologies, from children's health to Aboriginal health, and from performance indicators to dispute resolution. Then there are the reports submitted by various task forces and meetings with representatives of physician or nursing organizations. It's all grist for the mill, making for an ongoing series of very busy one- or two-day meetings of ministers, deputy ministers, and their senior officials. The Canadian Intergovernmental Conference Secretariat provides extensive logistical support for all these conferences. Health Canada, for its part, sees itself as a 'facilitator' and/or a 'coordinator' on health issues with a Canada-wide dimension (according to an unofficial document submitted in August 2000 to the Senate committee chaired by Senator Kirby).

In June 1992, the federal, provincial, and territorial deputy ministers of health unanimously decided to adopt a new advisory committee structure to replace the fifty-odd committees and subcommittees of various types that existed since 1990. This new structure was reduced to four advisory committees: one on public health, another on health human resources, a third on health services, and a fourth on health information, which subsequently became the Canadian Institute for Health Information. A few others have been added since, most as a result of SUFA (e.g., on health infrastructures – electronic means, privacy protection – and on performance indicators and accountability). For each of these broad sectors, of course, there are various working groups, which can be official or simply ad hoc (from 100 to 150 groups, for example the one on mental health indicators). These committees report back to the Conference of Deputy Ministers of Health. The plan was to fund them on a federal-provincial basis, with the provinces assuming a greater share of the funding (80–20), which can cause problems if a large province such as Quebec refuses to take part.

All of these working groups will be generating and sharing information, analysing in greater depth specific issues, seeking the best possible solutions and suggesting alternatives. No province, I was told during interviews, would have enough resources to develop expertise in all these sectors. I was also told that a broader agreement can be reached on matters of a more technical or clinical nature, where the *evidence* plays a larger role, by contrast with issues of a more political nature. An example is the campaign against tobacco use. It is easier to agree on the solutions for this health problem than on health funding, which is a political problem with fiscal implications.

In the area of health, however, consensus is often reached both at the deputy minister level and at the ministerial level. For example, ministers can reach an agreement on which broad policy directions to take, but must also take into account the public's expectations. This may lead to tensions between the consensus achieved at the lower (administrative) level and at the higher (political) level, where jurisdictional issues, government priorities, resource availability, and the expectations of the electorate and of given groups in society must all be taken into account.

In this dynamic sector, ministers usually meet once a year, deputy ministers usually twice, and committees many times per year. The committees are required to report back to deputy ministers at least twice a year. In fact, in 1999 alone deputy ministers held twenty meetings, some by teleconference; they met eighteen times in 2000; and thirteen times in 2001.

All in all, the rules and modus operandi of the structures put in place allow for dialogue on various issues, solutions and ways of doing things; this, in turn, makes it possible to reach consensus. Often, various parties offer the same diagnosis for a problem and share the same solutions, for example a holistic approach to primary care reform. It then becomes a matter of finding the required flexibility to implement these solutions. In other words, service delivery will take different forms in different provinces. The problem – if there is one – will surface at the political level, where consensus is made public, since that is when government authorities must factor in the political consequences of their actions. Thus, Quebec does not always want to be officially associated with a consensus, because it seeks to protect its jurisdictional autonomy. We might want to recall the general preamble to the news release on health issued at the end of the First Ministers' meeting in Ottawa in September 2000; released by the Canadian Intergovernmental Conference Secretariat (2000):

Nothing in this document shall be construed to derogate from the respective governments' jurisdictions. The Vision, Principles, Action Plan for Health System Renewal, Clear Accountability, and Working Together (i.e. the five key points in the news release) shall be interpreted in full respect of each government's jurisdiction.

This brings us to the crux of the problem facing intergovernmental relations: How can Ottawa, using its spending power, respect areas of provincial jurisdiction? In the final analysis, will it simply 'facilitate' consensus or simply 'coordinate' provincial undertakings, or will it be a major player in the health sector? The ambiguity persists. It is likely underlying the current Quebec-Ontario-Alberta axis that seems to be taking shape in the health area. The Social Union Framework Agreement sought to dispel this ambiguity by officially recognizing the federal government's spending power, but Quebec refused to go along out of a concern for jurisdictional encroachment.

An Assessment of Interstate Federalism

We should begin by establishing what the Canadian public thinks of intergovernmental cooperation. In a 2001 survey commissioned by the Centre for Research and Information on Canada (CRIC), two things stood out in terms of the approach needed to make the country work better. First, in each province, increased cooperation between Ottawa and the provincial government was seen as the best way to make the federation work better. However, it should be noted that support for cooperation was weaker in Quebec (62 per cent) and higher in Western Canada (71 per cent), the other regions falling somewhere in the middle (CRIC 2002, 22–4). In previous years (1998–2000), the picture was similar: more than six Quebeckers in ten (63 per cent) considered intergovernmental cooperation a high priority, while more than seven out of ten Canadians outside Quebec (73 per cent) shared that view, based on data obtained from previous CRIC surveys.

Second, while intergovernmental cooperation emerged as the favoured option to make the federation work better, it does not preclude Ottawa from transferring additional powers to the provincial governments. Here again, Quebeckers stand apart from residents of other provinces: in 2001, 42 per cent saw this option as a high priority, while Canadians outside Quebec gave it much lower support (from 18 per cent in Ontario to 30 per cent in the West). In other words, if intergovernmental cooperation appears to be a preferred option for making the Canadian federation work better, it is not a panacea that would obviate the need to make other changes, such as the transfer of powers.

The Effects on Federalism and Change

Beyond formal amendments to the Constitution and beyond the

interpretations made by the courts to address the shortcomings of intrastate federalism, intergovernmental cooperation mechanisms have undoubtedly allowed for greater flexibility and adjustments in the workings of the Canadian federation.

We should begin by clarifying a key point. People often tend to contrast intergovernmental cooperation with a distribution of powers based on 'watertight compartments,' each order of government being allocated exclusive powers, as is the case in Canada, but also in Switzerland and Belgium (Watts 1999, 37). Such a vision rests on the idea that, if each order of government enjoys exclusive powers, it can act independently in its areas of jurisdiction without the need to cooperate with other governments.

This classic vision of dualistic federalism, to use the term coined by K.C. Wheare (1963), has pretty much fallen out of favour today, replaced by so-called cooperative or interdependent federalism. To some, this suggests that the Canadian federation cannot avoid the 'mutual interdependence' of the modern world, and that the 'mutual independence' or watertight compartments of the past have become increasingly dysfunctional in a world of growing interconnectedness (Lazar 1998, 27). This notion of inevitable interdependence has served to justify the federal spending power and Ottawa's many encroachments into areas of provincial jurisdiction. What some provinces refuse to do, Quebec included, is link interdependence and encroachment by the federal government (via its spending power), whereas the two can be dissociated, as evidenced by the numerous cooperation agreements struck among the provinces. In other words, intergovernmental cooperation is justified by the necessary 'mutual interdependence' in the contemporary world, but it does not justify the use of the federal spending power in areas of provincial jurisdiction. This is the source of many conflicts in today's Canadian federation.

With this clarification made, even though the Constitution sets out watertight jurisdictions, it goes without saying that the lines separating the various jurisdictional areas are not always clear. For example, the employment insurance rules established by the federal government impact on and can even conflict with the provinces' social welfare policies. While each order of government operates in its areas of jurisdiction, there is room for intergovernmental cooperation. Similarly, conflicts may arise between the regulation of trade and commerce, an area of federal jurisdiction, and the regulation of labour relations, which falls under the provinces' authority. Hence the need for intergovernmental cooperation. When all is said and done, the compartments are not always as 'watertight' as one might claim, and even if they were, mutual interdependence still requires governments to cooperate with one another – although this does not justify Ottawa's intrusion in areas of provincial jurisdiction.

In such instances, intergovernmental cooperation mechanisms can hamper change, in that they seem to serve to justify actions by the federal government that one or more provinces would not accept. If they are used to legitimize encroachments by Ottawa or to allow it to impose conditions, they can indeed become a major impediment to change, since they would be seen as a tool for subordinating provinces to the federal government. Any form of subordination, whatever the mechanism used, is rightly perceived as contrary to the very foundations of federalism.

This point was stressed by Premier Lucien Bouchard in August 1996 when he explained Quebec's refusal to go along with the provinces on the social union. In his words, the Government of Quebec cannot 'become involved in intergovernmental decision-making processes that would subject it to standards to which Quebec would not have consented, in areas coming under its jurisdiction' (qtd. in Noël 2000a, 35, my translation).

In addition, and as we have seen earlier, the agreement on labour training – or, to be more precise, on the labour market – led to the recognition of asymmetry, with five provinces fully assuming this power while others opted instead for a form of comanagement with Ottawa. This is by no means an impediment to intergovernmental cooperation. Thus, during fiscal year 2000–1, Quebec took part in about ten conferences on the labour market, at both the federal-provincial and the provincial-territorial levels, involving senior officials, deputy ministers, or ministers. The asymmetry of these agreements does not stand in the way of intergovernmental cooperation; on the contrary, it can even encourage the sharing of information on various aspects. The same can apply to asymmetry in standards. In fact, several analysts (Burelle 1995; McRoberts 1997; Dufour 2002) argue that asymmetry can be a viable option for the Canadian federation, especially to satisfy Quebec's demands.

It was precisely this point that proved to be SUFA's major stumbling block in the case of Quebec: the federal government refused to recognize the right to opt out with financial compensation, thereby precluding the possibility of giving future consideration to genuine asymmetrical formulas in the social sector. One author who analysed SUFA suggests, however, that Quebec should 'take advantage of Western Canada's current focus on provincial autonomy as an opportunity to promote asymmetrical federalism as a potential solution to both the Quebec problem and Western alienation' (Dufour 2002, 20).

I fear, however, that the federal government is seeking to counter through various means any form of situational or ad hoc alliances that Quebec might form with one or more provinces. It is almost as if Ottawa feared that recognizing asymmetry in the social area (and particularly in the health sector) would lead to changes in the major principles underlying the Canada Health Act and to the establishment of social programs differing too much from one province to the next, which might prove an impediment to mobility. What's more, Quebec has developed an often unique expertise over the past decade in social policy reforms, and its non-participation in SUFA deprives other provinces of this expertise, as it deprives Quebec of the others' experiences (Vaillancourt 2002). The latter observation illustrates clearly that asymmetry in programs, more than uniformity, should more readily elicit cooperation among the provinces, because they likely feel a lesser need to cooperate when they are all doing the same thing.

Some see the social union going down an entirely different path: it encourages uniformity by discouraging provincial innovation independently from Ottawa and the other provinces. 'Throughout the document,' argues John Richards, 'lurks the danger of *la pensée unique* – reliance on a single policy response to any given problem' (2002, 6). Uniformity can be an effective tool for strengthening national unity, but it leaves no room for diversity. In reality, social union amounts to unity in principle but diversity in practice. Here again, an excessive emphasis on unity of principles can inhibit change, even if there is recognition of possible diversity in concrete application. Could there be recognition of asymmetry even in the definition of standards?

When assessing SUFA's winners and losers, Harvey Lazar (2000b) argues that the provinces lost by straying from some of the positions they defended as part of the Saskatoon consensus, including their stance on the opting-out clause. But they gained in that Ottawa accepted decision-making rules, which give the provinces a formal – albeit modest, as Lazar points out – role in the exercise of the spending power, something which they had lacked previously (115). However, Quebec appears to be the biggest loser, since the ability to opt out with full compensation, which was part of the Saskatoon consensus, is nowhere to be found in SUFA. For Quebec, this has always been a core demand. Ottawa, for its part, seems to have come out the big winner, since it met most of its objectives, including official recognition of its spending power, increased mobility within Canada, greater transparency and accountability on the part of the provinces, and only modest constraints on its spending power. In return, it pledged to invest more money in the social sector – which it would have done anyway given its budget surpluses – and to set up a dispute resolution mechanism, which still has to materialize three years later. By launching initiatives to manage the Millennium Scholarships, the purchase of medical equipment, or the one – since abandoned – aimed at supporting infrastructure investments, Ottawa has certainly not made itself overly transparent, but far less accountable.

Turning our attention to health and leaving aside the Social Union Framework Agreement which oversees this sector, we can see that, from the myriad studies by committees and working groups, agreement can emerge more easily on technical and scientific issues. Moving up to the deputy ministers and ministers, negotiations have often led, even at this more politicized level, to agreements on a host of subjects. As evidence, we need only read the news releases issued at the conclusion of these meetings. For example, the First Ministers' meeting held in Ottawa in September 2000 ended on a number of commitments on health promotion, primary care, homecare and community care, pharmaceuticals management, development of health information technologies, investment in equipment and health infrastructure, and health system performance reporting. The news release issued following the provincial-territorial premiers' meeting in Vancouver in January 2002 also announced numerous points of agreement among the participants and, most important, the creation of a Premiers' Council on Canadian Health Awareness aimed at improving Canadians' access to information and 'enhancing public awareness of the challenges of and solutions for the future of health care.'

In all likelihood, the most important issues are not linked to the technical or scientific aspects of this sector. Rather, they come from two other sources. The first is well known and involves health funding. To solve this problem, increased funding is contemplated, but we must bear in mind that health takes up the largest chunk of provincial budgets. This pressure on provincial budgets could be alleviated, however, by larger transfers from the federal government. Another source of problems is the way Ottawa approaches intergovernmental relations.

The notion of an *equal* partnership, evoked by Lazar (1998, 2000a) in his definition of collaborative federalism, could smooth out a number of difficulties. Yet it all comes down to an equal partnership, and many decisions announced in federal budgets do not reflect this partnership. Similarly, the current disagreement on dispute resolution mechanisms clearly shows that it is still difficult to act as equal partners. Too often, unilateralism seems to win out over a true partnership of equals.

Federalism, as has already been pointed out, is based on the dual notion of unity in the entire federation and a recognition of the diversity characterizing the federated entities. Intergovernmental cooperation mechanisms can be expected to reflect this duality. On the one hand, the introduction of mechanisms (including, for example, an Internal Trade Secretariat) and the results of negotiations reflect the *cooperative* aspect of federalism in which the central government and the provinces, or the provinces amongst themselves, can reach agreements, even if only after numerous compromises and even if, occasionally, that agreement is based on the lowest common denominator. On the other hand, in view of the prevailing diversity, the provinces can be expected to try to preserve their distinctiveness, which translates into different policies reflecting the needs and preferences of their citizens. Federalism appears, then, to be more *competitive* in essence, which is also reflected in federal-provincial or interprovincial negotiations.

The ITA is a good example of this duality. The cooperative aspect was reflected in an agreement, arrived at through painstaking negotiations and signed by all the parties, and in the fact that to date, the parties have abided by the decisions of dispute panels (in 1999 and in 2000; a third case, dealing with margarine colouring, is underway involving Quebec). The competitive aspect refers to the many legitimate objectives defended by one or the other party to the negotiations and by the many exemptions found in the Agreement. In other words, if the goal is closer economic integration and an unfettered internal market (cooperation), then the need to ensure economic development that also responds to a wide diversity of regional imperatives (competition) cannot be ignored.

Since federal-provincial relations are often marred by disputes over jurisdictions that a party holds or would like to obtain and over one party's willingness to respect the other's jurisdiction, it goes without saying that negotiations between provinces and the central government are usually based on competition between them and usually focussed on the potential effects of an agreement on the distribution of powers. Thus, each order of government likes to emphasize that a given agreement does not affect the distribution of powers set out in the Constitution. This is the case for the ITA, whose Article 300 states the following:

> Nothing in this Agreement alters the legislative or other authority of Parliament or of the provincial legislatures or of the Government of Canada or of the provincial governments or the rights of any of them with respect to the exercise of their legislative or other authorities under the Constitution of Canada. (Internal Trade Secretariat 2002a)

Similarly, at the beginning of the news release, emphasis is placed on respecting the areas of jurisdiction assigned to each order of government: the aim is to underscore a problem or a potential problem. If Ottawa wants to impose standards or guidelines (even under its spending power) in areas of jurisdiction belonging to the provinces, a number of provinces are going to rebel, Quebec chief among them. Gagnon and Erk cite the notion of 'federal trust' in an attempt to resolve this issue. According to them, this notion assumes a lack of clear consensus on issues, but requires a sense of *trust* among partners in the federation, so that they can work together in good faith (Gagnon and Erk 2002, 324–6).

This is also echoed by Harvey Lazar, who argues that the absence of a clear mission statement or overarching vision for the future of Canadian fiscal federalism makes it harder for the different orders of government to predict how their partners will behave and thus undermines the trust necessary to ensure effective cooperation between these governments (Lazar 2000a, 5, 22).

For partners to be able to reach agreements, they obviously must be able to trust each other and feel that everyone can work together in good faith. This 'good faith,' especially for Quebec, has been severely tested in the past. The coalition of eight provinces opposed to patriation in 1981 eventually fell apart; the pact made by the ten provinces on the contents of Meech disintegrated; the Saskatoon consensus reached by the ten provinces came unglued, leaving Quebec out in the cold – inevitably, all these elements undermine trust and cast doubt on the parties' 'good faith.'

Another factor that impacts on change is the 'joint decision trap.' According to this notion, imported from Europe, there could be high costs associated with a collaboration model that attaches a great value to consensus. This can lead to policies that represent 'the smallest common denominator' (Simeon 2001, 60). In the context of the Canadian federation, this is clearly a danger that can lead to inaction (Lazar 1998, 31). But it should be pointed out that while there have been some obvious failures with intergovernmental cooperation (Meech, Charlottetown), there have also been agreements, like the ITA and the labour market agreement. The most fundamental danger, in my view, lies not so much in the search for consensus as in the signing an agreement that does not unite all the provinces, particularly when the same province is the one being excluded. The resultant political schism is probably more harmful than signing agreements based on the smallest common denominator, since this type of agreement can always be enhanced after the fact. As pointed out by Bakvis and Skogstad (2002, 12), the phenomenon whereby nine provinces reach a consensus among themselves and with Ottawa, isolating Quebec or leaving it to negotiate a separate agreement with Ottawa, has been called '9-1-1 federalism': this is indeed emergency federalism, which cannot serve as a day-to-day model of how the Canadian federation is supposed to work.

One more factor could weaken federal-provincial relations. The recent attempt to judicialize relations between Quebec and Ottawa can only further reduce the chances for accommodation. It is not so much the Supreme Court's Opinion in the Quebec Secession Reference as Bill C-20, the so-called referendum clarity act (and Quebec's reply, Bill 99). The Opinion is fairly moderate, leaving grey areas that the Court did not wish to clarify – precisely to allow for discussion in the political arena (on a clear question, a clear reply, decision-making rules, the focus of the negotiations). The more people try to codify the grey areas, the less room there is for political debate, negotiations, and an eventual agreement. The legal route always points to an impasse or, at least, the perception by one of the parties involved that an impasse has been reached. This, in turn, brings discussions and negotiations to an end.

The Effects on Democracy

In the absence of a true forum for provincial representation in central institutions and as part of a parliamentary system characterized by the concentration of power in the executive branch (Savoie 1999), we have to ask ourselves whether linking intergovernmental relations and democracy does not constitute an oxymoron (Simeon and Cameron 2002, 278–95). Indeed, everything is pointing in this direction.

First, federal-provincial negotiations are conducted in secret, which does not encourage public debate. Yes, the media report on the most important meetings and outline areas of agreement. But the specific agenda for these meetings is rarely divulged. This makes it hard to measure the distance travelled between what was on the agenda and the results achieved as they appear in news releases. Moreover, a lot of meetings, especially administrative ones, take place out of the public gaze. The intent of these closed-door meetings, I was told during interviews, is to avoid creating overly high expectations among the general population and interest groups, expectations which would not be met in the short term. Sometimes, a number of meetings must be held before a consensus can emerge on a particular subject. In other words, intergovernmental relations do not really lend themselves to direct democracy, the fear usually being that citizen involvement and the majority rule prevailing in this form of democracy might worsen conflicts between majority and minority, between those on the 'inside' and those on the 'outside,' between Quebec and the rest of Canada.

The representative democracy characterizing Canada is founded on the idea that the people's representatives, and more specifically their governments, must be accountable for their decisions and their management. This democracy must therefore be based on two main operating principles: transparency and accountability. *Transparency* implies that the public will be informed of the subject of intergovernmental meetings, at least those held at the political level, and of the results obtained. *Accountability* implies that the public will be informed of the responsibility link of each order of government and that the decisions arrived at, if not the negotiations, will be submitted to public discussion.

The democratic deficit alluded to in Europe's case could be applied to Canada's intergovernmental relations. In both cases, negotiations are conducted behind closed doors and dominated by the executive branch, comprising members of the government and senior officials, including those of central agencies. It would likely be counter-productive to conduct negotiations in the public eye. Governments, as I was told during interviews, want to be able to discuss the most difficult issues and most controversial subjects in complete confidence among themselves. They fear that being too open to the public will lead to paralysis rather than consensus. That is why they prefer publicly discussing these topics only when the time is right. In the event that negotiations drag on, progress reports could be issued.

Above all, it is important to establish a *clear* responsibility link. It is difficult to maintain accountability when responsibilities are shared and governments spend funds that they are not responsible for raising (Simeon 2001, 60). To reiterate what was said at the outset, interdependence and cooperation among governments do not imply that each party's roles and responsibilities are intermingled or muddled. On the contrary, cooperation must be based instead on a clear division of responsibilities. This is required in order to avoid having governments constantly finding themselves on the defensive and pitted as adversaries. A clear distribution of responsibilities will ensure that the parties interact in a complementary fashion.

The use of the spending power by federal authorities serves only to further muddle the responsibility link of each order of government. A transfer of tax points or of any other adequate source of funding, coupled with greater respect for each government's jurisdictional areas and a clarification of its roles, can only result in increased transparency about its responsibilities and, hence, improved accountability to the electorate.

This necessary clarification of roles should therefore lead to increased accountability. As John Richards (1998) points out, a single order of government should generally be responsible for a particular field of social policy, and it should raise the necessary revenues through its own taxation sources. This would allow its constituents, better informed about their government's responsibility for social programs, to punish or reward it at the polls (72, 82–92). In the meantime, the responsible governments would have to be accountable to elected bodies and parliamentary commissions, even if it means finding a better way (e.g., the *interpellation* procedure that opposition MNAs can use in Quebec) to involve legislators in the debates on intergovernmental issues.

More and more, the Canada of today is characterized by less deference towards the elites and calls for greater citizen participation, as is also the case in other democracies (Nevitte 1996). In addition to responsible democracy, there is deliberative democracy. Citizens and groups must be given the opportunity to deliberate further, to become involved in the discussions surrounding intergovernmental relations and in parliamentary commissions. They must also be informed about the items on the agenda, the subjects under discussion, the distribution of responsibilities, and the results obtained. More specifically, the administrative committees and working groups should find appropriate means of incorporating into their work the results of consultations with concerned groups and outline this in their reports to their political masters.

Susan Philips (2001) uses the term 'instrumental federalism' to describe the new approach that seems to emerge in intergovernmental relations. For her, this type of federalism has three main elements: it puts the emphasis first on problem-solving, then on engaging citizens in the policy process, and last on using outcome-based measurement and public reporting to ensure greater accountability of governments. Citizen involvement in the political process is, in fact, provided for under SUFA, as is greater government transparency and accountability.

However, examining SUFA's record on this over the first three years, Philips concludes that it has been 'miserable,' seeing as how the provinces have no incentive to tie their own citizen engagement activities to SUFA (they interact with citizens and have developed partnerships with organizations that deliver services and the citizens who use them). Rather, it is the federal government which has an interest in encouraging citizen engagement in view of the need to strengthen its ties with the population, without going through the provinces.

She also describes the difficulty of involving volunteer groups or associations, to wit: there is no true peak representing an entire sector, and there is poor vertical integration of local, provincial, and national associations (Philips 2001, 14). Consequently, volunteer associations have often had a hand in their own exclusion from the political process.

In a nutshell, the intergovernmental relations process should constitute a trilateral (rather than a bilateral) relationship, involving dialogue among Ottawa, the provincial governments, and the public (Cameron 1994, 443). This in no way means that all the discussions must take place in public.

And What of Interprovincialism?

Several provinces are amenable to cooperating among themselves on a number of subjects. They normally do so on an equal footing, either to develop increased cooperation or to resolve thorny issues. For example, Quebec and Ontario premiers signed the Agreement on Public Procurement and Construction Labour Mobility in December 1993 and the Opening of Public Procurement for Quebec and Ontario in May 1996. This goes to show that the ITA did not resolve all of the problems that could arise between the two provinces.

Quebec also signed agreements with Manitoba, Saskatchewan, and Ontario in the field of education, as well as agreements calling for cooperation and exchanges in education and culture with Ontario, New Brunswick, and Prince Edward Island. Some of these agreements come with an additional protocol touching on other sectors, like tourism, health and social services, the environment, and science. In short, the provinces have reason to cooperate in several areas and, if need be, formalize this cooperation by signing memoranda of understanding.

This interprovincial cooperation also takes the form of numerous meetings bringing together all the provinces or the provinces and the territories represented by the sectoral ministers and deputy ministers. The annual conference of provincial (and now territorial) premiers is probably the best known and most widely covered by the media. Honoré Mercier, former premier of Quebec, convened the very first interprovincial conference in 1887 (Veilleux 1971, 31). There were many items on the agenda: adjustments in the subsidies granted to the provinces, limitation of the right of disallowance, status of lieutenant-governors, Senate reform, and so on.

This formula then fell out of favour, only to be reintroduced by Jean Lesage, also a former premier of Quebec. The first annual conference of provincial premiers, in its current form, was held in Quebec City in December 1960. Since then, it has taken place every year in a different province, according to the premier whose turn it is to chair the meeting. During the first conference, the premiers agreed that any decisions taken over the course of their deliberations would not be binding, and that their talks would provide an opportunity to exchange viewpoints, would be informal and would be held behind closed doors (SAIC 1960).

One of the main differences between interprovincialism and federal-provincial relations lies in the fact that the former arouses less mistrust in the beginning. Agreements are concluded between partners who see themselves more as collaborators than as opponents and who willingly agree to work together in a horizontal relationship free of any form of subordination. This does not mean, however, that there are no rivalries between provinces, based on economic wealth, demographic weight, or policy approaches. But a fundamental concept has governed inter-provincial relations, especially since the 1980s: the *equality* of the provinces (Cairns 1991).

Federal-provincial relations arouse more mistrust, especially on the part of certain provinces such as Quebec (and this has not been confined strictly to PQ-led governments), Alberta, and Ontario. Yes, federal-provincial agreements are concluded among partners, but partners who often see one another as rivals and who therefore perceive their relationship to be as much an adversarial as a complementary one. The feeling that seems to colour the discussions is not one of equality among the parties, but of *vertical* links, ultimately translating into a form of subordination to which several provinces are resistant. This does not mean that everything must be analysed from this angle, but simply that it is harder to conclude agreements between the provinces and Ottawa when, on the one hand, a vertical dimension imposes itself on the discussions and, on the other, the stakes are high and a lot of money is involved.

As for interprovincial relations, while the stakes can be high, as in the case of conflicts between Quebec and Ontario on labour mobility in the construction industry, disputes can be eased if the parties grant each other mutual concessions on an equal basis. Also, provinces can live side by side, and even as squabbling brothers or sisters, but it is harder to accept living under the everwatchful and reproachful eye of an older sibling. Whether this accurately reflects the reality of the situation matters little, in that the perception of this reality counts as much as reality itself.

Conclusion

In a society, legitimacy is based on the belief that existing political institutions are the most appropriate for that society, and that they fulfil the role expected of them. Seen in this light, the Canadian Senate has lost all legitimacy in terms of its representative role for federated entities. At this point, the provinces feel that any reform of the Senate has no chance of going through, as is the case with any constitutional reform. Accordingly, provincial governments prefer to represent themselves and have their voices heard directly at federal-provincial conferences rather than through the Senate, even a renewed Senate.

The same is true of the party system. The current fragmentation of Canada's party system reflects a deep dissatisfaction with traditional parties. But this dissatisfaction can be mitigated by the extent of the support enjoyed by the governing party. If it has Canada-wide support, there is less conflict; if it fails to win this support, however, the situation is exacerbated as regions are excluded from power and must turn to their provincial governments to defend their interests (Simeon 2001, 59–60).

These situations happen repeatedly in Canada, which points to the shortcomings, if not the failure, of the institutions in place as tools of intergovernmental cooperation. Consequently, solutions must be sought elsewhere.

In May 1964, Quebec Premier Jean Lesage outlined his vision of cooperative federalism in Moncton. In his view, it had to respect the provinces' autonomy and responsibilities:

> Cooperative federalism is not just about obtaining the provinces' support for centralizing policies. As far as Quebec is concerned, it marks instead the dawn of a new era in federal-provincial relations and the dynamic adaptation of Canadian federalism. Federalism should manifest itself in three ways: 1) regular cooperation when decisions are made about new policies; 2) ongoing consultation in implementing various policies; and 3) handing over to the provinces the financial resources they need to fulfil their increased responsibilities. (SAIC 2001, 29, my translation)

Nearly forty years later, these remarks still apply. Regular cooperation, ongoing consultation, and the necessary financial resources remain on the provinces' political agenda. What Premier Lesage was contemplating, therefore, was truly cooperative and collaborative federalism.

Every time Ottawa acts on its own by making direct payments to individuals or organizations in areas of provincial jurisdiction, as in the case of the Millennium Scholarships, several provinces, including Quebec, denounce the unilateral action by the federal government, insisting that it should either refrain from intervening in this sector or do so in consultation and cooperation with the provinces. And every time Ottawa forces the provinces to act in a given sector by using its spending power, many provinces call on the federal government to respect their jurisdiction and adhere to the spirit of collaborative federalism.

Collaborative federalism implies that the federal, provincial, and territorial governments act collectively. Seen in this light, 'national' policies that will result from this collective action can easily be conceived from the standpoint of diversity as opposed to uniformity. While it is possible to define a set of common, general objectives, the paths taken to meet these objectives can diverge considerably. Ultimately, one could say that collaboration appears less necessary when there is uniformity and more necessary when there is diversity. Moreover, since the provinces agree with the five broad principles underlying the Canada Health Act, one could envisage provincial laws that would include these principles without the need for a federal statute. Such a 'revolution' would clearly indicate that the provinces have primary responsibility for dispensing health care.

Today's collaborative federalism stresses *equality* between Ottawa and the provinces (Simeon 2001, 56). This is crucial for cooperation to exist. True collaboration means that the players involved act as genuine partners on a level playing field. If there are occasions when the parties see themselves as adversaries, this simply means that one party must convince the other, and that both have to talk some more to reach a consensus. In either case, collaboration cannot succeed within a framework of hierarchical or subordinating federalism. Subordination implies a form of submission. If, in spite of everything, there is collaboration, it is forced collaboration. A truly collaborative federalism can only succeed when there is equality between partners.

This notion dominates interprovincial or provincial-territorial relations. It is reflected, for example, in annual conferences of provincial premiers chaired by one of them on a rotating basis – an indication that they are on an equal footing. We need to achieve the same at federal-provincial conferences: nothing stands in the way of these being convened and chaired by a premier (or sectoral minister, as the case may be). This 'mini-revolution' would much better reflect the very spirit of collaborative federalism, namely, equality in diversity.

In short, more than putting the interstate mechanisms in place, which may be adequate, it is the *mindset* that must be changed. We need to work on people's attitudes and on the individuals in place, which is a much harder task than inventing new mechanisms.

NOTE

1 Five interviews (with seven people) were conducted in Ottawa and Quebec with federal and provincial officials between March and April 2002. All interview subjects spoke on the condition of anonymity.

REFERENCES

Bakvis, Herman. 1991. *Regional Ministers: Power and Influence in the Canadian Cabinet*. Toronto: University of Toronto Press.
Bakvis, Herman, and Grace Skogstad. 2002. 'Canadian Federalism: Performance, Effectiveness, and Legitimacy.' In *Canadian Federalism: Performance, Effectiveness, and Legitimacy*, ed. Herman Bakvis and Grace Skogstad, 3–23. Don Mills, ON: Oxford University Press.
Bégin, Monique. 2002. *Revisiting the Canada Health Act (1984): What Are the*

Impediments to Change? Montreal: Institute for Research on Public Policy, 30th Anniversary Conference (Ottawa), 20 February.

Binette, André. 2000. 'Principes.' In *L'union sociale canadienne sans le Québec: Huit études sur l'entente-cadre*, ed. Alain-G. Gagnon, 49–89. Montreal: Éditions Saint-Martin.

Burelle, André. 1995. *Le mal canadien. Essai de diagnostic et esquisse d'une thérapie.* Montreal: Fides.

Cairns, Alan C. 1992. *Charter versus Federalism: The Dilemmas of Constitutional Reform.* Montreal: McGill-Queen's University Press.

– 1991. *Disruptions: Constitutional Struggles from the Charter to Meech Lake*, ed. Douglas E. Williams. Toronto: McClelland and Stewart.

– 1977. 'The Governments and Societies of Canadian Federalism.' *Canadian Journal of Political Science* 10(4): 695–725.

Cameron, David R. 1994. 'Half-Eaten Carrot, Bent Stick: Decentralization in an Era of Fiscal Restraint.' *Canadian Public Administration* 37(3): 431–44.

Canadian Intergovernmental Conference Secretariat. 2001. *CICS.* 'Conference Information 2001.' http://www.scics.gc.ca. (6 April 2002).

– 2000. *CICS.* 'Conference Information 2000.' http://www.scics.gc.ca. (6 April 2002).

Carty, R. Kenneth, William Cross, and Lisa Young. 2000. *Rebuilding Canadian Party Politics.* Vancouver: UBC Press.

Centre for Research and Information on Canada (CRIC). 2002. *Portraits of Canada 2001.* Ottawa: CRIC Papers.

Clarke, Harold D. et al. 1991. *Absent Mandate: Interpreting Change in Canadian Elections.* 2d ed. Toronto: Gage.

Commission sur le déséquilibre fiscal. 2002. *Rapport. Pour un nouveau partage des moyens financiers au Canada.* Quebec City: Government of Quebec.

Covell, Maureen. 1991. 'Parties as Institutions of National Governance.' In *Representation, Integration, and Political Parties in Canada*, ed. Herman Bakvis, 63–127. Toronto: Dundurn Press.

Doern, G. Bruce, and Mark MacDonald. 1999. *Free-Trade Federalism: Negotiating the Canadian Agreement on Internal Trade.* Toronto: University of Toronto Press.

Dufour, Christian. 2002. *Restoring the Federal Principle: The Place of Quebec in the Canadian Social Union.* Montreal: Institute for Research on Public Policy.

Dupré, J. Stefan. 1985. 'Reflections on the Workability of Executive Federalism.' In *Intergovernmental Relations*, ed. Richard Simeon, 1–32. Ottawa: Minister of Supply and Services Canada.

Elazar, Daniel J. 1987. *Exploring Federalism.* Tuscaloosa: University of Alabama Press.

Elkins, David J. 1991. 'Parties as National Institutions. A Comparative Study.'

In *Political Parties in Canada. Representation, Integration and Political Parties in Canada*, ed. Herman Bakvis, 3–62. Toronto: Dundurn Press.

Gagnon, Alain-G. 2000. 'Introduction: L'opposition du Québec à l'union sociale canadienne.' In *L'union sociale canadienne sans le Québec: Huit études sur l'entente-cadre*, ed. Alain-G. Gagnon, 11–17. Montreal: Éditions Saint-Martin.

Gagnon, Alain-G., and Can Erk. 2002. 'Legitimacy, Effectiveness, and Federalism: On the Benefits of Ambiguity.' In *Canadian Federalism: Performance, Effectiveness, and Legitimacy*, ed. Herman Bakvis and Grace Skogstad, 317–30. Don Mills, ON: Oxford University Press.

Gibbins, Roger. 2001. *Shifting Sands: Exploring the Political Foundations of SUFA.* Montreal: Institute for Research on Public Policy, Policy Matters Series.

Internal Trade Secretariat. 2002a. 'The Agreement on Internal Trade. Original Text of the Agreement on International Trade. Chapter Three, Article 300. *The Agreement on Internal Trade.* http://www.intrasec.mb.ca/en (22 March 2002).

– 2002b. 'Implementation of the Agreement. Progress to Date.' *The Agreement on Internal Trade.* http://www.intrasec.mb.ca/eng (6 April 2002).

– 2001. *Strengthening Canada: Challenges for Internal Trade and Mobility.* Winnipeg: Proceedings of the National Conference on Internal Trade (Toronto).

King, Preston. 1982. *Federalism and Federation.* Baltimore: Johns Hopkins University Press.

Knopff, Rainer, and F.L. Morton. 1992. *Charter Politics.* Scarborough, ON: Nelson Canada.

Lazar, Harvey. 2000a. 'In Search of a New Mission Statement for Canadian Fiscal Federalism.' In *Canada: The State of the Federation 1999/2000. Toward a New Mission Statement for Canadian Fiscal Federalism*, ed. Harvey Lazar, 3–39. Montreal: McGill-Queen's University Press.

– 2000b. 'The Social Union Framework Agreement and the Future of Fiscal Federalism.' In *Canada: The State of the Federation 1999/2000. Toward a New Mission Statement for Canadian Fiscal Federalism*, ed. Harvey Lazar, 99–128. Montreal: McGill-Queen's University Press.

– 1998. 'Non-Constitutional Renewal: Toward a New Equilibrium in the Federation. In *Canada: The State of the Federation 1997. Non-Constitutional Renewal*, ed. Harvey Lazar, 3–35. Kingston, ON: Institute of Intergovernmental Relations.

MacDonald, Mark R. 2002. 'The Agreement on Internal Trade: Trade-Offs for Economic Union and Federalism.' In *Canadian Federalism: Performance, Effectiveness, and Legitimacy*, ed. Herman Bakvis and Grace Skogstad, 135–58. Don Mills, ON: Oxford University Press.

Mandel, Michael. 1989. *The Charter of Rights and the Legalization of Politics in Canada.* Toronto: Wall and Thompson.

McRoberts, Kenneth. 1997. *Misconceiving Canada: The Struggle for National Unity.* Toronto: Oxford University Press.

– 1985. 'Unilateralism, Bilateralism and Multilateralism: Approaches to Canadian Federalism.' In *Intergovernmental Relations*, ed. Richard Simeon, 71–129. Ottawa: Minister of Supply and Services Canada.

Monahan, Patrick. 1987. *Politics and the Constitution: The Charter, Federalism and the Supreme Court of Canada.* Agincourt, ON: Carswell.

Nevitte, Neil. 1996. *The Decline of Deference.* Peterborough, ON: Broadview Press.

Noël, Alain. 2001. *Power and Purpose in Intergovernmental Relations.* Montreal: Institute for Research on Public Policy.

– 2000a. 'Étude générale sur l'entente.' In *L'union sociale canadienne sans le Québec: Huit études sur l'entente-cadre*, ed. Alain-G. Gagnon, 19–48. Montreal: Éditions Saint-Martin.

– 2000b. *Without Quebec: Collaborative Federalism with a Footnote?* Montreal: Institute for Research on Public Policy.

Osberg, Lars. 2000. 'Poverty Trends and the Canadian "Social Union."' In *Canada: The State of the Federation 1999/2000. Toward a New Mission Statement for Canadian Fiscal Federalism*, ed. Harvey Lazar, 213–31. Montreal: McGill-Queen's University Press.

Pelletier, Réjean. 2000. 'Constitution et fédéralisme.' In *Le parlementarisme canadien*, ed. Manon Tremblay, Réjean Pelletier, and Marcel R. Pelletier, 47–87. Ste-Foy: Presses de l'Université Laval.

– 1999. 'Responsible Government: Victory or Defeat for Parliament?' In *Taking Stock of 150 Years of Responsible Government in Canada*, ed. Louis Massicotte and F. Leslie Seidle, 53–72. Ottawa: Canadian Study of Parliament Group.

– 1998. 'From Jacques Parizeau to Lucien Bouchard: A New Vision? Yes, But ...' In *Canada: The State of the Federation 1997. Non-Constitutional Renewal*, ed. Harvey Lazar, 295–310. Kingston, ON: Institute of Intergovernmental Relations, Queen's University.

Philips, Susan D. 2001. *SUFA and Citizen Engagement: Fake or Genuine Masterpiece?* Montreal: Institute for Research on Public Policy.

Quebec. Secrétariat aux affaires intergouvernementales canadiennes (SAIC). 2001. *Positions du Québec dans les domaines constitutionnel et intergouvernemental de 1936 à mars 2001.* Quebec City: Government of Quebec.

– 1960. 'Historique des Conférences annuelles des premiers ministres des provinces tenues au Québec – 1960' (Historic Annual Premiers' Conferences – 1960). http://www.mce.gouv.qc.ca/e/html/e0422002.html (22 January 2002).

Richards, John. 2002. *The Paradox of the Social Union Framework Agreement.* Toronto: C.D. Howe Institute Backgrounder.

– 1998. 'Reducing the Muddle in the Middle: Three Propositions for Running the Welfare State.' In *Canada: The State of the Federation 1997. Non-Constitutional Renewal*, ed. Harvey Lazar, 71–104. Kingston, ON: Institute of Intergovernmental Relations, Queen's University.

Robson, William B.P., and Daniel Schwanen. 1999. *The Social Union Agreement: Too Flawed to Last*. Toronto: C.D. Howe Institute Backgrounder.

Royal Commission on the Economic Union and Development Prospects for Canada. 1985. *Report*. Vol. 3. Ottawa: Minister of Supply and Services Canada.

Savoie, Donald J. 1999. *Governing from the Centre: The Concentration of Power in Canadian Politics*. Toronto: University of Toronto Press.

Schwartz, Bryan. 1995. 'Assessing the Agreement on Internal Trade: The Case for a "More Perfect Union."' In *Canada: The State of the Federation 1995*, ed. Douglas M. Brown and Jonathan W. Rose, 189–217. Kingston, ON: Institute of Intergovernmental Relations, Queen's University.

Simeon, Richard. 2001. 'Recent Trends in Federalism and Intergovernmental Relations in Canada: Lessons for the UK?' In *The Dynamics of Decentralization. Canadian Federalism and British Devolution*, ed. Trevor C. Salmon and Michael Keating, 47–61. Montreal: McGill-Queen's University Press.

Simeon, Richard, and David Cameron. 2002. 'Intergovernmental Relations and Democracy: An Oxymoron If There Ever Was One?' In *Canadian Federalism: Performance, Effectiveness, and Legitimacy*, ed. Herman Bakvis and Grace Skogstad, 278–95. Don Mills, ON: Oxford University Press.

Smiley, Donald V. 1980. *Canada in Question: Federalism in the Eighties*. 3rd ed. Toronto: McGraw-Hill Ryerson.

Smiley, Donald V., and Ronald L. Watts. 1986. *Intrastate Federalism in Canada*. Ottawa: Minister of Supply and Services Canada.

Supreme Court of Canada. 1998. *Quebec Secession Reference*. 2 S.C.R. 217.

Tremblay, Guy. 2000. 'Le pouvoir judiciaire.' In *Le parlementarisme canadien*, ed. Manon Tremblay, Réjean Pelletier, and Marcel R. Pelletier, 339–61. Ste-Foy: Presses de l'Université Laval.

Vaillancourt, Yves. 2002. *Le modèle québécois de politiques sociales et ses interfaces avec l'union sociale canadienne*. Montreal: Institute for Research on Public Policy.

Veilleux, Gérard. 1971. *Les relations intergouvernementales au Canada 1867–1967. Les mécanismes de coopération*. Montreal: Presses de l'Université du Québec.

Watts, Ronald L. 1999. *Comparing Federal Systems*. 2nd ed. Montreal: McGill-Queen's University Press.

Wheare, K.C. 1963. *Federal Government*. 4th ed. London: Oxford University Press.

5 Roles and Responsibilities in Health Care Policy

ANTONIA MAIONI

Health Care and the Division of Powers[1]

The division of powers enumerated in the Constitution Acts of 1867 and of 1982 set the parameters of the federal arrangement in Canada. These documents reveal a tension between a centralizing tendency implied in the economic and residual powers allocated to the federal government, and the decentralizing effect of the wide-ranging responsibilities accorded to the provinces. This tension has been exacerbated since 1867 for a variety of reasons, including judicial interpretations favouring the provinces and the passage of the 1982 Canadian Charter of Rights and Freedoms. Nevertheless, periods of intergovernmental cooperation did lead to important policy initiatives, including the programs that form the core of the welfare state in Canada.

Health care is a prime example of this dynamic. There are few specific references to health care in the Constitution Act, 1867, but, since then, conflict between levels of government over health matters has intensified with the growth of provincial power in areas of jurisdiction that became much more important than envisioned in the Constitution. (However, this does not mean, as some have suggested that, had the Constitution been written in 1982, the federal government would have had power over health care; the emphasis on subsidiarity in the European Union, for example, shows this.) Indeed, in 1867, health concerns were considered private rather than public matters, within the bounds of family responsibility and charitable institutions or religious communities, and government intervention was primarily limited to matters of public health (Guest 1997). Nevertheless, as the responsibilities of the modern State expanded over time, the enumeration of provincial responsibilities yielded a wider interpretation in the health sector (Stevenson 1985). Section 92(7) of the Constitution Act allows provincial legislatures to enact laws for the 'Establishment, Maintenance, and Management of Hospitals, Asylums, Charities and Eleemosynary Institutions,' through section 92(13), 'Property and Civil Rights in the Province,' and through section 92(16), 'Generally all Matters of a Merely Local or Private Nature in the Province.'

Despite the fact that, formally speaking, health policy is considered to be primarily within the bounds of provincial jurisdiction, the federal government also occupies an important political space in the health policy arena. Part of this space is related to the federal government's constitutional responsibilities for public health matters under section 91(11) and for the general welfare of specific classes of people (referred to as 'Indians' and 'aliens,' as well as federal inmates and members of the armed forces). In addition, although the federal government cannot legislate directly in provincial health systems, it does have a larger scope of financial resources at its disposal, such as the provisions of section 91(3) for the 'Raising of Money by any Mode or System of Taxation.' Through a series of constitutional amendments, however, jurisdictional space has been created for the federal government in other social policy areas, namely, unemployment insurance (1940) and concurrent jurisdiction for old age pensions (1951 and 1964).

While the federal government's involvement in health care has been primarily confined to the use of the federal spending power, the allocation of money has an obvious impact on provincial health policy (see Tuohy 1989). Two examples of the federal spending power are relevant for health care. The first is the use of transfer payments, whereby federal funds are used to help defray part of the costs of a provincial program. The original shared-cost programs in hospital and medical insurance are examples of this, as are more recent block-funding arrangements, such as the Established Programs Financing (which funded health care and postsecondary education, after 1976), and the Canada Health and Social Transfer (which covers health, education, and social assistance since 1995). Equalization payments, the second element of the federal spending power, are not targeted directly at program funding but instead flow directly into provincial general revenues. The rationale for equalization payments is to assist provinces with less powerful economies in providing similar levels of health care and other services to their populations. In addition to these two forms of subsidies to the provinces, the federal government also spends 'directly' in health care through its responsibility for First Nations, the Inuit, and military personnel in Canada, as well as through its programs in health promotion, protection, and research.

The Definition of Federal and Provincial Roles in Health Care

Ironically, the period in which *roles* were most clearly defined was the period in which the *responsibility* for health care was not exercised. In historical terms, the era in which federal and provincial roles were most clearly defined was at the beginning of the twentieth century, a period of so-called classical federalism (Mallory 1965; Robinson and Simeon 1999). During the first three decades of the century, two forces were responsible for the endurance of 'watertight compartments' between federal and provincial roles: the fact that governments had not taken on a major role in financing health and social services; and the fact that the Judicial Court of the Privy Council in London upheld several provincial complaints against federal intrusion or expansion into provincial jurisdictions. (See the Appendix to this chapter for a full chronological listing of events.)

The absence of appropriate levers for coordinated action became problematic, however, during the Great Depression of the 1930s. The federal government may or may not have had the political will to move forward on social policy, depending on how one interprets the Conservative government's 1935 Employment and Social Insurance Act or the Judicial Committee of the Privy Council's ultra vires ruling against it in 1937 (Smith 1995). What is clear is that provincial governments lacked the fiscal capacity to do so. For example, the British Columbia (Liberal) government passed health insurance legislation in 1936, but it failed to implement it because, without the financial help of the federal government, the province could not afford to do so (Naylor 1986).

A new era of 'cooperative federalism' was heralded by the Royal Commission on Dominion-Federal Relations (the Rowell-Sirois Commission). Reporting in 1940, the Commission suggested the federal government did have a fiscal role to play in social policy, by virtue of its spending power, but reiterated the provinces' primary responsibility in developing their own health care, education, and welfare systems (Smiley 1962). But cooperation in health policy would take considerably more time to develop, and involved substantial political struggles. Although the federal role in health care was actively promoted within the Department of National Pensions throughout the war years, in the 1943 Marsh Report and the 1944 Throne Speech, none of this led to concrete policy development (Maioni 1998). Although the federal government convened the 1945 Dominion-Provincial Conference on Reconstruction as a forum for discussion on concrete proposals for social reform (including health care), some provinces were vocal in their opposition to federal 'interference' (in particular Quebec and Ontario), and Prime Minister Mackenzie King had serious reservations about encroaching on provincial jurisdiction and engaging in fiscally expansive social commitments. Paul Martin (Sr.) did convince him to support the 1948 National Health Grants Program, but in the absence of other federal initiatives, provinces began to exercise their jurisdictional purview to innovate in health care. Two examples show how.

Saskatchewan's CCF government chose to 'go it alone' (Taylor 1987) in legislating the first public hospital insurance plan in North America in 1946; the Conservative government of Ontario, meanwhile, worked on pushing the federal government into sharing the costs of such a program. The demonstration effect of Saskatchewan, in tandem with some of the political pressure applied by Ontario at the 1955 Federal-Provincial Conference, contributed to the St-Laurent government's passage of the Hospital Insurance and Diagnostic Services Act of 1957. In this instance, provincial *push* led to federal *pull* in convening the provinces and in drawing them into an intergovernmental arrangement. This legislation set up an open-ended cost-sharing arrangement, in which the federal government reimbursed about half of the costs of provincial hospital insurance plans that were both *comprehensive* and *universal*. By 1961, all the provinces had hospital insurance plans in place that conformed to this new arrangement. Notably, Quebec was the last province to sign on after the 1960 Lesage victory; prior to this, the Union Nationale government had insisted hospital insurance remain a provincial – and more specifically, a private – matter.

Provincial experiment, intergovernmental negotiation, and federal incentives also provided the diffusion mechanism for public medical insurance. Two forces were at work here as well: first, Saskatchewan's NDP government introduced landmark legislation for public medical insurance in 1961 (although its introduction was delayed by a doctors' strike in 1962); then, the Royal Commission on Health Services (the Hall Commission) recommended in 1964 that the federal government, in effect, encourage this model throughout Canada. At the 1965

Federal-Provincial Conference, Prime Minister Lester Pearson convened the provinces to discuss plans for a new arrangement in which the federal government would share the cost of physician services only (not other health services) under a sliding-scale formula based on a Canada-wide average per capita cost of these services (see Soderstrom 1978, 162–5).

To ensure a measure of uniformity across the country, the Medical Care Insurance Act of 1966 stipulated that provincial programs would have to be *comprehensive, universal, portable,* and *publicly administered*. By 1971, every province had such a plan in operation, although not without having to clear several political hurdles. Provincial leaders in Alberta and Ontario objected to the diffusion of universal public health insurance. The Social Credit government in Alberta, for example, preferred its 'Manningcare' model for voluntary insurance plus public subsidies for the poor; Conservative premier John Robarts in Ontario referred to the federal policy as 'political fraud' (Taylor 1987). Successive Quebec governments attempted unsuccessfully to change the formula to one that allowed opting-out with compensation. Although there was widespread political and popular support for the Castonguay Commission's recommendations for universal insurance, the sticking point for Quebec was the extent to which the federal government could use taxation to fund programs within provincial jurisdiction (Desruisseux and Fortin 1999).

The hospital and medical insurance programs developed across Canada during the cooperative era were a high-water mark of federalism's power to shape effective social reform. This was encouraged by the fact that federal governments were able to convene and engage their provincial counterparts in the process of setting social policy. Fiscal responsibilities were relatively well defined at this point, and care was taken to ensure the perception of provincial autonomy. Provincial governments were beginning to develop their administrative capacities as provincial 'states,' most fuelled by the growing public sector responsibility for health, education and social services.

The emergence of a more activist exercise of social policy by *both* the federal government and the provinces also had to do with specific political ideas that were implicit in the post-war world view: Keynesian ideas about the role of the State in the economy, and the legacy of reconstruction that centred on the transition from warfare state to welfare state across the industrialized world. This was bolstered in Canada by the social-democratic influence of the Left and centre-left, which stressed that health care is a public good, that governments have an obligation to ensure universal coverage and equitable access, and that the federal (central) government belongs in the health policy arena as a guardian of the 'right' to health care. Federalism was the agent through which these ideas were diffused, although the social-democratic impetus was already evident in some cases (the CCF-NDP Saskatchewan) or growing stronger (e.g., the Lesage administration in Quebec); but in other cases (e.g., Alberta), the federal purse was able to trump contending ideas and alternatives. An additional idea was implicit in the federal Liberal government: that social benefits, including health benefits, contributed to regional equity in Canada and reflected a 'common Canadian citizenship' (Banting 1998).

By insisting on these conditions, and on the portability of benefits for all Canadians, the federal government was attempting to avoid the development of a crazy-quilt of health insurance programs. Thus, the goal was not to impose uniformity in the playing field, since provincial plans demonstrate varying degrees of diversity, but rather to ensure that the provinces played by the same 'rules of the game' and that Canadian taxpayers' money would be used to help finance publicly accountable health insurance systems that ensured some sort of 'equality' of social rights among Canadian citizens, regardless of their province of residence.

Fiscal Arrangements in the 1970s

The short history described above points to the federal government's initial role in health policy: that of a catalyst, convener, and negotiator in federal-provincial cooperative efforts in health care. The federal government used its spending power as a fiscal incentive to diffuse the publicly financed health care model throughout Canada, giving ammunition to those governments who supported the idea, and an inducement to those who did not. It did so despite the opposition of powerful interests (including the insurance sector, business, and the medical profession), of several provincial leaders, and from within the cabinet. In other words, the federal government deployed a substantial amount of political will to promote a progressive (social-democratic or centre-left) model of public-hospital and medical insurance.

Why would the federal government engage itself in this way? It is true that the popularity of public insurance was relatively high, but polls in the 1950s and 1960s showed that Canadians were still divided on private versus public insurance. The 'consensus' would come later, in part due to the initial success of the public programs in the provinces. In effect, the federal government considered health insurance as an important social benefit and recognized that not all provinces had the fiscal capacity to sustain such programs. In opting for the public model, the federal government paid attention to the Hall Commission's recommendations and the Saskatchewan experiment, in addition to progressive elements within the federal Parliament itself.

In a period of relative fiscal buoyancy, the political benefits for the federal government were substantial: essentially, it could 'claim credit' for what became an increasingly popular social benefit. However, as fiscal constraints closed in, and as the inflationary potential of an open-ended funding arrangement was recognized, the federal role became more difficult to sustain. It sought therefore to disengage itself from part of this commitment, while at the same time 'avoiding blame,' a political strategy that is often easier in federal systems as compared with non-federal systems (Weaver 1986). Fiscal tensions between the provinces and the federal government over social programs began almost immediately with the recessionary fiscal climate of the early 1970s. After the 1973–6 Social Security Review (an exercise which included provincial consultation), the federal government inaugurated a change in the fiscal transfer formula. In 1977, cost-sharing was replaced with a new per-capita cash and tax-point formula under the Established Programs Financing (EPF) arrangement (for health care and postsecondary education). Ostensibly, this arrangement lessened federal oversight (the end of federal audits for determining costs to be shared) and allowed the provinces greater flexibility in setting spending priorities. However, it also meant that the provinces were now responsible alone for increases in health care spending, and for allocating the EPF transfers between health care and postsecondary education.

The federal government, in closing the open wicket for health care, left considerable flexibility in the hands of the provinces as to how to spend the money, but no effective way of monitoring how they did so nor any visible recognition for its fiscal contribution to health care. The EPF arrangement did not have specific conditions attached to it; the prevailing 'rules' of the hospital and medical insurance legislations were still presumed in effect and applicable to the *cash* portion of the block transfer (Smith 1995). Emmett Hall's 1979–80 Commission of inquiry concluded that provinces were using federal contributions for health care purposes but that, in allowing extra-billing and user fees, there was a risk to the long-term viability of public health insurance

(Hall's Royal Commission report in 1965 had made similar observations) (Taylor 1991).

The Canada Health Act

The Canada Health Act (CHA) of 1984 (RSC 1985, c. C-6) was a response to these concerns and a political effort to regain federal visibility in the health policy arena. It was contested by the provinces for both reasons. Essentially, the new legislation amalgamated the existing federal hospital and medical care insurance acts, introduced a mechanism through which the government could unilaterally impose financial penalties on the provinces, and restated the existing conditions into five principles: universality of coverage, comprehensiveness of services, portability of benefits, public administration, and equal access to care on 'uniform terms and conditions'. This last provision was new and explicitly designed to ban extra-billing and user fees through the imposition of deductions to cash transfers. While the first four of these broad principles existed in previous legislation, the CHA emphasized that the 'primary objective' of federal involvement in health policy was to 'facilitate reasonable access to health services without financial or other barriers.' In addition, for the first time, the federal government requested recognition from the provinces in the health care area: section 13 of the CHA spells this out by requiring that provincial governments 'give recognition' of federal contributions in public documents, advertising, or promotional information.

Even though the legal scope of the CHA is explicitly limited to the cash transfers the federal government is prepared to deploy, the symbolic scope of the CHA goes much farther. The Act increased the federal government's political space in the health policy arena, by designating its role in a 'Canadian' health care system that could be defined as something greater than the sum of its parts. Through the CHA, the federal government institutionalized its presence in health policy. And, as 'policies restructure politics' (Pierson 1993), the CHA shaped the political playing field in health care by setting the boundaries of health reform. The existence of the CHA has led to a situation in which the federal government has become 'embedded' in the public mind as a standard-bearer and protector of Canadians' health care; much like the State is 'embedded' in society through its past policy decisions (Cairns 1986).

This went substantially further than the spirit of the 1957 and 1966 legislation. As in 1966, the federal spending power was deployed as a fiscal incentive to bolster public health insurance. But, unlike the situation in 1966, the process by which this came about was widely criticized. There had been no convening of provincial governments on the matter nor did the Act contain a dispute resolution mechanism that allowed for provincial input. In theory, the mechanism governing this process works in a bilateral fashion, but in practice it resembles more a unilateral process in which decisions are made by the federal government. Each province is required to submit an annual report, including a financial statement that details how its health care plan conforms to CHA principles. Under section 14 of the CHA, if the federal minister of health decides that a provincial health care plan has 'ceased to satisfy any one of the criteria,' he or she is empowered to report to the cabinet and direct the finance department to make deductions from transfer payments. There is a consultation process through which the minister informs the province and allows time for discussion, but the final enforcement decision is his or hers alone. In some cases, provincial governments have conferred with the federal government before implementing certain practices, thus voluntarily modifying them to avoid financial penalties. Regardless of whether there is a dispute or not, however, the federal minister of health is seen to act as 'judge and jury' of the provinces (Ministerial Council on Social Policy Reform and Renewal 1995).

Fiscal Arrangements and the Social Union

The CHA is an example of the federal government's role in *setting* health care policy, but it was enacted at the same time that the federal government was *disengaging* itself further from fiscal responsibility. In other words, the federal government attempted to 're-establish federal power' while at the same time displace fiscal responsibilities to the provinces (Hawkes and Pollard 1984). From 1984 onward, the federal government's fiscal commitment to provincial social programs continually declined, from the limits on EPF payments to the transformation, in 1996, of federal contributions into the Canada Health and Social Transfer. Even in the context of the fiscal crisis that gripped the country, this was a singularly bold attempt to effect social reform. As in the mid-1970s, this decision came in the wake of an economic recession and after an inconclusive review of social security programs; unlike that precedent, however, there had been little provincial input or forewarning of the 1995 budget speech. This was seen as a unilateral action without the engagement of the provinces and widely decried by provincial governments attempting to address their own fiscal shortfalls in the 1990s.

Was the federal government setting health policy through the CHST? It may have been sending a signal to the provinces to get their fiscal houses in order and rein in health care costs, but for many provinces, the 'shock' of adjustment proved to be destabilizing for their health care systems. Overall, from the mid-1980s to the mid-1990s, the lack of fiscal transparency allowed the federal government to claim credit as the 'guardian' of a popular social policy (the famously cited 'sacred trust,' in Prime Minister Mulroney's words) while at the same time avoid blame for the types of costs associated with readjustment in health care payments and delivery in the provinces.

Technically speaking, the federal government could deploy its spending power as it saw fit. But the crux of the matter, for many, was this: could the federal government continue to reap the benefits of its role in health care while reducing its responsibility to pay for the costs associated with maintaining a public health care system in the provinces? In other words, was it legitimate for the federal government to 'set' policy (by providing the start-up through cost-sharing) and then assume the provinces would develop the capacity to pay for these very expensive programs? For others the question was the extent to which budget decisions actually threatened the federal government's ability to set policy by undermining its enforcement capacity for existing standards in the Canada Health Act (Banting 1995).

While intergovernmental conflict has been the norm in areas involving the distribution – and redistribution – of money, provincial government resentment grew throughout the 1990s. The perception of federal intransigence and the unilateral changes imposed through the CHST, the ideological disposition of activist Conservative governments in Ontario and Alberta, the legacy of 'megaconstitutional' politics which had empowered provincial premiers as political leaders, and the 'unity crisis' engendered by the Quebec referendum on sovereignty all seemed to build momentum towards change in intergovernmental affairs and, in a sense, legitimized the quest for provincial autonomy. During this period, federal and provincial governments seemed to be moving along parallel tracks on issues of health reform, rather than engaging in the cooperative model of the past. Much of the tension was related to the proprietary role the federal government staked in the moral 'high ground' of public debate, while provinces were increasingly beleaguered by the problems 'on the ground' in the health care sector.

The refusal of most provinces to participate in the National Forum on Health was evidence that considerable tension existed between levels of government in health policy. The NFH itself reported that although the federal government must ensure the integrity of the Canadian health system, there should be more institutionalized cooperation between governments, as well as an end to federal imposition of change on the provinces (National Forum on Health 1997). It was, in part, the provincial governments' perception of unilateral gamesmanship in social policy by the federal government that spurred provincial leaders (including Quebec) to discuss forging a new interprovincial 'social union'. The 1995 Ministerial Council's Report to Premiers reflected concerns about the federal government's unilateral actions, and recommended federal-provincial discussions to define the Canada Health Act, federal-provincial consultations to interpret the CHA and resolve disputes over its meaning, and a predictable funding base for health services through a guarantee that cuts in transfers to the provinces would not exceed federal expenditure cuts.

At the 1996 premiers' conference, a Provincial/Territorial Council on Social Policy Renewal was set up specifically to address the ways in which provinces could be more engaged in standard-setting and put an end to 'federal unilateralism.' The Council's 1997 report stressed the need for provincial input to identify and enforce 'shared' principles, establish procedural ground rules for intergovernmental cooperation, and develop new joint mechanisms for dispute resolution. Provincial and territorial ministers of health (with the exception of Quebec) signed on to a 'Vision' document in January 1997, observing that an effective partnership between the federal and provincial governments would entail 'adequate, predictable, and stable cash transfers' and new, formal mechanisms to ensure more transparency and less ambiguity in dispute resolution. At their August 1998 Saskatoon conference, it seemed the provinces (again including Quebec) had come to a historic entente about how to adapt intergovernmental processes to reflect provincial interests and needs (see chronology in Stilborn and Asselin 2001).

Throughout this remarkable process, the provinces were raising the notion that there could be a basis for cooperation without the presence of the federal government acting as a 'hegemon' (a concept borrowed

from international relations theory) – an idea that has particular resonance in terms of the CHA (Maioni 1999). The federal government
eventually entered into this process with the signature (minus Quebec)
of the Social Union Framework Agreement in February 1999. Although
broad in scope, the provisions of SUFA were relevant to health policy
and largely targeted defusing some of the intergovernmental tensions
in the health sector. The agreement acknowledged the need for more
transparency and consultation in intergovernmental policy-making,
including dispute resolutions.

The 1999 federal budget, unveiled one week later, demonstrated a
commitment to providing stable funding for health care in the provinces and introduced measures to eliminate interprovincial disparities.
But the SUFA did not fully reflect the interprovincial processes that led
to its development. The 1998 entente, with its provisions for opting out
of federal social spending programs, was not incorporated into the
SUFA – a decision that cost the process both Quebec's support and any
resolution of where the jurisdictional boundaries in health care lie
(Noël 2000). Obviously, the SUFA did not resolve matters, as in August
1999, the provincial premiers' conference focused on the sustainability
of health care funding, echoed the following year by their concerns
over the 'vertical fiscal imbalance' between the provinces and a federal
government with a budgetary surplus. The increased funding in the
1999 federal budget and the September 2000 health care funding agreement increased transfers to the provinces through the CHST, but still
left provincial leaders concerned about their fiscal capacity to meet
increasing responsibilities for managing health care costs.

Roles of Governments

Arguably, in comparative terms, Canada's health care system is among
the most decentralized of any industrialized country, or at least any
federal polity (Banting and Corbett 2002). In most other industrialized
countries, both federal and unitary, central governments are usually
responsible for a certain measure of fiscal harmonization and for some
kind of oversight to ensure social benefits to their citizens. Yet, by the
same token, in most of these countries, a private-market for health
care, including medically necessary services, exists to varying degrees.
The standards that 'tie' provincial health care systems together are at
once more fragile and more robust than in other industrialized countries: more fragile since they rest on a federal statute designed to pro-

vide negative incentives; and more robust in the sense that they do not allow for much experimentation with private-market mechanisms. In most federal systems, the standard-setting role of the federal government in health care is better entrenched, both constitutionally and historically.

Nevertheless, it is clear that provinces have the primary responsibility for setting health policy in Canada, both in theory and in practice. The recent release of several reports by provincial commissions of inquiry confirm that provinces have built up the administrative capacity and expertise needed to effectively manage health care systems. While it is true that the federal government is more involved in health care than it was forty years ago – that it has carved out a visible role in health policy – so too have provincial governments built up an active role in this policy area. Provincial governments are responsible for this most costly of program areas, and are faced with day-to-day realities on the ground of how to best respond in the short term to pressing problems in the organization and financing of services to their populations. Given the increasing pressures on the health care system – including demographic pressures, cost escalation in the pharmaceutical sector, and new technologies – it is understandable that provincial governments are concerned about their long-term capacity to pay for health care, particularly when balanced against the other pressing needs in social services and education.

Thus, health care policy can, and is, set by provincial governments. Provincial health care systems – and the insurance they provide to residents – are publicly administered by provincial ministries or regulated by their public agencies. Each province's health system is bounded by provincial statutes, not federal legislation. Provinces define what is medically necessary, negotiate fee schedules for payment to health care professionals, and set 'global budgets' for health care institutions. A cursory reading of provincial health statutes shows that, despite some differences in coverage, 100 per cent of the eligible population is covered for all medically necessary procedures – and so far, on equal terms and conditions. And every recent reform, from the closure of hospitals in major cities to Alberta's Bill 11, has been the result of a provincial policy decision for which provincial governments are accountable to their voters.

But this does not mean that the federal government is, or should be, irrelevant in health policy. Health care is a 'big ticket' item in the relationship between state and society, both in terms of the considerable commitment in financial resources and in terms of the direct personal impact on people's lives. The federal government can have an important role to play, *in concert with the provinces*, in engaging in the long-term vision exercise that is necessary to set the markers and determine the resources needed to ensure sustainable health care systems across Canada. In other words, the health system as a whole could benefit from a big picture view of health policy that includes an exchange of input and ideas. The federal government's most positive role in health care is as an *enabler* (rather than as enforcer) in ensuring that all Canadians can look forward to affordable, quality health care across provincial borders. The federal government can also continue to invest in its public health responsibilities through the promotion of population health and the social determinants of health in provincial health reform (see, for example, Glouberman 2001). Many of the recommendations in Quebec's Clair Report, for example, are based on an integrative model of health and social services that is explicitly concerned with health promotion and the continuity of care.

This does not necessarily mean that the federal government can 'guarantee' exactly the same health benefits to every citizen, because its role is not to micromanage the health care system. Indeed, the federal government cannot be the arbiter of individual patient case-loads. Nor does it mean that the federal presence in health care is synonymous with 'one size fits all' solutions in the provinces. But it does mean that the federal government has an important role in articulating and affirming publicly financed health care as an entitlement. To achieve this, the federal government must, in symbolic terms, be prepared to articulate and defend a coherent vision and, in practical terms, be prepared to offer the incentives for its affirmation in provincial health care plans. The symbolic pay-offs are considerable, but in order to reap these rewards, the federal government must be prepared to invest in the product.

Against this backdrop, the call for a health charter by the Canadian Medical Association is both ironic and interesting (*Globe and Mail* 2002). It echoes by almost forty years the 1964 Hall Report recommendation for a 'Health Charter for Canadians' based on government-sponsored, comprehensive, universal health services, which was roundly criticized by organized medicine at the time. But the implicit message that health care must become more centralized – that the federal government must in a sense 're-enforce' its role in health policy – may not be the best scenario to effect health care reform. Much of the rhetoric around the charter idea suggests that the federal government must 'protect' Canadians from their provincial governments – a perilous argument in democratic dialogue, even if only for symbolic effect. The other obvious point is that if practicable, how could such a charter be enforced? The Canada Health Act does not include such a mechanism, nor could a twenty-first-century federal government be expected to apply disallowance in the health policy area. In the European Union, for example, the Charter of Basic Rights includes the right of individuals to access health care under the conditions established by national legislatures, and health policy is jealously guarded by member states both in terms of financing and regulation decisions.

Mechanisms for Cooperation and Existing Fiscal Arrangements

The critical questions surrounding debates about cooperation and conflict in health care are: What is the role of each level of government in health care? What is the responsibility of each with respect to the health of individual Canadians? Conflict, in a democratic polity, is not necessarily a negative thing and conflict in health care, which involves the redistribution of resources and risk, is to be expected (Evans 1990). But conflict that paralyses dialogue and undermines public confidence is ultimately destructive, not only to the federation but to the quality of life of its citizens. It is unconscionable to use a vital issue like health care as a political football in intergovernmental gamesmanship, even more so when one stops to reflect that the football being bounced about represents real people's lives and well-being, not to mention their tax dollars.

Curiously, for a decentralized federation, Canada has few mechanisms for intergovernmental cooperation and conflict resolution in health care policy. Numerous intergovernmental health advisory committees already operate at the ministerial, deputy minister, and administrative levels. In addition, provincial health ministers meet formally twice a year and with their federal counterpart, following meetings of their deputy ministers, as part of the Federal/Provincial/Territorial health conference 'system.' While these exchanges have been important in policies related to targeted programs (such as tobacco control and blood supply issues) and to specific populations (such as women's and children's health), these intergovernmental committees and meetings have not become venues for addressing broad and pressing concerns related to health care financing and restructuring (O'Reilly 2001).

And, in recent years, first ministers' conferences have been dominated by war of words between provinces and the federal government over the cash crunch in health care. The drill, for the past few years, has been to use these instances of 'executive federalism' to publicize claims and apportion blame, intensifying the 'corrosive and long-distance hollering' (Romanow 2002) into up-close shouting matches and threats.

There has been movement, stemming from the recommendations of the SUFA, to consider a third-party mediation panel that would involve more provincial input in order to resolve disputes over interpretations of the Canada Health Act (Mahoney and Laghi 2002). But the ability to enforce the CHA, a federal statute, remains in the hands of the federal government, so the final decisions of the panel would not be binding. Nor does this initiative resolve the fact that Quebec has not signed onto the SUFA. Basically, dispute resolution through the SUFA is really only the tip of the iceberg of federal-provincial conflict in health care.

In effect, the focus of attention on the CHA as a lightning rod in health care debates diverts attention from the real and pressing needs for real reform in the health care sector across all the provinces. Critics describe the CHA as the roadblock to health reform while supporters liken it to the rampart against the deluge of privatization. But the CHA has no such magical powers. It is at the most basic level a set of negative incentives attached to federal fiscal transfers. The impact of these penalties has so far been minimal, meaning that they work more as a disincentive, or that their impact is better gauged through the 'political loop' of public backlash (see Stilborn 1997). Indeed, the principal architect of the Canada Health Act, former minister of Health Monique Bégin, argues that, while the CHA was instrumental in 'rooting' public health insurance in the Canadian 'psyche,' the time has come to consider revising the Act to address the problems of modern health care and the roadblocks in governance and implementation of health reform, and to remedy the 'adversarial and arbitrary' nature of the CHA enforcement process (Bégin 2002).

The political problem is not so much that the CHA exists, but the way it is used to shape the political debate around health care reform. In effect, intergovernmental discussions in health care have become stymied by the relentless spotlight on a statute that regulates fiscal transfer programs, making it difficult if not impossible to coherently address issues of governance and long-term sustainability in health care. Federal politicians have been wont to brandish it as the 'Ten Commandments,' using financial muscle to weigh in on provincial jurisdiction; while some provincial politicians have claimed that it stifles the capacity to address real issues and pursue innovative reform avenues. The focus on the CHA and its 'punishment' effects – both real and imagined – have created dysfunctional (some would say toxic) politics around health care in Canada.

While it can be argued that the emphasis on 'medically necessary' services has tended to siphon resources into acute care rather than global health, the CHA does not prevent provinces from funding home care or covering pharmaceutical costs, for example. Rather, the CHA's disincentives – through the emphasis on public administration and equal access – have for the most part been directed at private market alternatives. The entanglement of conflicts over what level of government is responsible for cost control, and the extent to which provincial health policy choices can be constrained by federal government preferences, has opened the political space for these alternatives to gather political momentum.

One of the solutions envisioned in the perceived democratic deficit in intergovernmental relations (Simeon and Cameron 2002) would be to allow for more 'citizen engagement,' a process by which governments encourage citizen participation in public policy making (Abele et al. 1998). The SUFA itself alludes to the involvement of Canadians in 'developing social priorities' through citizen engagement. Recent musings on engaging citizens in the health care system through 'policing' the Canada Health Act are not exactly in the same spirit. Nor should citizen engagement be a smokescreen to devolve further the responsibility for 'tough choices' that are ultimately the responsibility of publicly accountable policymakers (Lomas 1997). The Romanow Commission's use of consultation research to 'dialogue with citizens' may introduce a new frontier in citizen engagement by asking participants to envision and work through concrete scenarios for change. But for such practices to be truly effective, they will have to be accompanied by similar dialogues between senior government officials: dialogues that are not restricted to targeted issues (such as the Federal/Provincial/Territorial conference system), and dialogues that do not become monologues about money and power.

The Quebec government's Séguin Commission on fiscal imbalance between the federal government surplus and pressing provincial budgetary needs, recommends a more drastic change: abolishing intergovernmental conflict at its source by replacing conditional cash transfers under the Canada Health and Social Transfer by tax room for the provinces. In this scenario, the federal spending power would become a moot issue in health care, allowing the provinces greater fiscal capacity to set their agendas for health policy. The report is a scathing criticism of the federal government's fiscal neglect of the provinces, but its recommendations cut through the roles and responsibilities debate by suggesting provinces should have exclusive leeway in setting health policy. Although less of a concern for the Quebec government, an earlier version of these arguments put forward in the Ontario context also suggested that a social union could be preserved by replacing Ottawa's 'enforcer' role with an interprovincial 'convention' (Courchene 1996). But there is no certainty that provincial governments, with divergent ideological baggage and political priorities based on distinct social and economic conditions, would share the same norms about health care without some form of incentives.

For all the quibbles over resources in health care between the provinces and the federal government, political battles over health care have never been *only* about money. In the past sixty years, recurring lines of demarcation between the federal government and some provinces have included ideological battles about public and universal as opposed to private and voluntary health insurance (historically, the preference of fiscally 'conservative' governments in 'richer' provinces such as Ontario, Alberta, and British Columbia). The contested political space in health policy often has to do with the *type* of health care system one wants to encourage, and, more broadly, over the role of the *state* in health care altogether. Attempts to control public spending in health care and the subsequent escalation of conflict in intergovernmental relations over this issue have opened a window of opportunity for political and social actors that believe in less state intervention to question the legitimacy of federal standards and to justify attempts to explore other options for financing health care.

Provinces have functioned as laboratories of innovation in the past and continue to do so. Today, however, it is neither a relatively less well-off province with a social-democratic government, like Saskatchewan, nor a government pushing the state into modernity, as in Quebec, that is at the forefront of change in health care. It is not insignificant to note that the most innovative solutions being promoted in Canada today are those emanating from 'richer' provinces under more fiscally conservative governments with health reform agendas based on stretching the flexibility of the public model. In other words, the provincial governments that are most vocal about necessary changes to the fiscal order and the federal government's role in it are those that are least tied to its fiscal purse-strings. The exception is Quebec, where the current government has fewer ideological quibbles with the public model (solidarity and equality, not speed and quality, are the leitmotifs of the provincial Clair Commission report) and more constitutional baggage about policy sovereignty in health care. For Quebec, the jurisdictional issue takes precedence: the extent to which provinces can opt out with compensation from federal cost-sharing arrangements, and the extent to which a 'fiscal imbalance' between the provinces and the federal government threatens the provinces' ability to provide optimal health and social services to their residents.

Roles and Responsibilities

Federalism is a political arrangement by which power is constitutionally distributed between governments and in which the social and economic lives of citizens are affected by both these governments (Smiley 1987). In an uncluttered, ideal world one could suggest that federalism is a system of watertight compartments in which each sphere of government attends to its own jurisdiction. But the real world of Canadian politics is a messy place. In fact, there is more clarity around the assignment of *roles* in health care but less consensus on the apportionment of *responsibility*. With whom does accountability rest? Whose task is it to ensure the viability of the health care system?

There exist at least two misleading 'legends' about federalism and health care in Canada. The first is that there exists a 'national health insurance' or 'medicare' system in Canada. Both of these terms are imports from the United States and refer, respectively, to the historic and ongoing U.S. debates about extending universal coverage for health care services through federal legislation, and to the medical insurance for the aged program financed and organized by the federal government. In Canada, obviously, the federal government does not play such a role; there does not exist a 'Canadian health care system'; instead, we have provincially regulated health care systems financed by public revenues, with a federal fiscal contribution tied to certain standards of compatibility between the provinces. In this sense, the 'Canadian' health care model can be thought of as a mosaic of ten provincial and three territorial health insurance plans, resembling one another by certain 'norms'. Norms are standards of behaviour that reflect a certain code of conduct, but in order to be operative, norms have to be imposed in some manner: formally, through a power relationship in which an actor or set of actors can inflict reprisals or informally in ways that are not legally binding but suggest some kind of sanction. It is, at present, difficult to gauge to what extent the principles of the Canada Health Act are norms to which provincial governments, health care providers, and even individual citizens would ascribe to under different conditions than those in place today.

The second 'legend' is that health care is a purely provincial matter in which the federal government has no role to play. Health care has become one of the primary symbols of a modern State's involvement in society, literally 'protecting' citizens' well-being. In essence, involvement in health care represents a way in which the State can help establish the boundaries of social consensus. This, in turn, contributes to the legitimization of the State's role in the economic and social lives of citizens. Thus, arguments against federal 'interference' are based on assumptions about jurisdictional autonomy – which level of government should be responsible (such as those emanating from Quebec) – and on the limits of State involvement in citizens' lives – should governments be responsible in the first place (emanating from conservative and neo-liberal governments).

In the *Federalist Papers*, James Madison suggests that 'aggregate' interests are referred to the central government, while 'particular' interests remain in the purview of subnational or local governments. The real question this dichotomy raises is whether or not health care can be considered in the purview of provincial governments or incorporated into a larger vision of the public interest. If health care is an aggregate interest, then the federal government has a role, but also a responsibility, in ensuring that these services are available to its citizens. The health policy realm places an enormous responsibility on the modern State, one that many governments are finding difficult to sustain. The development of provincial health care systems along public, universal lines, would not have been possible across Canada without federal involvement. By the same token, the basic existing model is not sustainable – politically or fiscally – without federal involvement, both in its fiscal capacity and the use of fiscal levers to encourage the public model. Obviously, the provinces were not expecting the federal government to cover only the 'start-up' costs in this considerable undertaking, but rather expected a sustained commitment to these expensive programs.

If the end-game in health care is to retain its meaning as a public good, then the federal government would be better off putting more emphasis on encouraging consensus rather than enforcing rules. Part of this task involves evaluating alternatives and suggesting the boundaries of what is feasible and desirable in health care reform. Under what conditions can the federal government encourage innovations that are not entirely at odds with the basic premises of the public model? To what extent is more structured exchange of information needed in identifying, evaluating – and possibly diffusing – provincial recommendations from commissions of inquiry, new models of delivery, or experiments such as integrated care in Quebec, or health care systems in Europe and elsewhere? There are relatively large bodies of evidence to suggest that public health care systems do better in providing care and controlling costs, that health care systems focused on preventive and integrated care work better in keeping populations healthy, and so on. In order to retain a relevant role in health policy, the federal government should be willing to evaluate the available evidence in suggesting the markers and signposts and in helping to build the capacity for real health reform. To this end, a measure of 'political goodwill,' for lack of a better term, is necessary in reshaping the federal-provincial dialogue on health care.

Devolution and Accountability

Most provinces have decentralized the allocation of resources in health care through the creation of regional health boards (some elected, others appointed, still others a mix of the two). These initiatives were intended to devolve authority from provincial health ministries to regional or local bodies that would have some measure of discretion in allocating health care resources. This process was generally designed to encourage population-based funding and other allocative efficiencies, such as ensuring the optimal level of resource mix for a particular region (Dorland and Davis 1996). Although almost all provinces have instituted such regionalization through the creation or reorganization of existing local and regional health boards, these experiments have not all been successful in establishing efficiency. Part of the problem is that these boards are not always empowered to make important decisions, such as those related to physician fees and drug use. Questions have been raised as to just what kinds of decisions such boards are equipped to make: in terms of representation and accountability in the case of non-elected members, and in terms of expertise for elected members. In practice, for example, professionals often outweigh community representatives in terms of the influence exerted on the board. In addition, provincial governments also saw these initiatives as a form of 'community empowerment' designed to harness public support for health care reform and 'conflict containment' in the wake of public sector spending cuts and its consequences (Lomas, Woods, and Veenstra 1997). Indeed, most regional boards were created or became operative in the mid-1990s, just as provincial governments were faced with tough cost-cutting measures in the public health care sector.

In theory, such decentralization has the potential to 'democratize' the health care sector if citizens are being engaged in a process of influencing decisions about service delivery, including issues of allocation and rationalization. If important decisions are made affecting the delivery and use of health care for individuals and their families, then citizens ought to be informed and involved in making and supporting these decisions in their communities. But the rationale of the 'democratic wish' behind decentralization – that citizens can engage in public decision-making (Morone 1990) – is potentially problematic for at least three reasons: (1) specifically, because health care delivery and financing are part of a highly complex system that is difficult for non-experts to decipher; (2) more broadly, because effective engagement involves opening up a Pandora's box of new actors in the policy process, which can potentially widen the scope for conflict and make it difficult to achieve consensus; and (3) hypothetically, because attempts at inclusiveness can raise the potential for blame avoidance by governments and the offloading of accountability between governments and citizens.

Decentralization and health care are compatible only insofar as a balance can be struck between decision-making and accountability. Concepts such as citizen engagement and regional boards cannot become smokescreens for authoritative decisions about cost-control and scarce resources. Of broader concern is the risk that with a continual downloading of decision-making and accountability, local concerns may be served at the expense of the larger provincial – or even national – community (Maioni 2001).

Appendix:
Key Events in Health Insurance Legislation in Canada

1919 – Dominion Department of Health established (becomes Department of Pensions and National Health, 1928).

1928 – House of Commons Select Standing Committee on Industrial and International Relations studies 'sickness insurance.'

1932 – British Columbia Royal Commission on the State Health Insurance and Maternity Benefits (recommends compulsory health insurance for low-income workers).

1933 – Alberta holds a second Commission of Inquiry on the issue of establishing a provincial health insurance scheme. Winnipeg Medical Society launches 'doctors' strike' except for emergency care.

1934 – Canadian Medical Association endorses 'the principle of health insurance.'

1935 – Government of British Columbia presents a preliminary bill to the provincial Legislative Assembly calling for the creation of provincial health insurance.

   – Ontario government signs an agreement with the Ontario Medical Association to subsidize the cost of patients on relief; municipal medical relief plans are also implemented in cities in other provinces.

1936 – British Columbia Health Insurance Act passed (never implemented).

1939 – Voluntary medical insurance initiatives (Windsor Medical Services; Associated Medical Services in Toronto); Manitoba Blue Cross established.

1940 – The Report of the Royal Commission on Dominion-Provincial Relations (the Rowell-Sirois Report) recommends cost-sharing by federal government of health insurance to ensure fiscal capacity of provinces and to maintain similar standards throughout Canada.

1942 – Interdepartmental Advisory Committee on Health Insurance developed by Minister Ian Mackenzie and chaired by J.J. Heagerty, presents a draft bill for health insurance (via conditional grants-in-aid to the provinces).

1943 – House of Commons Special Committee on Social Security studies health insurance.

1944 – Prime Minister Mackenzie King delivers the Throne Speech, which calls for health insurance and family allowances as central part of post-war reconstruction.

   – Ontario (Progressive Conservative) Premier George Drew calls for a reconstruction conference with health insurance on the agenda.

- Alberta (Social Credit) adopts the Alberta Maternity Hospital Plan.
1945 – Dominion-Provincial Conference on Post-War Reconstruction discusses 'Green Book' proposals for social programs, including health insurance; some provinces oppose federal intervention in their jurisdiction.
˜1946 – Cooperative Commonwealth Federation (CCF) government led by Tommy Douglas introduces Saskatchewan Hospital Services Plan (implemented in 1947).
1948 – Federal Finance Minister Paul Martin, Sr., develops National Health Grants program (federal financial support to provinces).
  – British Columbia (Liberal Conservative Coalition) government develops hospital coverage.
1949 – Alberta (Social Credit) government begins establishment of hospital insurance via a municipal hospital plan (similar to Saskatchewan, but with patient contributions).
1951 – Canadian Medical Association (CMA) establishes the Trans-Canada Medical Service (TCMS) that included seven insurance plans on a provincial basis (by 1955, all provinces with 2 million beneficiaries).
1955 – Ontario (Progressive Conservative) government establishes Hospital Insurance Plan; at Federal-Provincial Conference, Ontario Premier Leslie Frost calls on Prime Minister Louis St Laurent to develop federal cost-sharing for hospital insurance.
1956 – Canadian Medical Association opposes universal hospital insurance.
1957 – In March, House of Commons (Liberal majority) passes Bill 165 on hospital insurance with a unanimous vote; in June, Prime Minister John Diefenbaker's (Progressive Conservative minority) revokes the majority province rule required to implement Bill 165.
1958 – On 1 July, the Hospital and Diagnostics Services Act of 1957 comes into effect (based on a 50-50 cost-sharing formula).
1960 – Prime Minister Diefenbaker appoints Royal Commission on Health Services, chaired by Emmett Hall.
  – In June, a referendum on medical insurance is held by the CMA as a means to protect the interests of its members, such as the right for physicians to make clinical decisions in patient care, without intervention or interference from a third party (the government).

1961 – All provinces have legislated hospital insurance and have entered into cost-sharing agreements with the federal government.

– Saskatchewan Premier Woodrow Lloyd (CCF) introduces a medical care insurance bill to the provincial legislature.

1962 – 1 July starting date for medical insurance in Saskatchewan leads to province-wide doctors' strike; 22 July, Saskatchewan physicians are ordered back to work by the provincial Superior Court.

1963 – Alberta Premier Ernest Manning (Social Credit) government introduces medical insurance plan (known as 'Manningcare') that offers subsidies for low-income earners to allow them to pay for voluntary coverage.

1964 – The final report of the Hall Commission recommends comprehensive health coverage for all Canadians.

1965 – The Canadian Medical Association expresses concern about these recommendations.

1966 – Ontario Medical Services Insurance Plan introduced to provide insurance to the medically indigent and to low-income earners.

– Health and Welfare Minister Allan MacEachen introduces Bill C277 to the House of Commons; Medical Care Insurance Act passed with a vote tally of 177–2.

1967 – Cost-sharing program for medical insurance comes into effect; Saskatchewan and British Columbia become the first two provinces to join the program.

1969 – Newfoundland, Nova Scotia, Manitoba, Alberta join the program.

1970 – Quebec passes legislation for medical insurance, after strike by specialist physicians; extra-billing is not permitted by law.

1971 – New Brunswick and Northwest Territories join the program.

1972 – Yukon joins the program.

1976 – At Federal-Provincial Conference, Prime Minister Pierre Trudeau proposes tax points and block-grant funding to replace cost-sharing programs for medical care.

1977 – The Established Programs Financing Act (EPF), based on per-capita transfers to the provinces tied to growth in GNP, passed to replace the 1972 Revenue Guarantee Act.

1979 – Progressive Conservative Prime Minister Joe Clark appoints Emmett Hall to chair the Health Services Review Committee; Committee recommends end to extra-billing.

1981 – Extra-billing is banned in British Columbia.

1983 – Health Minister Monique Bégin presents White Paper on 'Preserving Universal Medicare,' focusing on guarantees to access to health care services.

1984 – The Canada Health Act of 1984 becomes law; financial sanctions for provincial non-compliance with the five principles of the Act become effective immediately.

1985 – Saskatchewan doctors agree to end extra-billing.
     – The Ontario Health Care Access Act introduced in the legislature.

1986 – Province-wide physicians' strike launched in Ontario; Ontario Medical Association disputes the constitutionality of Bill 94 (Ontario Health Care Services Act).
     – Canadian Medical Association opposes Canada Health Act, as a violation of the *Constitution Act*, 1982; case is redirected to the Supreme Court of Canada.
     – Alberta bans extra-billing and proposes that the fee schedule be negotiated through binding arbitration.

1987 – Extra-billing end date for New Brunswick.

1989 – EPF transfers are scaled back to GNP increases minus three percentage points.

1990 – EPF transfers are frozen for five years.

1991 – The Health Action Lobby (HEAL) formed as a coalition of health and consumer organizations expressing concern over the erosion of the federal government's role in health care.

1994 – National Forum on Health appointed by Prime Minister Jean Chrétien.

1995 – Canada Health and Social Transfer replaces EPF and Canada Assistance Plan; substantial reduction in transfers to the provinces for social programs.

Mid-1990s – Important reductions in several provincial health budgets; hospital and bed closures; reduction of some services; salary caps for specialist services; regional boards implemented in most provinces.

1997 – Quebec introduces mandatory pharmacare plan.

1999 – Alberta Progressive Conservative government under Ralph Klein introduces Bill 11 (allows for contracting-out with private care facilities for minor elective surgery).
     – Saskatchewan Commission on Medicare (chaired by Ken Fyke) releases its report: *Caring for Medicare: Sustaining a Quality System*.

- Social Union Framework Agreement signed between federal government and provinces (except Quebec).
- Federal budget injects $11.5 billion in health care over five years.
2000 - Federal budget earmarks extra $2.5 billion in cash for provincial health care needs.
- Ontario Health Services Restructuring Commission (chaired by Duncan Sinclair) releases its report: *Looking Back, Looking Forward: A Legacy Report.*
2001 - Quebec Health and Social Services Commission (chaired by Michel Clair), releases its report: *Emerging Solutions – Report and Recommendations.*
- Commission on the Future of Health Care in Canada appointed, chaired by Roy Romanow (former premier of Saskatchewan).
2002 - Alberta Premier's Advisory Council on Health (chaired by Don Mazankowski), releases its report: *A Framework for Reform.*
- Romanow Commission releases its report: *Building on Values.*

NOTES

1 This section is based on Antonia Maioni, 'Federalism and Health Care in Canada,' in Keith G. Banting and Stan Corbett, eds., *Health Policy and Federalism: A Comparative Perspective on Multi-Level Governance* (Kingston: McGill-Queen's University Press, 2002). Some of the subsequent sections in this chapter draw in part from 'Health Care in the New Millennium,' in Herman Bakvis and Grace Skogstad, eds., *Canadian Federalism: Performance, Effectiveness, and Legitimacy* (Toronto: Oxford University Press, 2001).
2 The source for this chronology was the McGill Institute for the Study of Canada. *Public Health Insurance Through History. Virtual Exhibit.* 'Key Events.' http://www.misc-iecm.mcgill.ca/HCC/expo.html (July 2002).

REFERENCES

Abele, Francis, Katherine Graham, Alex Ker, Antonia Maioni, and Susan Phillips. 1998. *Talking with Canadians: Citizen Engagement and the Social Union.* Ottawa: Canadian Council for Social Development.
Banting, Keith G. 1995. 'Who R Us?' In *The 1995 Budget: Retrospect and Prospect,* ed. Thomas Courchene, 173–81. Kingston: Queen's University John Deutsch Institute for the Study of Economic Policy.

- 1998. 'The Past Speaks to the Future: Lessons from the Postwar Social Union.' In *The State of the Federation 1997: Non-Constitutional Renewal* ed. Harvey Lazar, 39–69. Kingston: Institute of Intergovernmental Relations, Queen's University.

Banting, Keith G. and Stan Corbett. 2002. 'Health Policy and Federalism: An Introduction.' In *Health Policy and Federalism: A Comparative Perspective on Multi-Level Governance*, ed. Keith Banting and Stan Corbett, 1–38. Kingston: School of Policy Studies.

Bégin, Monique. 2002. 'Revisiting the *Canada Health Act* (1984): What Are the Impediments to Change?' Ottawa, Institute for Research on Public Policy 30th Anniversary Lecture Series, 20 February 2002.

Cairns, Alan C. 1986. 'The Embedded State: State-Society Relations in Canada.' In *State and Society: Canada in Comparative Perspective*, ed. K. Banting, 53–86. Toronto: University of Toronto Press.

Conference of Provincial/Territorial Ministers of Health. 1997. *A Renewed Vision for Canada's Health System* (January).

Courchene, Thomas J. 1996. 'ACCESS: A Convention on the Canadian Economic and Social Systems.' Working Paper prepared for the Ministry of Intergovernmental Affairs, Government of Ontario, Toronto, August.

Desruisseux, Alain, and Sarah Fortin. 1999. 'The Making of the Welfare State.' In *As I Recall/Si je me souviens bien*, ed. The Institute for Research on Public Policy. Montreal: IRPP.

Dorland, John L., and S. Mathwin Davis. 1996. *Regionalization and Decentralization in Health Care*. Kingston: School of Policy Studies, Queen's University.

Evans, Robert G. 1990. 'Tension, Compression, and Shear: Directions, Stresses, and Outcomes of Health Care Cost Control.' *Journal of Health Politics, Policy and Law* (4): 101–28.

Globe and Mail. 2002. 'Dr. Henry Haddad's Welcome Prescription.' 8 April, A12.

Glouberman, Sholom. 2001. *Towards a New Perspective on Health Policy*. CPRN Study No. H/03. Ottawa: Canadian Policy Research Networks.

Guest, Dennis. 1997. *The Emergence of Social Security in Canada*. 3rd ed. Vancouver: UBC Press.

Hawkes, David C., and Bruce G. Pollard. 1984. 'The Medicare Debate in Canada: The Politics of New Federalism.' *Publius: The Journal of Federalism* 14: 183–98.

Lomas, Jonathan, John Woods, and Gerry Veenstra. 1997. 'Devolving Authority for Health Care in Canada's Provinces: An Introduction to the Issues.' *CMAH* 156: 371–7.

Lomas, Jonathan. 1997. 'Reluctant Rationers: Public Input to Health Care Priorities.' *Journal of Health Services and Research Policy* 2: 103–11.

Mahoney, Jil and Brian Laghi. 2002. 'Ottawa Wants Medicare Mediation Panel.'
   Globe and Mail, 13 April, A9.
Maioni, Antonia. 1998. *Parting at the Crossroads: The Emergence of Health Insurance in the United States and Canada*. Princeton: Princeton University Press.
– 1999. 'Decentralization in Health Policy: A Comment on the ACCESS Proposals.' In *Stretching the Federation: The Art of the State in Canada*, ed. Robert
   Young, 97–121. Kingston: Institute for Intergovernmental Relations, Queen's
   University.
– 2001. 'The Citizenship-Building Effects of Policies and Services in Canada's
   Universal Health Care Regime.' Canadian Policy Research Networks Discussion Paper No. F/17, September.
Mallory, James R. 1965. 'The Five Faces of Federalism.' In *The Future of Cana-
   dian Federalism*, ed P.-A. Crépeau and C.B. Macpherson, 3–15. Toronto: Uni-
   versity of Toronto Press.
Ministerial Council on Social Policy Reform and Renewal. 1995. *Report to Pre-
   miers*.
Morone, James A. 1990. *The Democratic Wish: Popular Participation and the Limits
   of American Government*. New York: Basic Books.
National Forum on Health. 1997. *Canada Health Action: Building on the Legacy*,
   Ottawa: Minister of Public Works and Government Services.
Naylor, C. David. 1986. *Private Practice, Public Payment: Canadian Medicine and
   the Politics of Health Insurance, 1911–1966*. Montreal: McGill-Queen's Univer-
   sity Press.
Noël, Alain. 2000. 'General Study of the Framework Agreement.' In *The Cana-
   dian Social Union without Quebec: Eight Critical Analyses*, ed. Alain-G. Gagnon
   and Hugh Segal, 9–35. Montreal: Institute for Research on Public Policy.
O'Reilly, Patricia. 2001. 'The Federal/Provincial/Territorial Health Conference
   System.' In *Federalism, Democracy and Health Care in Canada*, ed. Duane
   Adams, 107–29. Montreal: McGill-Queen's University Press.
Pierson, Paul. 1993. 'When Effect Becomes Cause: Policy Feedback and Politi-
   cal Change.' *World Politics* 45: 595–628.
Robinson, Ian, and Richard Simeon. 1999. 'The Dynamics of Canadian Federal-
   ism.' In *Canadian Politics*, 3rd ed. Edited by James Bickerton and Alain-G.
   Gagnon, 239–62. Peterborough, ON: Broadview Press.
Royal Commission on Health Services. 1964. *Final Report:* Volume I. Ottawa:
   Queen's Printer.
Romanow, Roy. 2002. *Notes for Remarks at McGill University.* Montreal: McGill
   Institute for the Study of Canada. http://www.healthcarecommission.ca
   (15 February).
Simeon, Richard, and David Cameron. 2002. 'Intergovernmental Relations and

Democracy: An Oxymoron If Ever There Was One?' In *Canadian Federalism: Performance, Effectiveness, and Legitimacy*, ed. Herman Bakvis and Grace Skogstad, 278–95. Toronto: Oxford University Press.

Smiley, Donald V. 1962. 'The Rowell-Sirois Report, Provincial Autonomy and Post-War Canadian Federalism.' *Canadian Journal of Economics and Political Science* 28(1) 54–69.

– 1987. *The Federal Condition in Canada*. Toronto: McGraw-Hill Ryerson.

Smith, Miriam. 1995. 'Medicare and Canadian Federalism.' In *New Trends in Canadian Federalism*, ed. François Rocher and Miriam Smith, 319–37. Peterborough, ON: Broadview Press.

Soderstrom, Lee. 1978. *The Canadian Health System*. London: Croom Helm.

Stevenson, Garth. 1985. 'The Division of Powers.' In *Division of Powers and Public Policy*, ed. Richard. Simeon, 71–123. Toronto: University of Toronto Press.

Stilborn, Jack, and Robert B. Asselin. 2001. *Federal-Provincial Relations*. Ottawa: Library of Parliament, Political and Social Affairs Division (93–10E).

Stilborn, Jack. 1997. *National Standards and Social Programs: What the Federal Government Can Do*. Ottawa: Library of Parliament, Political and Social Affairs Division (BP-379–E).

Taylor, Malcolm G. 1987. *Health Insurance and Canadian Public Policy: The Seven Decisions that Created the Canadian Health Insurance System and Their Outcomes*. 2nd ed. Montreal: McGill-Queen's University Press.

– 1991. *Insuring National Health Care: The Canadian Experience*. Chapel Hill: University of North Carolina Press.

Tuohy, Carolyn J. 1989. 'Federalism and Canadian Health Care Policy.' In *Challenges to Federalism: Policy-Making in Canada and the Federal Republic of Germany*, ed. W. Chandler and C. Zollner, 141–60. Kingston: Institute of Intergovernmental Relations, Queen's University.

Weaver, R. Kent. 1986. 'The Politics of Blame Avoidance.' *Journal of Public Policy* 6 (November): 371–98.

6 Health Care Politics and the Intergovernmental Framework in Canada

CANDACE JOHNSON

The idea of citizenship is expressed in many ways. Citizens and States exchange duties and services, rights and responsibilities, in order to create workable, sustainable political communities. In Canada, as in other countries, this exchange is made visible through social policy. Benefits are accorded through pensions, education, housing, and health care as compensation for, or to enable, participation in the military, the economy, and society. Such an exchange reflects, reinforces, and generates beliefs about the Good Society and delineates patterns of social inclusion and exclusion. For Canadians, some of the substance of citizenship is revealed in the health care policy arena. Canadians are proud of their universal health system and hold that it is a feature that distinguishes them from Americans. Further, Canadian citizens understand the citizenship bargain through which they exchange taxes for health insurance and have come to communicate this exchange in the language of rights. This 'rights-talk' has developed in tandem with, or perhaps as a result of, loss of confidence in the State's ability or willingness to maintain existing health care programs and develop new ones.

Thus, it is critically important to evaluate the State's role in health care and the ways in which it has enriched or diminished hospital and medical services insurance (commonly referred to as medicare). In the Canadian context, the evaluation focuses, inevitably, on questions of federalism. I will argue that the federal-provincial relationship has effected a stable and efficient set of arrangements for health care, but has not been completely successful in developing an effective system. In fact, the stability and efficiency of the system might undermine its effectiveness. On the one hand, medicare is effective because it embodies and makes tangible the five principles of the Canada Health Act – universality, accessibility, comprehensiveness, portability, and public administration. On the other hand, the stability of government-group relations and the efficiency that those relations produce are not conducive to dynamic policy change. Further, many reforms and improvements, namely, macro-level policy discussions, do not get done because of federal-provincial disagreement and deadlock. This is a significant problem given the new challenges to health systems around the globe.

The Creation of a Health Care System

The historical record shows that federalism has facilitated health care policy development in Canada. After a few 'false starts' in some of the Canadian provinces in the 1930s and 1940s, the Saskatchewan government implemented a public hospital insurance plan in 1947 (Maioni 1998, 73–7). It might have been the case that the provinces had no choice but to develop health programs on their own. In 1937, Prime Minister Bennett's New Deal Legislation, a national policy proposal to provide relief in the aftermath of the Depression, was declared ultra vires. The Judicial Committee of the Privy Council (JCPC) protected the provincial terrain of social policy from federal encroachment. Thus, a federal government willing to act in response to economic adversity and social decline was prohibited from doing so. The question might be asked: Would a different JCPC decision have created a different social policy landscape in Canada? Would the federal government have acted earlier to develop public health insurance programs without the inspiration of innovative provincial forerunners? But who knows? These questions cannot be answered. The provinces *did* lead the way in terms of progressive health policy. What remains to be seen is whether, in the face of much needed reforms, the provinces can be entrusted with the national vision that has been shaped, nurtured, and institutionalized over the past four or five decades and whether the provinces can implement reforms consistent with that vision.

In order to evaluate federal-provincial relations in the health care arena, it is necessary to identify the sources of tension in the relationship and determine the relevance of the intergovernmental framework. It is clear that the federal government has developed, in conjunction with the provinces, a national vision that reflects and comports with public sentiment. This vision is the product of a number of forces. First, it was evident following the Second World War that the existing federal grants-in-aid for specific purposes (such as tuberculosis control and hospital construction) were piecemeal and insufficient. Furthermore, the war effort was a demonstration of citizenship and responsibility, and the State was compelled to respond with a cadre of rights. Thus, federal action in 1957 and 1966 (national hospital insurance and national medical insurance, respectively) provided citizens with tangible health benefits and also declared the social dimensions of Canadian nationalism.

Such pan-Canadian action in a field of provincial jurisdiction was made possible through the federal spending power. The Canadian Constitution authorizes the federal government to spend in all policy areas, even those of exclusive provincial domain. Given the tangible benefits of universal health care, the national dimensions of the program, and the federal financial contribution to a policy area outside of its ambit, it was inevitable that health care would become a hotly contested intergovernmental issue.

Rights Reorientation

The Charter of Rights and Freedoms and the Canada Health Act inspired a new rights orientation in the field of health care (Redden 2002; Manfredi and Maioni 2002; and Flood 1999). The authority of full judicial review moved debate concerning constitutional matters beyond mere questions of jurisdiction. Thus, it no longer made sense to consider health care as an exclusively intergovernmental issue. It is important to recognize that the federal-provincial perspective is narrow, process-focused, and that the intergovernmental dimensions of health care intersect with debates related to rights, civil societies, and bioethical reflection. In my estimation, one of the most serious problems concerning the federal-provincial framework for health care is that the process of intergovernmentalism has crowded out many issues relevant to health care (such as rights, bioethics, and global distribution). The process, in some cases, seems to engulf the substance of the debate. Moreover, questions about the impact of federal-provincial relations on the sustainability of medicare are, to a certain degree, wrong-headed. The Canadian health care system is a creature of intergovernmental politics. Federal-provincial relations, both harmonious and discordant, have facilitated *and* constrained policy change.

Evidence of significant change in the Canadian health system comes in many forms. One of the most profound and interesting is the rights orientation that has developed over the past two decades. It is commonplace for people to speak for rights to various things, both fundamental and frivolous. To claim that one has a right to something is not to indicate its value. For example, one might believe that one has a right to smoke cigarettes on the street, although such behaviour has been prohibited in many communities. The maker of this claim might feel strongly about his or her asseveration, but likely would not believe that this 'right' is equivalent to the right to life, liberty, or free speech (although the right to smoke might follow from more fundamental rights). Thus, rights-talk is important because it delineates not value but cultural expressions of sentimentality and attachment. To be sure, the claiming of rights is, in large part, the expression of societal values. However, the daily rubric of rights reveals emotional excursions into citizenship, sentimental attachments to objects, services, and familiar patterns. In fact, instead of the proliferation of rights discourse further entrenching cold enlightenment rationality, it liberates it. Profuse rights-claiming might transcend rationality and serve as evidence of a postmodern configuration of citizenship.

For example, some people feel violated when their range of choices is impinged in any way. For example, not being able to buy a Coke on a university campus that has a contract with Pepsi. It is plausible that this is a violation of the right to freedom of expression. And while that seems to be stretching the boundaries of fundamental rights, it might not be possible to separate the irrelevant from the relevant. Similarly, the debate concerning health care rights requires the assessment of primary versus luxury services, values, and sentiments. On an intuitive level, health care convincingly follows from more fundamental rights. I have argued elsewhere that the right to health care is properly understood (philosophically and politically) to be a citizenship right rather than a human right (Redden 2002). The right to public health insurance in advanced industrialized democracies is not equivalent to rights to basic health services like immunizations, clean drinking water, and shelter.

Health care as a citizenship right is made visible through intergovernmental and constitutional politics. In 1984, the Canada Health Act (CHA) increased provincial responsibility for health care by enumerating the conditions for disbursement of federal funds and, more importantly, identifying the penalties for failure to comply with those conditions. It should be noted that the main problem with the CHA is not the stringency and unreasonableness of federal conditions, but that it allows the federal government to claim a shared vision as its own.

The Charter has inspired more (and different) litigation concerning health care. Whereas in the pre-Charter era most litigation concerning health care focused on physician-patient relationships (Flood 1999), in the post-Charter era the focus of litigation turned to matters relating to fundamental rights, equality, and access (see the *Eldridge* and *Waldman* cases in British Columbia, and the *Cameron* case in Nova Scotia). This reflected and further inspired change in the nature of rights claims. On the one hand, citizen-patients came to expect services delivered in absolute terms. After all, the language of rights is unequivocal. And the gravity of health care issues could not be denied by the State. On the other hand, the CHA and the Charter seriously altered the provincial role in health care by increasing the level of provincial responsibility in both symbolic-political and constitutional realms. Citizen-patients direct their rights claims against provincial governments, which bear sole constitutional responsibility for health care. Moreover, provinces have assumed greater financial responsibility for health care; they are carrying more of the fiscal burden as the proportion of federal government funding declines.

It is not possible to determine with any degree of certainty whether this increase in degree of provincial responsibility is positive or negative. And it is not as simple as deciding whether the federal role is illegitimate or whether the provinces are fatally constrained by federal legislation, constitutional arrangements, and an increasingly litigious society. To be sure, public-opinion polls show that Canadians want the federal government to continue to play a role in health care and uphold national standards (Merck Frosst Canada & Co. et al. 2000, 26). It is clear, however, that the provincial role has changed as a result of the CHA and the Charter (as well as other factors) while the federal role has remained, more or less, constant. This is problematic because it creates an imbalance of rights and responsibilities, which diminishes possibilities for reform. As provinces assume more financial and moral responsibility for health care policy, the federal role becomes questionable, which presents a serious constraint to necessary change.

Problems and Patterns: Fiscal Federalism

Recent tensions between the federal and provincial governments concerning health care are consistent with historical patterns. One of the most significant factors that affects the intergovernmental relationship is funding and the uncertainty created by changes in the structure of federal transfer payments. Because health care is a field of exclusive provincial jurisdiction and the federal government is involved in most health care policy only to the extent that it can convince the provinces to comply with national standards, much about the federal-provincial relationship can be understood through an investigation of fiscal federalism.

Hospital and medical insurance programs were funded initially through cost-matching grants. The federal government contributed approximately 50 cents for every provincial dollar spent on health care (for details see Barker 1988). The provinces were free to spend as they wished, provided that they spent on designated programs (like hospital construction). Thus the process was established at the outset whereby the federal government established priorities and made funding available to provinces so that those priorities could be operationalized. As health care programs developed and provincial expenditure budgets expanded, concerns arose about sustainability of the health care system and its fiscal capacity. The turbulent economic environment of the 1970s, precipitated by the OPEC price shocks in 1973, inspired serious change in all policy areas. For health care this meant the renegotiation of funding arrangements.

In 1977, the federal government replaced cost-sharing for health care with a block-grant system called Established Programs Financing (EPF). The new grant combined two policy areas – health care and postsecondary education – and set limits for transfers to provinces in both areas. This new arrangement ostensibly relaxed program conditionality – provinces had to spend on health care and postsecondary education and uphold the spirit of the universal system, but could now set their own priorities. The provinces viewed the change with guarded optimism, if not suspicion. While the increase in discretion was regarded as a victory for the provinces, it was feared that the new transfer payments, which allowed the federal government more control over spending, would be insufficient to cover escalating costs.

Ultimately, and predictably, the federal government would control spending levels by adjusting the EPF escalator against inflation. Beginning in 1986, the federal government applied the EPF escalator to the entire transfer, which set the increase in annual payments at GNP −2 per cent. The EPF transfer, which consisted of a block grant (cash component), a tax-point transfer (13.5 personal income tax points and 1 corporate income tax point), and an equalization component, was initially intended to become sustained through the tax points. In other words, as the yield of the tax points increased, it was estimated that the cash component would be reduced and eventually eliminated. However, the tax yield was much lower than expected, and the cash component diminished but remained.

This worked well for the federal government. Although the block component required outlays of (federal) cash, it effectively secured adherence to national standards. This meant that the federal government could reduce the EPF escalator and thereby reduce the cash component, while continuing to insist on its conditions. The provinces, of course, felt aggrieved by this arrangement and complained that the federal government should either increase funding for health care or relax conditions and broaden the idea of national standards.

This was a period of great tension in federal-provincial relations. The provinces would lose the battle over funding and national standards in two episodes of major policy change. Both were components of the trend of federal unilateral decision-making in health care policy, which explains, in large part, the intergovernmental discord. The first was the Canada Health Act (CHA), 1984, which reiterated the five principles of medicare that were identified in the EPF legislation and attached provincial compliance with these principles to financial penalties. That is to say that, prior to 1984, the provinces were expected to adhere to national standards but it was not clear what recourse the federal government would have if they failed to do so. In the context of ongoing funding disputes and extra-billing by physicians, which were symbolically damaging to Canada's most revered social program (Tuohy 1988), the CHA was the federal government's attempt to champion universal health care in the face of mounting challenges.

The second episode of policy change came in 1995 when the federal government replaced EPF with the Canada Health and Social Transfer (CHST). The CHST amalgamated funding for health care and postsecondary education (EPF) with funding for welfare programs (the Canada Assistance Plan). The CAP was Canada's last major shared-cost program and as such required substantial federal cash payments. The cash component of EPF, to which conditions were tied, was decreasing and was expected to run out completely by 2010 (Smith 1995, 328), which would have left only the tax-point portion of the transfer. While tax points were part of the transfer, they could not easily be withheld. This meant that the financial penalties for contravention of the CHA would be virtually impossible to impose. By combining EPF with CAP, the federal government increased the cash component of the CHST while it reduced the overall amount of the transfer by approximately $6 billion (Department of Finance 1999, 15). This posed serious challenges to the provinces which now had to establish priorities among three policy areas, rather than two, and meet growing demands in the social policy arena with fewer resources.

The story of fiscal federalism indicates that harmony and discord in federal-provincial relations for health care are linked, first and foremost, to funding issues. The provinces are concerned with autonomy in policymaking and securing enough money to adequately fund health care, and the federal government is concerned with cost control and compliance with national standards. The Canada Health Act, to some extent, ensures effectiveness through the stated conditions of payment. Efficiency in decision making, although impaired by two layers of governmental authority, is achieved, somewhat facetiously, through federal unilateralism. And stability in funding levels (although there has been slow decline, which has caused greater uncertainty for the provinces) is secured through negotiated funding arrangements, public opinion, and medical profession-state relations. Thus, as Carolyn Tuohy argues in *Accidental Logics* (1999), the Canadian health system has remained relatively stable through turbulent times.

However, the other side of the efficiency coin is this: stability can be a constraint to much needed change. As noted in the introduction, federal-provincial disagreement in the field of health care consumes a significant amount of creative energy. This means that there are many reforms, improvements, and innovations that do not receive adequate consideration. With an inordinate amount of attention devoted to intergovernmental processes, disputes, and historical patterns and grievances, many macro-level discussions, through which policy is created and understood, are rendered irrelevant by more immediate concerns. A more harmonious federal-provincial relationship might be more supportive of such discussions and thereby lead to more widespread and successful innovation in the system.

In the sections below, I explore three issues that cannot easily be accommodated by the federal-provincial framework under examination here. The first is social rights and the development of policies aimed at diversity. These issues exemplify the conception of health and equality as transcendent of geographical spaces. The second is civil society – realization through public policy and structural change of the need to engage citizens and their communities in decision-making.

Such engagement might alter the structure of intergovernmental politics. And the third is bioethical reflection. Deliberations about distribution, what the State ought to provide for citizens, and how humans ought to treat one another constitutes the substance and essence of health care debates. In this discussion, I explore four main conceptual distinctions. Some of these distinctions, or deliberative fields, can be accommodated by existing federal-provincial structures, while others are non-spatial in that they transcend borders.

Social Rights and the Challenge of Difference

Canada's health care system has undergone a number of substantial changes throughout the late twentieth and early twenty-first centuries in each of the provinces. Many of the reforms have (1) attempted to reconcile commitments to universality with challenges of difference and diversity, (2) engaged citizens and their communities in health care decision making (and thereby strengthened civil society), and (3) recognized the global impact and universality of bioethical and human rights issues. Such developments are clear examples of the decline in relevancy of T.H. Marshall's social rights thesis and the need to define new relationships among the government, the economy, and society. All three of these dimensions intersect with intergovernmental arrangements.

T.H. Marshall explains in *Citizenship and Social Class* (1964) that social rights developed in Britain in the twentieth century in response to the extant inequalities and the needs of the State following the Second World War. The development of civil and political rights in the eighteenth and nineteenth centuries, respectively, guaranteed formal procedural equality for British citizens. However, it became abundantly clear that the substance of British citizenship was plagued with inequality (largely tied to economic factors) and that national security was best served by enabling citizens to fulfil their duties to their country. Well-functioning military and industrial sectors were dependent upon a healthy and educated populace. Social rights in the form of welfare schemes, health services, and education provisions, which were distributed equally among all British citizens regardless of social class or income level (i.e., welfare state programs), would guarantee 'the right to a modicum of economic welfare and security to the right to share to the full in the social heritage and to live the life of a civilized being according to the standards prevailing in the society' (78).

The main benefit of social rights development is that equality is established and maintained through social programs that go beyond rhetoric to deliver tangible benefits. In Canada, economic inequality, combined with patterns of urbanization and advancements in medical technology, declared the need (in the early decades of the twentieth century) for State action in health care (Dickinson 1993). Such action began at the local level with plans to hire municipal doctors (Taylor 1987) – communities paid a stipend to a doctor who made a commitment to practice within their area. By the time that people were experiencing serious economic hardship in the 1930s, it was clear that this patchwork approach was insufficient. The grass-roots initiative was assumed by some provincial governments and the Canadian Medical Association (CMA). It was in the interests of provincial governments (which had constitutional jurisdiction for health care) and doctors (who needed to get paid for their services) that public health plans were created.

The history of public health insurance in Canada was been well documented and explained elsewhere (Taylor 1987; Maioni 1998). The point that I would like to make here, and I will return to it in the next section, is that grass-roots participation – the engagement of civil society – is only possible when it is authentic, that is, when it reflects a genuine set of needs and interests and not a manufactured one. Pre-welfare state grass-roots mobilization was extraordinary in that action was imperative, whereas in the post-welfare state era, citizens have already decided or accepted that federal and provincial governments are responsible for health care decision-making.

In the literature, the current defenders of social rights and the welfare state tend to be convincing (Armstrong and Armstrong 1996; King and Waldron 1988). However, the choices that governments face are much more complex than the binary option of statist or market approaches. It is practically inarguable that welfare state programs have brought about a measure of equality in many advanced capitalist democracies. Yet while social class and socio-economic status remain central to analyses of inequality, governments and their societies must find ways to deal with a much broader, sometimes overlapping and sometimes competing, range of inequalities. Differences based on gender, sexuality, race, and ability, in short ascription and identity, complicate the welfare state's promise to deliver unity through universal social programs.

The possibility of a 'third way' (Giddens 2000a, 2000b), which cuts a hopeful path between the welfare state and the postmodern angst of seemingly irreconcilable differences, market forces, and globalization, is intriguing. In fact, it might continue the tradition in Canada, which began with the Charter of Rights and Freedoms in 1982, of understanding how rights and entitlement to social services affect both individuals and groups. The Charter recognizes that while equality among individuals is a priority for any liberal democracy, the basis for claiming equality might be difference or that equality might not be possible without respect for difference. As such, the Charter, in theory, resists the trend that has plagued American social policy: realization in practice of formal commitments to individual equality with recognition for group marginalization and difference only insofar as those groups are excluded from the formal commitments. Canada, by contrast, includes as part and parcel of its formal commitments, recognition for group difference. Michael Ignatieff explains that '[c]onstitutional change might have begun with Prime Minister Trudeau's desire to anchor Canadian equality in the equality of individual rights. But by the time the process had finished, Canadians had insisted that individual rights were not enough: guarantees for collective language rights, women's equality, multicultural heritage, and Aboriginal land claims had been forced into the Charter' (Ignatieff 2000, 7).

Health and Difference

It is generally accepted that differences such as gender, language, and age have varying and significant impacts on health. The issues presented by the realities of increased life expectancy are new and complex. Life-extending technologies raise difficult questions about length of life vs quality of life trade-offs. The need for home care and pharmacare options is pressing for this population. And the bioethical dimensions of organ transplants, end-of-life issues (distribution of scarce resources to terminal patients, do-not-resuscitate orders, and euthanasia) and family restructuring (to care for aging relatives) make impossible simple responses in the form of the usual appeals to universality.

Governments have developed limited pharmacare programs and have increased spending on home care, although there is little coordinated policy for the latter initiative. In 1998, public home care expenditures reached the $2.1 billion mark, an increase of $1.1 billion or 104 per cent from 1990–1 (Health Canada 1998). The National Forum on

Health (1997) recommended that Canada adopt a more deliberate and coordinated approach to ethical reflection. The Values Working Group of the NFOH found that there are few well-developed research networks among organizations and institutions concerned with bioethics (NFOH 1997, 21). However, many of the (federal) recommendations of the NFOH have not been implemented, and it remains to be seen whether a more systematic discussion concerning health care ethics will ensue. (The Canadian Institutes for Health Research might provide some structure for this objective.)

In addition, there has been much attention at all levels given to the distinct challenges and concerns of women's health. Since 1996, the federal government has sponsored the creation of five national centres for excellence in women's health. These centres, located in different parts of the country, reflect the federal government's commitment to exploring health issues for women and to implement its gender-based analysis policy (Health Canada 2000). The need for policies and perspectives that recognize women's sex and gender differences as they affect health encompasses medical research, health services distribution, bioethics, and lifestyle factors. Thus it is a step beyond universality as sameness of treatment and provision for all patients regardless of difference.

Different individual Canadian citizens and different groups of Canadian citizens experience access to health care in different ways. For example, the English-speaking population in Quebec found its access to health services seriously affected by the closing of many English hospitals and the reducing or removing of bilingual services from many others in the province. While hospital closures have been a staple of most provincial reform agendas, the Quebec government's decision to close English hospitals presented a distinct affront to access. Closing a hospital in a rural area might have meant that patients must drive to the nearest urban centre to receive care. But closing English hospitals that provided service in English not only compromised access, it eliminated it (Commissioner of Official Languages 1998, section 2).

Similarly, in 1997 in British Columbia, the provincial government decided to discontinue funding for interpretation services for patients with hearing disabilities (the *Eldridge* case). The Canada Health Act (1984) stipulates that:

12. (1) In order to satisfy the criterion respecting accessibility, the health care insurance plan of a province

(a) must provide for insured health services on uniform terms and conditions and on a basis that does not impede or preclude, either directly or indirectly whether by charges made to insured persons or otherwise, reasonable access to those services by insured persons. (chap. C-6)

However, prior to *Eldridge*, accessibility had only been enforced to prohibit user fees and extra-billing practices. That is to say, that the federal government withheld from its transfer payments to provinces the user fees levied by clinics or monies extra-billed by physicians. The penalties for other transgressions are more difficult to exact. How much can be withheld from a province that fails to provide the means to access, such as interpretation services? What are the other punitive options?

This difficulty of reconciling national standards with provincial policy prerogatives is nothing new in the Canadian health care arena. However, this case is unique because it was not argued on the terrain of federal legislation (i.e., the issue was not whether the B.C. government's decision contravened the Canada Health Act) but as a constitutional matter. Colleen Flood (1999) explains that

[p]rior to *Eldridge*, the existing case law was clear that the Charter did not apply to hospitals on the grounds that the government did not exert sufficient control over these institutions to qualify them as 'government' ... However, in *Eldridge*, the Supreme Court of Canada found that the Charter *did* apply to a hospital's decision not to fund translation services for deaf patients. (36)

Thus, the *Eldridge* case is significant because the appeal to the Charter expands notions of health care rights to formally include individuals and groups, equality and difference. It also signifies a new era of legal reinforcement of provincial responsibility and increased rights-claiming by citizen-patients (see Rioux 1999). It also demonstrates that public policy issues can become formal rights issues and, as such, acquire status not alterable by either federal or provincial governments.

The study of inequality as it relates to health has been the concern of epidemiologists (see, for example, Wilkinson 1994; Farmer 1999). However, there has been very little consideration given to the intersection of health and inequality by those interested in political questions (with the major exceptions of Evans, Barer, and Marmor 1994; Daniels, Kennedy, and Kawachi 2000). This is surprising because the study of politics is the study of power and resources and how each is distributed among groups and individuals in a given population. Perhaps because formal political commitments to political equality have been the hallmark of modern liberal democracies, issues concerning inequality have not been fully recognized or addressed. However, the post-war commitments to social rights and the securing of political equality through social programmes are somewhat outdated. The challenges of difference and inequality cannot be appropriately met by the existing intergovernmental arrangements in Canada.

Of course, there have always been policies in place to deal with diversity and marginality. The federal government recognizes its responsibility for Native populations and the health needs that are unique to those populations through the Non-Insured Health Benefits Program. Despite the appearance of a single, universal health system in Canada, each province has created, and continues to develop, its own health system. As the population ages, provincial governments make arrangements for health services for seniors that are not available to the general population. And the changing dynamics of disease and treatment have prompted governments to provide drug benefits for patients who require prohibitively expensive medications (pharmaceuticals administered outside of hospitals are not covered by provincial health insurance plans). Finally, the entire system, or network of systems, is built on the notion that physicians will provide individual patients with whatever program of care they deem to be 'medically necessary.' In all of these ways, the Canadian health system already recognizes diversity and difference. However, the centrality of the intergovernmental framework contributes to static patterns. While the processes and products of fiscal federalism have created a stable health system, they have, at the same time, reduced most policy questions to intergovernmental ones. To be sure, health policy is made in an intergovernmental context of federal-provincial negotiation. But questions about the future of health care in Canada go (and ought to go) far beyond the mechanics of transfer payments.

Strengthening Civil Society

In the 1990s, provincial governments in Canada undertook various reform efforts. One feature that most of them (all, with the exception of Ontario) had in common was the decentralization of health care decision-making. Provinces created regional or community level units (called regional health authorities or regional and community health boards) through which citizens could participate directly in the shaping of health policy for their area. In Saskatchewan, these community governance structures became exercises in democracy – some of the board members were elected by their constituents – and in other provinces, such as Nova Scotia, board members were appointed by officials in the Department of Health (for a full examination of devolution in the Canadian provinces see Lomas, Woods, and Veenstra 1997a–d). The goals of this type of reform initiative were diverse and have been realized to widely varying extents. However, it can be concluded that one of the main aims of community governance structures was to strengthen civil society.

Although there is no consensus on what 'civil society' means, and provincial governments did not describe their populations as 'civil societies' in the reform literature, the term is applicable to evaluations of citizen engagement in health care decision-making. The main question surrounding the term 'civil society' seems to be the degree to which citizens' groups and communities are distinct from the activities of government. Civil-society organizations are assumed to be somewhat autonomous and provide views from 'outside' the State. These organizations include non-profit and community-service organizations, such as HIV/AIDS activist and service groups. Although the definition of civil society remains elusive, the term has been used generally in recent literatures to stand for the ideas of autonomy, outside perspectives, citizen engagement, and community empowerment (see Cohen and Arato 1994; Keane 1999). Community governance structures in reorganized health care systems present opportunities (again, to varying extents) for citizen participation and representation of community needs. Thus, they promise to lead to better-informed policy decisions, as well as to stronger civil societies. They were also important components of the trend (in the 1980s and 1990s) towards democratic administration (Albo 1993), increased 'consumer' awareness, and empowerment in regard to public policy (Pierre 1995).

Notions about civil society fit into the intergovernmental framework in that they are created and sustained by provincial governments. Citizen engagement through community-governance structures was (and, in some cases, still is) a popular policy tool. Provincial governments can employ community health authorities to provide information, solicit input, and make decisions. However, the people who are empowered through these structures are both federal and provincial citizens. They are not public servants of one order of government or another, nor are they trained to negotiate policy in the context of fiscal federalism. Rather, they are members of deliberative bodies, moral agents, makers of claims, raisers of questions, and purveyors of expectations. As a layer of government they are, at the same time, meta- and subprovincial.

One of the most promising or potentially transformative effects of engaging citizens in health care decision-making is that a strengthened civil society with institutional support can provide some counterbalance to the dominance of the medical profession. Elite decision-making for health care in Canada accounts for much of the stability of the health care system. Carolyn Tuohy (1999) explains that 'through the 1970s and 1980s, the playing out of the logic of the single-payer system gave the Canadian system extraordinary structural and institutional stability' (204). While this stability is favourable in many ways, it might have the negative effect of developing patterns of policy decisions that are resistant to change. Exercises in community engagement provide opportunities for alternative or excluded visions and create new avenues for policy explorations.

While it is difficult to evaluate Canada's health system against health systems in other countries, an opportunity for comparison might be afforded by the United States. In 1997, the U.S. federal government introduced the State Children's Health Insurance Program (SCHIP). As in Canada, health care is the responsibility of the individual states, and the federal government may establish funding for programs and the conditions upon which that funding is disbursed. The U.S. federal government produced guidelines for the SCHIP but realized that each state would necessarily implement a very different version of the program. To recognize this in practice, but maintain national standards, the federal government solicited formal proposals from each state. These proposals included details about program goals, spending targets, additional funding sources, the profile of low-income, uninsured children, and justifications in cases where a state's plan diverged from the federal prescriptions. Hence, each state had to formally apply for federal money and prove that it had met the conditions of the program and was in compliance with national standards *before* it received the money (see Centers for Medicare and Medicard Services 2002).

A similar process might give the Canadian federal government more control over funding and program conditionality at the same time that it might give the provinces increased latitude for experimentation and innovation because provincial plans or proposals are made public and approved at the outset. Further, public debate on the applications might bring out more voices, thereby contributing to and expanding 'active' or participatory modes of citizenship.

While this suggestion might inspire rethinking Canadian funding mechanisms for health care, it needs to be stated that cross-country comparisons (in search of reform possibilities) are limited and difficult. The United States does not have a universal health system. Entitlement to health insurance is linked to employment rather than citizenship. Many people acquire insurance through their employers. Those who meet their state's eligibility requirements for social assistance also qualify for federal health coverage (Medicaid). Senior citizens are entitled to health insurance through another federal program (Medicare). And approximately 45 million Americans have no health insurance coverage. Social policy in each country, and health care in particular, reflects very different values concerning citizenship (the obligations of the State and the rights of citizens) and the Good Society.

Bioethical Reflection

The foregoing discussions of diversity and civil society intersect with intergovernmental debates (historical patterns of negotiation and tension, fiscal federalism), but the former cannot be understood fully within the context of the latter. That is to say that federal-provincial decision making for health care has been able to accommodate diversity while maintaining universality and has, to some degree, successfully institutionalized competing voices through community-governance structures. However, the federal-provincial relationship, mainly conceived as a set of formal fiscal arrangements, is focused on the process of health care debates, not their substance. This renders an efficient and stable set of arrangements somewhat ineffective.

This is particularly problematic for the final issue to be considered: bioethical reflection. In this section I explore four models or sets of compatible ideas. The first two fit within spatial models, which means that deliberation is contingent upon an understanding of geographical spaces: citizens and strangers, and bodies, states, and universals. The third makes a distinction between political priorities and international human rights imperatives and, as such, begins to move beyond the spatial model and into the realm of normative discourse. The fourth is a non-spatial model that considers the complex ethical terrain of medical technology. All four address important substantive health care issues as they relate to access, distribution, and citizenship.

It is becoming clear that health can no longer be conceived as only a domestic social policy issue:

> The relationships among medicine, public health, ethics, and human rights are now evolving rapidly, in response to a series of events, experiences, and struggles. These include the shock of the worldwide epidemic of human immunodeficiency virus and AIDS, continuing work on diverse aspects of women's health, and challenges exemplified by the complex humanitarian emergencies of Somalia, Iraq, Bosnia, Rwanda, and Zaire. (Mann 1999, 439).

The new realities of infection and inequality implicate all populations and call for global action. Health can be conceived as a human rights issue in many ways, all of which are related to the basic human right to dignity (Mann et al. 1999). As I explain below, the understanding of health as a human right depends on the definition of human rights – what is deemed fundamental to humanity and what is considered to be a 'perk' of membership to one political community or another.

Bioethical discussions are linked to human rights discourse. Both are concerned with questions of 'ought.' As a global community, what ought we to respect about one another by virtue of our shared humanity? What offences are so egregious that they ought to be labelled human rights violations? What ought to be done for a particular patient in a particular circumstance? What options ought to be available for terminally ill patients? What health services ought to be provided by the State for its citizens? Bioethical questions range from particular, patient-specific concerns to broad issues concerning distributional equity.

By focusing attention on health care and bioethics as issues for both citizenship and global human rights action, several important distinctions can be made. The first is the distinction between populations 'inside' the State (citizens) and populations 'outside' the State (refugees, migrants, or temporary workers). All nation-states distinguish between citizens and non-citizens for the purpose of allocating resources. In Canada, all citizens, landed immigrants, and conventional refugees are entitled to public health insurance whereas non-citizens must secure private insurance. However, there is another layer of inclusion and exclusion. Among the citizens of a State, some have entitlements that are not made available to others. In the United States, senior citizens are entitled to public health insurance (Medicare), but for all other citizens health insurance is linked to employment. And in both Canada and the United States, many citizen-patients are marginalized due to their difference and regardless of their formal entitlements. For example, such reproductive rights issues as birth control, abortion, and NRTS (new reproductive technologies like in vitro fertilization) reveal patterns of inequality within societies. Dorothy Roberts (1997) explains (regarding race and regulation) that,

> [e]ven though there are restrictions on white mothers, it's a fundamentally different kind of regulation ... A perfect example is sterilization. In the seventies, a group of feminists opposed to waiting periods and rigid informed consent procedures for sterilization. Women of color said, 'Let's put limits on sterilization because doctors are guilty of abuse.' But this just didn't register with some of the mainstream reproductive rights groups that had been pushing for greater access to sterilization for white, middle-class women. While poor black women were, in some cases, forcibly sterilized, sometimes without their knowledge, let alone consent, white women had a hard time getting sterilized. (78)

The point to be made is that bioethical issues, and hence health as a human rights issue, are complex indicators of inequality. And that human rights abuses (such as forced sterilization) can be hidden by freedom-enhancing rights claims (access to abortion and NRTs) of relatively privileged segments of society (white women).

The second is the distinction between particular (patient-specific), domestic (state specific), and universal bioethical deliberation. Bioethics, as the field of ethical questions as they relate to the body, is sometimes very narrowly applicable and sometimes very widely applicable. For example, the decision of a particular hospital to provide an expensive and complicated lung transplant to an elderly cancer patient will take into consideration all information and ideas relevant to that particular case. And the decision will not necessarily establish policy concerning all future transplant patients. The next patient to require a lung transplant will be considered on the merits of his or her own case. Domestic or state-specific deliberation concerns the distribution of health resources in a state. Thus this type of deliberation is the substance of citizenship. Should citizens be entitled to publicly funded cosmetic surgery, as in Argentina, should citizens be entitled to a comprehensive range of 'medically necessary' services, as in Canada, or should citizens be responsible for securing their own insurance, as in the United States?

And the third is the distinction between negotiation concerning political priorities and international human rights imperatives. Human rights issues for health care include matters pertaining to provision, access, and bioethics. The first matter, provision, is the most basic. In many developing countries, public health services such as clean drinking water and immunizations are not made widely available. And in wartime, disaster, and refugee situations, many people go without adequate food and shelter. Because these matters are linked to the issues of development and war, it is practically inarguable that they constitute human rights violations (they are clearly human security issues). It seems fundamental that every human being has access to the most basic medications and services. International humanitarian organizations such as Doctors Without Borders (DWB) and the International Red Cross are committed to the promotion of health as a human rights issue and provide support for populations in need. For example, DWB had been working in Afghanistan to ensure that marginalized sections of the population had access to health services. Such a project involves sensitivity to cultural and political factors that affect health. Women in Afghanistan were forbidden to receive care from a male practitioner, yet in many areas there were no female physicians or nurses. DWB placed female practitioners in such underserviced areas so that women could receive care.

The issue of access covers everything from user charges for health services in Canada to the 45 million people in the United States with no health insurance coverage to the legacy of Apartheid in South Africa (Chapman and Rubenstein 1998). These 'violations' might be more appropriately labelled citizenship breaches because they are directly linked to citizen-State relationships in each country. However, these violations or infringements or gaps in coverage may also be conceived as human rights issues. While in each of the three countries mentioned above most people have access to clean drinking water and childhood immunizations, the rights to life and liberty are seriously impaired if citizens are too ill to access them. Health is central and not adjunct to social, political, and cultural life. All three of these distinctions can be conceived as borders that are policed and transgressed by diverse populations.

Finally, the issue of modern bioethics (as it relates to the applications of medical technology rather than basic access and allocation) is relevant to advanced industrialized democracies. There is great distance between the need for or right to clean drinking water and the right to doctor assisted suicide or in vitro fertilization. The language of rights has been invoked to bolster all three claims, yet there seems to be an intuitive ordering of each claim as a human rights issue. That is to say that the first passes as a human rights issue quite easily due to the immediacy of the need and its direct effect on quality of life. The two bioethical issues noted subsequently are more complex and reflect higher order 'needs.' Whether the issues of provision, access, and bioethics are different in degree or substance remains an open question. Do all noted patterns of inequality count as human rights violations? Is the person who cannot gain access to an abortion in the United States (because she is a recipient of Medicaid or has no health insurance and cannot afford it) equal in terms of disadvantage, loss of dignity, and quality of life to the person in earthquake-shattered Columbia who has no clean drinking water and no option for medical care? Do these claims have to be equivalent in order to constitute human rights issues?

Conclusion

My purpose in raising issues concerning rights, civil society, and bioethics is to demonstrate that health care is an incredibly dynamic policy field that is often rendered static by the limitations of the intergovernmental framework. While it is important to maintain respect for intergovernmental arrangements for health care, it should be recognized that the inertia of federal-provincial relations constrains policy change. Discussions of citizenship rights (in the form of entitlements to health care) transcend questions of jurisdiction and funding. Bioethical concerns are both universal and particular and will need to be addressed at the global level, in communities, and in hospitals. Change in medical technology, citizenship, and domestic politics alters the delicate balance of obligations and commitments in a federal state. And, in the case of health care in Canada, the provinces are left to create new understandings, bargains, and programs for citizens.

It is possible that by acknowledging this imbalance of rights and responsibilities among federal and provincial governments and citizens, clarity can be established, and from this clarity a new intergovernmental relationship can be built. To be sure, intergovernmental politics can accommodate (and has accommodated) issues of distributional equity. Intergovernmental politics has addressed problems concerning allocation of health resources and might be able to provide a model for future negotiation on the terrains of bioethics and rights. However, as currently understood and applied, the intergovernmental perspective is inappropriately narrow. The process of federal-provincial decision-making for health care overshadows many issues relevant to health care and eclipses substantive policy issues.

REFERENCES

Albo, Gregory, David Langille, and Leo Panitch. 1993. *A Different Kind of State? Popular Power and Democratic Administration.* Toronto: Oxford University Press.

Armstrong, Pat, and Hugh Armstrong. 1996. *Wasting Away: The Undermining of Canadian Health Care.* Toronto: Oxford University Press.

Barker, Paul. 1988. 'The Development of the Major Shared-Cost Programs in Canada.' In *Perspectives on Canadian Federalism,* ed. R.D. Olling and M.W. Westmacott, 195–219. Scarborough, ON: Prentice-Hall.

Centers for Medicare and Medicaid Services. 2002. *State Children's Health Insurance Program.* http://www.cms.hss.gov/schip (June).

Chapman, Audrey R., and Leonard S. Rubenstein, eds., 1998. *Human Rights and Health: The Legacy of Apartheid.* Washington, DC: American Association for the Advancement of Science.

Cohen, Jean-Louis, and Andrew Arato. 1994. *Civil Society and Political Theory.* Cambridge, MA: MIT Press.

Commissioner of Official Languages. 1998. *Annual Report 1997.* Part IV: The Official Language Community. Minister of Public Works and Government Services, Canada. http://www.ocol-clo.gc.ca/e4.html (24 December 2001).

Daniels, Norman, Bruce Kennedy, and Ichiro Kawachi. 2000. *Is Inequality Bad for Our Health?* Boston: Beacon Press.

Department of Finance. Budget 1999. *Building Today for a Better Tomorrow: Federal Financial Support for the Provinces and Territories.* Ottawa: Department of Finance.

Dickinson, Harley. 1993. 'The Struggle for State Health Insurance: Reconsidering the Role of Saskatchewan Farmers.' *Studies in Political Economy* 41 (Summer): 137–8.

Evans, Robert G., Morris L. Barer, and Theodore R. Marmor, eds., 1994. *Why Are Some People Healthy and Others Not? Determinants of Health of Populations*. New York: Aldine De Gruyter.

Farmer, Paul. 1999. *Infections and Inequalities: The Modern Plagues*. Berkeley: University of California Press.

Flood, Colleen. 1999. 'The Structure and Dynamics of Canada's Health Care System.' In *Canadian Health Law and Policy*, ed. J. Downie and T. Caulfield, 5–50. Toronto: Butterworth.

Fox, Renée. 1999. 'Medical Humanitarianism and Human Rights: Reflections on Doctors without Borders and Doctors of the World.' In *Health and Human Rights: A Reader*, ed. Jonathan M. Mann, Sofia Gruskin, Michael A. Grodin, and George J. Annas, 417–35. New York: Routledge.

Giddens, Anthony. 2000a. *The Third Way and Its Critics*. Cambridge, UK: Polity Press.

– 2000b. *The Third Way: The Renewal of Social Democracy*. Cambridge, UK: Polity Press.

Hall, Emmett. 1964. *The Royal Commission on Health Services* (Report). Ottawa: R. Duhamel, Queen's Printer.

Health Canada. 2000. *Health Canada's Gender-based Analysis Policy*. Ottawa: Health Canada.

– Policy and Consultation Branch. 1998. *Public Home Care Expenditures in Canada 1975–76 to 1997–98*. Ottawa: Health Canada.

Ignatieff, Michael. 2000. *The Rights Revolution*. Toronto: House of Anansi Press.

Keane, John. 1999. *Civil Society: Old Images, New Visions*. Princeton: Princeton University Press.

King, Desmond, and Jeremy Waldron. 1988. 'Citizenship, Social Citizenship and the Defence of Welfare Provision.' *British Journal of Political Science* 18: 415–43.

Lomas, Jonathan, John Woods, and Gerry Veenstra. 1997a. 'Devolving Authority for Health Care in Canada's Provinces. 1. An Introduction to the Issues.' *CMAJ* 156: 371–7.

– 1997b. 'Devolving Authority for Health Care in Canada's Provinces. 2. Backgrounds, Resources and Activities of Board Members.' *CMAJ* 156: 513–20.

– 1997c. 'Devolving Authority for Health Care in Canada's Provinces. 3. Motivations, Attitudes and Approaches of Board Members.' *CMAJ* 156: 669–76.

– 1997d. 'Devolving Authority for Health Care in Canada's Provinces. 4. Emerging Issues and Prospects.' *CMAJ* 156: 817–23.

Maioni, Antonia. 1998. *Parting at the Crossroads: The Emergence of Health Insurance in the United States and Canada*. Princeton: Princeton University Press.

Manfredi, Christopher, and Antonia Maioni. 2002. 'Courts and Health Policy: Judicial Policy Making and Publicly Funded Health Care in Canada.' *Journal of Health Politics, Policy, and Law* 27: 213–40.

Mann, Jonathan M. 1999. 'Medicine and Public Health, Ethics and Human Rights.' In *Health and Human Rights: A Reader*, ed. Jonathan M. Mann, Sofia Gruskin, Michael A. Grodin, and George J. Annas, 439–52. New York: Routledge.

Mann, Jonathan M. et al. 1999. 'Health and Human Rights.' In *Health and Human Rights: A Reader*, ed. Jonathan M. Mann, Sofia Gruskin, Michael A. Grodin, and George J. Annas, 7–20. New York: Routledge.

Marshall, T.H. 1964. *Class, Citizenship and Social Development*. New York: Doubleday.

Merck Frosst Canada and Co., POLLARA Research, Coalition of National Voluntary Organizations, Canadian Medical Association, Canadian Nurses Association, Canadian Association of Community Care, Canadian Home Care Association. 2000. Health Care in Canada: A National Survey of Health Care Providers and Users. Montreal: Merck Frosst.

National Forum on Health (NFOH). 1997. *Canada Health Action: Building on the Legacy.* Synthesis Reports and Issues Papers, Volume 2. Ottawa: National Forum on Health.

Pierre, Jon. 1995. 'The Marketization of the State.' In *Governance in a Changing Environment*, ed. Guy Peters and Donald Savoie, 55–81. Montreal: McGill-Queen's University Press.

Redden, Candace Johnson. 2002. 'Health Care As Citizenship Development: Examining Social Rights and Entitlement.' *Canadian Journal of Political Science* 35: 103–25.

– 1999. 'Rationing Care in the Community: Engaging Citizens in Health Care Decision Making.' *Journal of Health Politics, Policy, and Law* 24: 1363–89.

Rioux, Marcia. 1999. 'An Appeal to the Charter of Rights and Freedoms.' In *Do We Care? Renewing Canada's Commitment to Health*, ed. Margaret A. Somerville, 144–7. Montreal: McGill-Queen's University Press.

Roberts, Dorothy. 1997. *Killing the Black Body*. New York: Pantheon. Excerpt reprinted in *Ms.* Magazine, April/ May 2001.

Smith, Miriam. 1995. 'Retrenching the Sacred Trust: Medicare and Canadian Federalism.' In *New Trends in Canadian Federalism*, ed. François Rocher and Miriam Smith. Peterborough, ON: Broadview Press.

Taylor, Malcolm. 1987. *Health Insurance and Canadian Public Policy: The Seven Decisions that Created The Canadian Health Insurance System*. Montreal: McGill-Queen's University Press.

Tuohy, Carolyn Hughes. 1999. *Accidental Logics: The Dynamics of Change in the*

Health Care Arena in the United States, Britain, and Canada. New York: Oxford University Press.

– 1988. 'Medicine and the State in Canada: The Extra-Billing Issue in Perspective.' *Canadian Journal of Political Science* 21(2): 268–96.

Wilkinson, Richard G. 1994. 'The Epidemiological Transition: From Material Scarcity to Social Disadvantage.' *Daedalus* (Fall): 61–78.

7 The Conditions for a Sustainable Public Health System in Canada

LOUIS M. IMBEAU, KINA CHENARD, and
ADRIANA DUDAS

The aim of this chapter is to answer the following question: How does a political environment geared to balancing budgets, paying down the debt, and cutting taxes impact on the preservation or sustainability of ·the health system? We will proceed in three stages. First, we address the notion of the health system's sustainability and demonstrate that it depends on the system's financial, organizational, and epistemic capacities to respond to the health needs of current generations without compromising the system's ability to meet the needs of future generations. Second, we describe Canada's political and economic environment and show that the forces at work and the international context have undermined at once the system's financial capacity and its organizational and epistemic capacities. Third, we ask ourselves what could have justified such an attack on the health system's capacities. We show that, by stressing the financial capacity of organizations, the prevailing economic theory neglects the organizational and epistemic aspects of the health system's capacity, and that there are other economic theories that take these aspects into account. In conclusion, we argue that there are certain threats to the preservation of the Canadian health system, identify a few principles that should be followed in order to enhance its sustainability, and formulate recommendations that can help to achieve this.

The Sustainability of the Health System

Currently, there are two opposing schools of thought in the health world: a capacity perspective, which Moreau, Berthod-Wurmser, and Béchon (1992, 205) call the OECD vision, and a needs perspective, which the same authors identify as the WHO vision. These competing viewpoints can be found in that portion of the specialized literature devoted to defining the concept of sustainability. Indeed, two meanings of this concept share centre stage in this debate, with each bringing a different perspective to health and the health system.[1] The first meaning is built on a biological analogy. It sees sustainability as *the ability to last*. In French, this term is defined in the *Petit Larousse* as 'viable: ce qui *peut* vivre' (viable: that which is *able* to stay alive), and speaks to the central notion of an organism's *ability* to live or survive, a definition that was reproduced in a recent publication of the Canadian Medical Association (CMA). Obstetrics, for example, speaks in terms of a 'viable' fetus, that is, a child capable of living and developing outside the mother's womb.

The second meaning of sustainability is built on an ecological analogy and views the concept as one of sustainable development. According to the Brundtland Commission, sustainable development is 'development that meets the *needs* of the present without compromising the ability of future generations to meet their own needs' (Harrison 2000, 2). Thus, the ecological analogy stresses two important dimensions: needs and intergenerational equity. So we have two perspectives, which, far from conflicting, complement each other. A sober analysis of the sustainability of Canada's health system requires that we take into account the system's capacities, Canada's health needs, and intergenerational equity.

The Capacities of the Health System

The current discourse on the health system focuses to a great extent on its funding, testifying to the indispensable role of financial capacity as a cornerstone of a system's sustainability. Indeed, no organization can survive without financial resources. The goods and services it consumes cost money. But there are other capacities that are also essential to a health system's survival and development.

A social system cannot exist without organizational capacity, in other words, without the resources required to ensure cohesive decision-making structures. By this we mean the rules or standards that define the roles that each of the actors is required to play within the organization and the actors' conformity to these standards. Standards and conformity to standards produce a division of labour and a cohesiveness that ensure the quality of the services offered by the organization. The division of labour produced by these standards dramatically increases the scope of what the system can do. The cohesiveness that these standards create among the members of the organization ensures that a cohesive product is offered. Division of labour and cohesiveness are, in the final analysis, the main sources of efficiency.

In addition to the financial and organizational capacities, there is the epistemic capacity – without this, no health system is feasible. This capacity has to do with the knowledge and competencies acquired through formal training or through experience and learning and provides the actors with a framework for assessing the situation to which they must react in order to identify which course of action to take. This framework refers both to technical knowledge acquired through scientific research and to normative knowledge acquired through experience.

Thus, we have three types of capacity that ensure the system's sustainability. There are two things we should point out here. First, each of these capacities is essential in preserving the system. A health system cannot survive in the absence of financial, organizational, or epistemic capacities. If one is missing, the entire system comes crashing down. Second, these three types of capacity are not independent of one another. If one is changed, there can be a major impact on the others. Thus, financial, organizational, and epistemic capacities are essential and closely linked. But why seek to preserve a health system if not to meet the health needs of the public? If one is to have a useful discussion on the sustainability of the health system, one must first discuss needs.

Health Needs

A sustainable health system is one that meets the health needs of the population. At first blush this may appear simple, but it is not. What, in fact, is a health need? For a long time we have distinguished between essential needs (those having to do with nature) and non-essential needs (those having to do with culture). Jean-Jacques Rousseau, for example, distinguished natural needs from artificial needs and John Maynard Keynes made a distinction between absolute and relative needs. Although attractive from an intellectual standpoint, this distinction is of little use to us because when it comes to defining health needs in terms of demand for care, the nature-culture distinction becomes blurred. When all is said and done, the needs-based demand for health care is a question of cultural artefact. To prove this point, let us deconstruct the notion of state of health according to the arguments of economist Sophie Béjean.

State of health is often defined in terms of morbidity. The process starts when the patient evaluates his or her own health. This evaluation, based on a psychological thought process and a social conception of health and illness, determines the perception this individual has of his or her need for medical services. This perceived morbidity is transformed into diagnosed morbidity through the coding carried out by the medical profession and the health apparatus. Diagnosed morbidity represents 'the outcome of a supposedly objective scientific procedure ... In the end, it appears to be a reflection more of the institution, the health apparatus or the physician formulating this diagnosis than of the state of health it is supposed to describe' (Béjean 1994, 109, our translation). Indeed, diagnosed morbidity, as the physician's coding, can differ greatly from perceived morbidity as well as objective morbidity, since the discomfort felt by the patient can go unrecognized by the physician, just as an illness might not be felt by the patient.

And so the process of moving from need to demand for health services involves three steps: first, the morbidity felt by the patient is expressed; second, this need is codified by the physician (diagnosed morbidity); third, the physician translates this diagnosed morbidity into demand for care. Objective morbidity is a long way away from demand for care. A series of factors come into play between the two, including the psychological and social representations of illness and health on the part of the patient and the physician, the pressures brought to bear by the health system on the physician in terms of service availability, advances in medical and pharmaceutical research and the physician's knowledge of these, and so on. State of health and, even more so, demand for health care are not simply a product of nature. They are social constructs in which the health system is directly involved. Consequently, any modification of the system's financial, organizational, or epistemic capacities is likely to influence the demand for health care. This is what economists call supply inducing demand.

Intergenerational Equity

In addition to capacities and needs, the sustainability of a health system involves intergenerational equity. There are two questions we must ask ourselves: Do we have obligations to future generations? Are we responsible for the impact that the decisions we take today have on our grandchildren and perhaps on theirs? If we accept that all human beings will continue, in the future, to have rights concerning the availability of adequate health care, some of the decisions we take today might violate these rights, regardless of who these future human beings will be. Thus, these people could argue that they have been deprived of the right to health on account of the policies adopted in the past. Consequently, certain decisions made today might be bad for future generations, from an ethical standpoint.

There are two things we need to consider here. The first has to do with health system funding, a topic that has occupied centre stage in the recent discourse surrounding the efforts to eliminate Canada's deficit. Is it fair for us, the current generations, to benefit from a series of health services while future generations get stuck with the bill for these services in the form of the annual deficit and public debt? Borrowing to pay health costs is tantamount to shifting the burden of payment onto those who will have to pay off the debt, a sort of a negative inheritance. From the standpoint of intergenerational equity, there is no question that the health system must be funded through taxes, and the temptation to borrow must be resisted. When it comes to investments, however, debt financing is acceptable from the perspective of intergenerational equity. But investments are not confined to real estate and equipment.

This brings us to our second consideration: What are our responsibilities towards future generations in terms of the organizational and epistemic capacities of the health system they will be inheriting? The level of health we enjoy and the quality of health services of which we can avail ourselves today are the product of the efforts made by past generations. Had Pasteur and his contemporaries not made their discoveries in the field of microscopic life, Flemming would have been unable to discover penicillin. Had Semmelweis and his contemporaries not discovered the role of hygiene in transmitting what they called puerperal fever, we would not have succeeded in bringing the perinatal death rate down to almost zero. The quality of the care from which future generations will benefit depends in large part on the investments we make today in the organizational and epistemic capacities of the health system. In this regard, we can view the extensive cuts in nursing staff – aimed at 'restoring' fiscal health – as a disinvestment in the health system's organizational and epistemic capacities. From the point of view of intergenerational equity, these measures were deleterious because, all things considered, failing to protect these investments constitutes negligence on our part, and our inaction could come back to haunt future generations.

Towards an Integrated Perspective

The preceding discussion should convince us of the futility of contrasting the capacities perspective with the needs perspective. Each of these two visions tells only part of the story. If we want to see the big picture, we must adopt an integrated vision whereby the sustainability of the health system depends on the financial, organizational, and epistemic capacities to adequately meet the health needs of today's generations without adversely affecting future generations. This way of looking at things suggests that the definition of demand for health care depends in large part on the health system's capacities, and that intergenerational equity requires that we look beyond deficit- and debt-related considerations to integrate protection of the organisational and epistemic capacities of Canada's health system. From that angle, one is justified in asking what impact an environment characterized by fiscal discipline, debt repayment, and tax relief might have on the future of Canada's health system. That is the question we will now address.

The Political and Economic Environment

Canada's recent history is marked by two major events that turned the country's political and economic environment upside down. The first escaped public attention. In 1991–2, international credit rating agencies downgraded the Government of Saskatchewan's rating several times in succession, to the point where the provincial government almost failed to meet its borrowing needs. This brush with bankruptcy was seen as a wake-up call by balanced-budget crusaders in the federal and provincial governments. The ensuing campaign to wipe out the deficit profoundly transformed Canada's budgetary and fiscal landscape. Under the pretext of 'fiscal discipline,' provincial bureaucracies were co-opted into advancing the political agenda of those who supported reducing the State's role in society through privatization of Canada's health system. The second event affected the vast majority of Canadians. In the referendum of 1995, 49.5 per cent of Quebeckers supported sovereignty. This brush with constitutional crisis was seized on by many as an opportunity to do battle with the defenders of provincial autonomy. On the pretext of 'national unity,' the federal bureaucracy was co-opted into advancing the political agenda of those who advocated a stronger central government.

Both of these political events facilitated the adoption of measures that, officially, sought to restore fiscal health with a view to strengthening, over the long term, the financial capacity of the federal and provincial governments to assume their functions adequately. In actual fact, however, the measures seriously damaged the financial, organizational, and epistemic capacities of the health system. To understand the serious implications of this climate of fiscal discipline, debt repayment, and tax reduction, it is necessary to shed light on the agendas that came out of these two events – the first originating in the international context and the second in Canada's domestic political situation. We will begin by discussing the international context before examining the substance and effects of the privatization agenda and of the stronger central government agenda.

International Context: Governments Faced with Fiscal Crisis

Government efforts at reducing deficits, cutting taxes, and paying down the debt must be seen within the international context of recurrent budgetary deficits and the growing public debt in all the industrialized nations. But make no mistake: economists do not all speak with one voice concerning the importance and potential effects of this situation. Indeed, in its report on fiscal discipline in the American federal system, the Advisory Council on Intergovernmental Relations (1987) indicates that normative discourse concerning deficits can be grouped into five schools of thought:

1 *The deficit is an illusion*, some economists argue. According to them, if the public sector used the same accounting rules as the private sector, the American federal deficit would become a surplus.
2 The deficit 'problem' is an illusion. The deficit has no significant impact on interest rates and inflation rates.
3 Large recurrent deficits represent a significant economic problem. But this is a recent phenomenon, resulting from the convergence of a number of political events, and the political system will likely solve this problem shortly through administrative changes, changes in the

majorities holding power, or pressure brought to bear by stakeholders and the public.

4 Deficits are a problem resulting from how the decision-making process is structured. Solving this problem requires certain limited reforms in the rules governing decision making.

5 Deficits result from a major structural defect that requires radical reform.

In this battle of rhetoric, it was the most alarmist positions that prevailed in the court of public opinion, the result being that in the 1990s, fiscal discipline and control of public finances became a priority objective in most OECD countries. In Sweden, for example, the 'rebuilding program' initiated in 1994, aimed at ending the cycle of budgetary deficits, reduced the overall level of transfers to households while at the same time increasing the tax burden. In the United Kingdom, fiscal belt-tightening has been one of the main factors affecting the shift in social policy in recent years. Switzerland and the United States also embarked upon a process aimed at balancing the books over the medium term, while the Maastricht Agreement saw the countries of the European Union pledge to limit their deficits. In most of the cases, the belt-tightening imposed a reduction in spending on social programs and, in particular, on public health programs. Indeed, these programs take up a large part of the budget, and it is often argued that restoration of fiscal health would be impossible without reducing health spending.

On this front, Canada does not stand out from the other OECD countries. The need, already recognized prior to the 1990s, to moderate health spending stemmed from both the convergence of outside pressures and from four internal factors:

1 The growing portion of the provinces' overall budget that is earmarked for health: the opportunity costs associated with such an increase translate into a reduction in the resources allocated to other public services such as education and housing.

2 The recession of the early 1990s reduced the provinces' fiscal capability.

3 The observation that a rise in health spending would not bring about a corresponding improvement in public health, especially when considering such indicators as infant mortality rate or life expectancy at birth.

4 Canada's ranking in relation to other countries in terms of health
   spending. In 1987, the OECD ranked Canada first for the volume of
   per capita health spending among countries with a public health
   system.

It is not surprising that, in a context such as this, those calling for
privatization of Canada's health system were able to gain visibility for
their agenda.

The Privatization Agenda

For all intents and purposes, the 1990s saw the federal and provincial
governments adopt a right-wing agenda. For one thing, they now
share the conviction that balancing the budget is an absolute priority,
and their experience in eliminating the deficit has convinced them that
they are able to impose this fiscal agenda. For another thing, they seem
to have gained the certainty that cutting taxes and paying down the
debt are essential to economic growth. The combination of these two
elements destabilized the health system by undermining its financial,
organizational, and epistemic capacities to the point where the system's sustainability is now in doubt.

The period between 1992 and 1997 saw a reduction in program
spending. In the wake of the scare experienced by the Government
of Saskatchewan in 1992, the federal and provincial governments
adopted one by one a series of draconian spending reduction measures
aimed at eliminating their deficits. The result: the combined deficit of
public administrations in Canada, which had sat at nearly $60 billion
in 1993, had completely disappeared by 1997 (figure 7.1). By 2001, only
British Columbia and Nova Scotia were still grappling with a significant deficit. Among the nineteen leading OECD countries, Canada rose
during this period from the fourth to the first quartile in terms of fiscal
balance. It is now one of the five countries with the highest annual
budget balance (Richards 2000).

The fiscal restraint that made this possible affected almost every sector of activity. In Quebec, for example, only the budget of the Ministère
de la Famille et de l'Enfance escaped the budget cuts of 1995–7. The
budget of the Ministère de la Métropole was chopped by 67 per cent,
the budget of the Ministère des Transports by 40 per cent, and those of
the Ministères du Conseil exécutif, du Revenu, et des Régions et
affaires autochtones by more than 30 per cent. Health spending was

Figure 7.1
Budget balance of public administrations in Canada, 1961–99

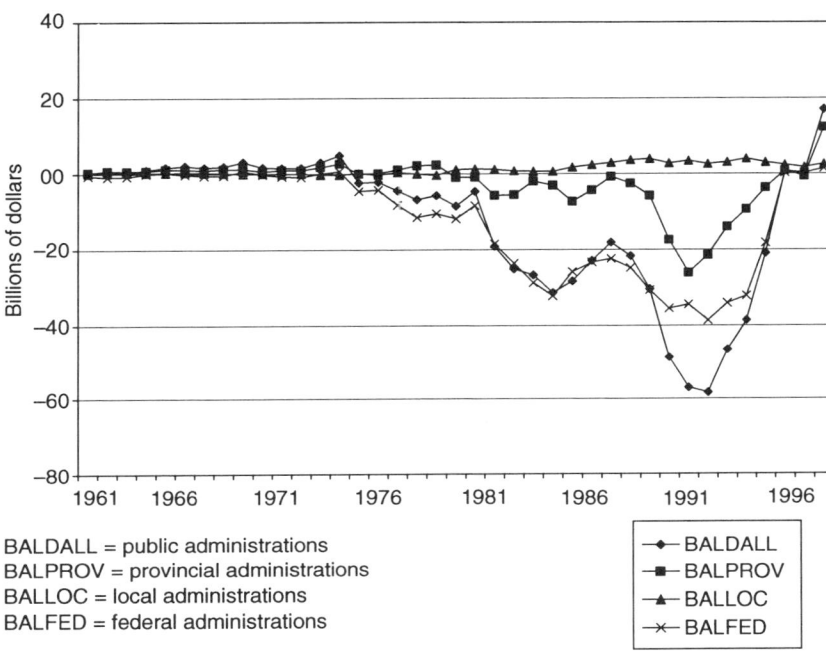

BALDALL = public administrations
BALPROV = provincial administrations
BALLOC = local administrations
BALFED = federal administrations

◆	BALDALL
■	BALPROV
▲	BALLOC
✕	BALFED

Source: Statistics Canada, CANSIM II Database, Matrices 6554, 6555, 6556.

cut by 4 per cent, or $521 million. In absolute terms, the other hardest-hit sectors were education (−$1,078 million) and transportation (−$621 million). A similar picture could be painted for most of the provinces during the 1992–1997 period.[2]

Not only did the governments in place at the time prioritize balanced budgets by slashing their spending, but they also imposed this priority on their successors by passing 'anti-deficit' laws – some of them Draconian. Starting in 1993, six provinces passed laws limiting the capacity of future provincial governments to introduce budgets that showed a deficit. Some of these statutes required balanced budgets annually, while others required balanced budget plans over the medium term. Some also included concrete measures to pay down accumulated debt. The Manitoba legislation even provided for penalties in the event of budgets that showed a deficit: cabinet members' annual salaries would be reduced by 20 per cent the year after the government ran the deficit, and by 40 per cent if the deficit continued. It also required that any income, sales, or payroll tax increases be approved by a referendum (Millar 1997). In short, a series of legislative measures lent weight to the idea that balancing the budget had become an absolute priority.

Thus, governments showed that they were capable of imposing the measures required to achieve their fiscal balance objectives. Because, even though the budget cuts caused considerable pain, they generated little in the way of public reaction. Massive downsizing in the public and parapublic sectors was met with barely a murmur from the unions. Compared with the 1970s, union mobilization was anemic. The nurses' unions in Saskatchewan and Quebec, which defied the provincial legislation, quickly fell back into line in the face of the provincial governments' resolve.

In addition to the budget cuts and anti-deficit legislation, Ottawa and all the provinces proclaimed tax cuts (Ort and Perry 1999), and most of the governments that achieved budget surpluses earmarked a portion for debt repayment. In other words, in addition to cutting their spending, government also reduced their revenues. The official rhetoric to the effect that the budget cuts were ad-hoc measures and that the attendant decrease in services was temporary proved to be less than truthful. Attacking government revenues made a return to previous spending levels difficult, if not impossible.

These fiscal restraint policies disrupted the health system by directly affecting its financial capacity to meet the needs of the public. Provincial governments' health envelopes had increased by an average of 9.7 per cent a year between 1976 and 1991. But starting in 1992, the provinces began to reduce their investments in health, such that between 1993 and 1996, their per capita spending on health declined year by year, from $1,700.90 per person in 1992 to $1,651.72 in 1996 (a decrease of 2.9 per cent). Starting in 1997, the trend reversed itself, but by 2001, health spending had yet to regain the pace of the increases it had seen from 1976 to 1991 (see table 7.1). The severity of these fiscal-restraint measures varied from province to province but all, with the exception of Newfoundland, saw their spending on health decrease in absolute terms. For example, Alberta reduced its spending by 8.9 per cent in 1994, standing clearly apart from the other provinces with a severity index of 17.7 points, situating it 2.6 standard deviations above the pro-

Table 7.1

Year-by-year changes in health spending by provincial governments, in current dollars per capita, by province (as a percentage)

	1976–91[a]	1992	1993	1994	1995	1996	1997	1998–2001[b]	Severity[c]
Alberta	9.7	4.6	-2.6	-8.9	-6.2	3.3	8.6	9.5	17.7
Saskatchewan	10.7	-1.5	-6.2	1.1	1.8	2.1	6.4	7.1	7.7
Nova Scotia	10.0	1.0	-3.1	-3.5	1.6	0.8	17.4	4.9	6.6
Ontario	10.0	3.4	-2.2	-0.6	-2.3	-0.4	0.6	6.6	5.5
Quebec	9.1	2.9	1.2	0.8	-0.4	-4.0	2.3	5.1	4.4
Prince Edward Island	9.3	3.0	3.4	-3.3	0.5	3.8	-0.1	6.8	3.4
New Brunswick	10.6	3.2	0.9	2.8	3.7	-0.2	-1.8	7.6	2.0
Manitoba	9.8	4.2	-1.1	-0.2	1.7	0.6	2.6	8.0	1.3
British Columbia	9.9	5.6	3.0	3.2	0.2	-0.5	1.5	7.0	0.5
Newfoundland	9.4	2.2	0.0	3.5	3.8	1.3	5.8	8.6	0.0
Canada[d]	9.7	3.4	-0.7	-0.3	-1.1	-0.8	2.6	6.7	4.9

[a] Average annual change for the period 1976–91. Calculated by the authors.
[b] Average annual change for the period 1998–2001 (the data for 2000 and 2001 are projections). Calculated by the authors.
[c] Restraint severity index: sum of negative year-over-year changes (as a percentage), 1992–7. Calculated by the authors.
[d] Weighted average, except for severity index.
Source: Canadian Institute for Health Information, 4 January 2002, table 10.

vincial mean. Newfoundland and British Columbia were the provinces with the least severe budget cuts during this period.

The budget cuts had a domino effect on the system's epistemic capacity (one of the effects being a dead loss of expertise through the early retirement of the most experienced nursing staff) and its organizational capacity (for example, changes in the roles and responsibilities of the remaining staff; decline in stakeholder motivation; numerous changes in organizational routines; restructuring; closing of hospital beds; shorter hospital stays; reduced access to operating rooms; structural changes in the decision-making process brought on by regionalization). In a nutshell, the entire organizational and epistemic capacity of Canada's health system took a direct hit.

This has cleared the way for the privatization of health care in Canada. As Yannick Villedieu (2002) points out,

> We have to ask ourselves in whose interest it is to devalue the public health system? Who stands to gain from systematically denigrating and depreciating it? We must find out who in the blazes could profit from what basically looks more like a plot or even an ideological conspiracy – the campaign for privatization – than a methodical demonstration of an inexorable failure of the public health system. (260, our translation)[3]

Budget cuts have thrown the system into disarray, bringing enormous pressure to bear on the quality and quantity of services. Tax cuts and debt repayment have limited governments' capacity to pump new money into the system in order to ease the crisis. The conclusion seems obvious: since the current system is not working well and governments lack the financial means to solve the problem, the health system must be overhauled, new sources of financing must be found ... in a word: privatization. This is how the agenda of the advocates of the health system privatization was implemented by the provincial governments, even though, paradoxically, it strengthens the hand of those supporting a stronger federal role at the expense of the provinces.

The Stronger Central Government Agenda

The provinces' intensive deficit-elimination campaign coincided with the trauma of the federalist camp's near defeat in the Quebec referendum of 1995. At the time, many felt that Ottawa needed to take forceful action to prevent this situation from recurring. The elimination of the

Figure 7.2
Financial funding of provincial social programs since 1957

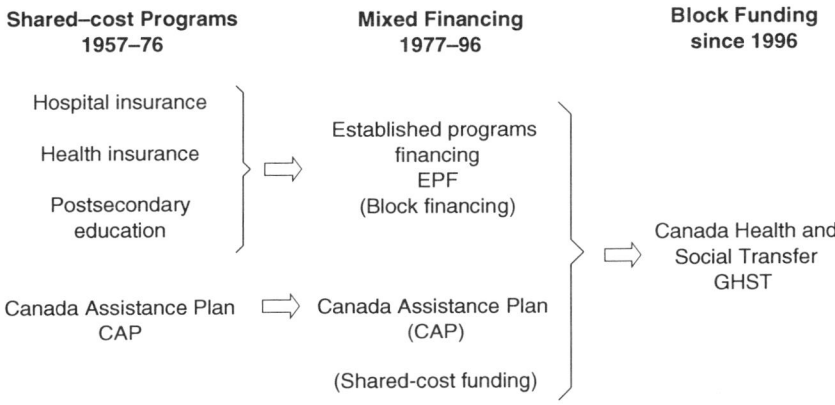

Source: Commission sur le déséquilibre fiscal (2001, 8).

federal deficit would give them the opportunity they sought, since a large portion of the federal budget consisted of financial transfers to the provinces. Reducing these transfers and changing distribution rules would weaken the provincial governments – not to mention improve the federal government's bottom line.

Ottawa's efforts to regain control over the growth in health and social spending are not new. Indeed, since 1957, the federal government has made significant changes in the funding of provincial social programs, changes affecting the structure of the transfers as well as the funding levels (figure 7.2).

The changes in the structure of the transfers were carried out in three stages. From shared-cost programs (in which the program costs were shared equally between the federal government and the provinces), there was a gradual shift to block funding (whereby Ottawa determined how much it would give to the provinces, irrespective of costs). When Canada's major social programs were created (hospital insurance, health insurance, income support, and so on), the provincial governments gave up part of their constitutional jurisdiction in the area of health and social services in return for federal funding. Thus, the programs' structures and content were defined in an agreement between the federal and provincial governments, with each level of government providing 50 per cent of the funding – Ottawa's share coming in the form of cash transfers to the provinces and the transfer of tax points. The sum of these transfers was therefore based on the costs of the programs implemented. This funding formula was reformed for the first time in 1976. From that point on, federal transfers in the fields of health and higher education would no longer be based on program costs but rather on a block transfer, calculated on the basis of the costs at the time.

Starting in 1977, block transfers were used to fund health and higher education programs, and funding for the Canada Assistance Plan was provided on a shared-cost basis. In 1996, a second reform of the system of federal social transfers to the provinces transformed the final portion of shared-cost funding into block transfers, giving birth to the Canada Health and Social Transfer (CHST). Ever since then, federal transfers for social programs have been determined by a decision made by Ottawa (and Ottawa alone) and no longer made on the basis of the costs of the programs. The law makes no provision for any formal cost-indexing formula or any mechanism for taking into account changes in program costs. Although the federal government's commitment was originally linked to the costs of the services rendered, this is no longer the case.

Changes in funding levels occurred more gradually. Federal health transfers amounted to 26.9 per cent of provincial health care costs in 1977–8. This share gradually fell, reaching 16.3 per cent just before the introduction of the CHST. The deep cuts accompanying this change brought Ottawa's share of the funding to 10.2 per cent in 1998–9 – a drop of 62 per cent over 22 years (see figure 7.3). During the same period, the total cost of health services in Canada in constant 1997 dollars increased to $87.24 billion in 1999 from $42.9 billion in 1978, an increase of 103 per cent.

The changes in the structure as well as the level of the federal funding for provincial health programs gave Ottawa more leeway and upped the budgetary pressure on the provincial governments. By separating its contribution from the growth in health costs, the federal government gave itself the power to set the level of its contribution. What a perfect opportunity for proponents of a stronger central government to weaken the provinces! The provinces bore the brunt of the budget cuts while Ottawa reaped the benefits in the form of healthy surpluses. In other words, the electoral cost of the fiscal restraint policies was not paid by the authors of these policies.

Figure 7.3
Federal health transfers as a percentage of provincial health costs

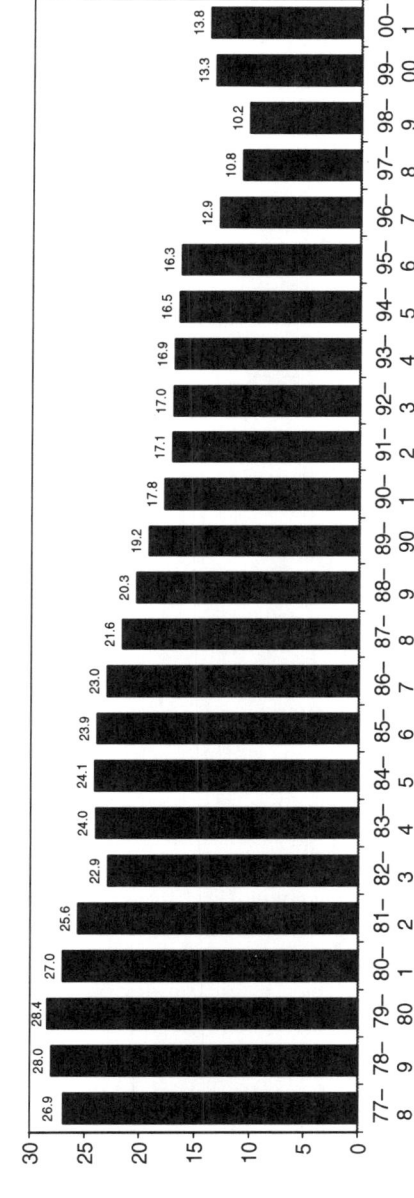

Source: Ontario Ministry of Health and Long-Term Care (2000, 19).

The verbal sparring between the two camps on the question of restoring the federal transfers to their pre-deficit-cutting levels is a good illustration of this. The big guns on the federal side insist that the federal contribution must include the value of the tax points transferred to the provinces over the years, thereby increasing Ottawa's share of health funding and reducing the shortfall, since the growth in the value of these tax points has more or less kept pace with the development of the economy. It seems clear, however, that the tax points' inclusion is nothing more than a rhetorical sleight of hand. If this truly must be taken into account to determine Ottawa's actual share, why stop at the fiscal arrangements of the 1960s and 1970s? Why not go back to the fiscal arrangements at the time of the Second World War, when the provinces undertook a massive transfer of their taxation power to the federal government? As then Ontario premier Leslie Frost pointed out during the federal-provincial conference of July 1960, shared-cost programs – like transfer programs in general – constitute a system by which Ottawa whets the provinces' appetite with their own money, money they lost since the Second World War fiscal arrangements (Perry 1997, chap. 14). Today, proponents of a stronger central government are using the budgetary situation of the provincial governments and the fiscal breathing room Ottawa created by cutting its transfers to the provinces in order to push their agenda, which consists in raising the federal government's profile with voters and providing federal officials with greater powers in the field of health.

The discussions concerning Canada's health system are set against an economic and political backdrop such that, in addition to the explicit agenda of health system reform to ensure greater efficiency, there are hidden agendas on the part of stakeholders who are pursuing a number of political objectives. First, there are the objectives of those in favour of dismantling the welfare state. These people want to take advantage of the health system reforms to privatize as much of the system as possible. Second, we have the supporters of stronger federal powers vis-à-vis the provinces. They too want to take advantage of the reforms, with a view to weakening the provincial governments and thereby entrenching Ottawa's hegemony in the Canadian political system. The direct impact of this dynamic is a weakening of the health system's financial capacities as well as its organizational and epistemic capacities to meet the health needs of today's generations and ensure the system's survival in the interest of future generations. From that vantage point, the sustainability of a public health system in Canada is by no means assured.

But at this point in our reflection, we have to stop and ask ourselves the following: How could fiscal discipline have served as the sole justification for such an attack on the sustainability of Canada's health system? Or, as a corollary to that question, How could the objectives of protecting the system's financial capacity have made us lose sight of the organizational and epistemic capacities? The next section is devoted to this fundamental question.

The Teachings of Economic Theory

The main threat to the sustainability of a public health system in Canada lies in the fact that we are overly concerned about financial capacity to the detriment of the system's organizational and epistemic capacities. In this section, we argue that to realize the importance of a system's organizational capacity, one must move beyond the prevailing economic theory (i.e., neo-classical theory) and embrace agency theory. And in order to take into account epistemic capacity, one must complement agency theory with convention theory. We therefore present the basis of each of these theories, as well as the approaches they propose to the question of sustainability of a public health system in Canada.[4]

Neo-classical Theory

The first characteristic of the neo-classical theory is its use of the postulate of substantial, calculating, and individualistic rationality of economic agents. The neo-classical theory is based on a second postulate, that of market coordination of individual behaviours. This assumption has four main implications: (1) individual decisions come together to form supply and demand; (2) prices adjust themselves until individual decisions become compatible in the whole; (3) the place where these decisions come together is the market; and (4) businesses, public organizations, or other aggregates of people are considered as individuals, each pursuing a sole objective. The consequence of this fourth implication is that we take no account of the relationships among the persons composing the aggregate.

Several analyses of the health system are based on this model. They present the patient as a consumer who 'demands' health services or as an investor who would like to increase his or her health capital; the doctor as an individual businessperson who 'supplies' health services; and the hospital as a business that produces health services in response to the 'demand' from doctors and patients, or as a 'bureau' represented by a bureaucrat looking to maximize his or her discretionary budget. This approach, which is the basis for recommendations aimed at privatizing health care, holds that the optimum allocation of health resources will be achieved if patients, doctors, and hospitals are allowed to choose the goods and services they want to demand or supply. Through the free interaction of supply and demand, the market would be able to produce an optimum set of health goods and services without waste.

The simplicity of the neo-classical theory and the conviction of its adherents that they speak the truth make it a very effective tool of persuasion. But the neo-classical model is not without its problems. One of these problems has to do with the nature of the market. The model assumes a market of perfect competition, which all serious observers agree is a fiction. Several alternative formulations have been proposed, but there is no consensus regarding the nature of the market. Another problem is that the autonomy of the demand is negated by virtue of the asymmetry of information between patient and doctor. As we have seen, it is the latter who determines, through his or her diagnosis, the nature of the demand. Demand is therefore induced by supply. In addition, neo-classical theory states that behaviours will be coordinated in the interplay between supply and demand through prices, which result from this interplay. But the decisions that engage the health expenditures are dissociated from financial responsibility, and the fees are administered by the State. So the role played by prices is greatly reduced.

Furthermore, considering the hospital as an individual actor (business or bureaucracy) conceals the fact that what is seen as the choice or behaviour of the hospital is not the result of a rational calculation but of the interaction between the members of these organizations, individuals who share neither the same interests nor the same information. The artifice of presenting the hospital as a unique entity conceals more than it reveals. Finally, defining in monetary terms the resources to be allocated focuses attention on financial capacity to the detriment of organizational and epistemic capacities. In short, the neo-classical model is seriously flawed and does not by itself suffice to guide public decisions.

When all is said and done, the applications of the neo-classical theory to health systems usually consist in 'highlighting, *in a pragmatic manner*, the inefficiency of the public sector in comparison with an ideal private sector, seen *in purely theoretical terms*' (Béjean 1994, 68, our translation and emphasis). In the context of the inevitable political adjudication between the various interests involved, this theoretical discourse often becomes an ideological discourse whose function is to lend an air of rationalism and 'truth' to the proposals of the privatization camp.

Agency and Incentives Theory

In response to these limitations of neo-classical theory, the agency (or contracts) and incentives theory proposes opening the black box and analysing what is going on inside of it while stressing that information is a source of profit for the person holding the information. The main way in which this theory parts company with neo-classical theory is that it abandons the theoretical fiction that the organization behaves as a single, profit-maximizing individual. The theory of agency and incentives is built on three postulates: (1) decisions are made in an environment of uncertainty; (2) there is asymmetry of information (certain actors control information); and (3) there is a divergence of interests among the actors (individual interests do not always coincide with the collective interest). On this basis, the relationships among the actors in an organization are seen as relationships of agency – that is, relationships in which one of the parties, the *principal*, delegates his or her decision-making power in a sector of activity to another party, the *agent*. The latter possesses information which the former does not. This asymmetry of information gives a major advantage to the agent, who can often impose his or her agenda by choosing what information to reveal to the principal; thus, he or she can hide information about his or her own behaviour. The principal might therefore doubt the effort that the agent will make to satisfy the principal's interests. This is what we call 'moral hazard.' The agent might also conceal information about the features of the health product (cost, quality, likelihood of accident), which can lead the principal into making bad decisions (choosing goods or services that do not meet efficiency objectives). This is what we call 'the risk of adverse selection.' By not revealing the 'truth,' the agent leads the principal into attempting to reappropriate the information, hence the issuing of incentive contracts that try to reconvince the agent to reveal the truth: performance contracts, bonuses or penalties geared to results, and so on.

In the area of public policy, the most important aspect of this theory is how it demonstrates that regulation of the public health system must not be based on prices or constraints but on incentives. The objective is to ensure that agents behave in the principal's interest, not because they are obligated to do so, but because it is in their own interest to do so. In fact, some health system reforms conform to the recommendations stemming from agency theory; for example, the introduction of budget allocation rules which reward managers or care providers on the basis of the outcomes of their actions. This is the most useful approach in terms of justifying the recommendations of the supporters of a stronger federal role. The federal government, as 'principal,' is entitled to exert control over the provincial governments, as 'agents,' to avoid the 'moral hazard' of seeing the provinces adopt policies after the fact that are inconsistent with its priorities.

But the agency and incentives approach poses at least three problems. The first of these problems is shared with the neo-classical approach: the 'heroic postulate of substantial rationality,' which requires of the actor a phenomenal and unrealistic calculating capacity (Simon 1978, our translation). Indeed, the effectiveness of incentive contracts is tied in with the principal's and agent's capacity to 'calculate' the long-term results of all the possible scenarios and to choose the one most conducive to his or her well-being. Human beings simply do not have the cognitive capacities needed to make such an assessment of their choices in terms of their results. There are at once too many uncertainties to gain an accurate understanding of the reality involved and too much information for the human brain to process completely, hence the necessity for simplification mechanisms.

The second problem is that the postulate of substantial rationality holds that self-interest guides all decisions and denies the existence of philanthropic, ethical, or equitable behaviour among the various actors. But we know that not only do these behaviours exist but they are also very prevalent in the field of health. If we exclude them from the analysis, we risk overlooking an essential dimension of a system's organizational capacity: eliciting conformity to standards.

The third problem is that the theory identifies 'good guys' and 'bad guys' in the organization. The 'agent' is the bad guy who refuses to reveal the truth and the 'principal' is the good guy who is only seeking the truth. The theory's positive applications are less likely to pose this problem, since they view all relations inside an organization as relationships of agency. Thus, the same actor – a hospital administrator, say – is the agent in the department-hospital relationship, but the principal in the hospital-doctor relationship. The normative analysis of agency does not always bother with these subtleties and is sometimes quick to identify a guilty party, an 'agent' (bureaucrat, physician, or even provincial government) who knowingly conceals information to serve his or her (or its) self-interest. When this type of discourse prevails, how can the trust and motivation at the heart of the health system's epistemic capacity be maintained? Three problems, then, which call for a new theoretical approach based on procedural rationality: convention theory.

Convention Theory

Convention theory is quite different from agency and incentives theory in that it rejects the postulate of substantial rationality in favour of procedural rationality. This makes it possible to take into account a patient's emotional rationality, a physician's adherence to a code of professional ethics, and equity as a founding principle of the coverage system for illness risk. It also makes it possible to take into account the knowledge acquired through the learning process inside organizations and the trust relationships on which this knowledge is based. All these characteristics contribute to a system's epistemic capacity.

The actor conceived by the conventionalist approach is neither *homo sociologicus*, whose behaviour would be predetermined by the norms and customs he or she acquired during the socialization process, nor *homo oeconomicus*, who would be completely motivated by a desire to maximize his or her own utility. This individual is somewhere in the middle. His or her behaviour is guided by convention rules – 'systems of mutual expectations of competencies and behaviours' (Salais 1989, 213, qtd. in Béjean 1994, 268, our translation). Conventions are meta-rules, some explicit and codified (e.g., codes of ethics or control processes by professional associations), others implicit and sometimes spontaneous (e.g., trust relationships, which often develop between administrators and administered in the budgetary process), which take shape over a long process of interaction among the actors in an organization and which serve as a 'collective cognitive device' (Favereau 1989, 1993, qtd. in Béjean 1994, 270, our translation), allowing for a saving of information costs. Given the flood of information submerging the members of an organization and their cognitive limitations, convention rules come into being to simplify the processing of this information by establishing routines and defining roles for the main actors involved. Thus, conventions are part of an organization's resources, since they increase its epistemic capacity (capacity to respond to uncertainty) and its organizational capacity because, built by a trust-based learning process, they strengthen its cohesion.

Convention theory, as applied to health economics, identifies two conventions at the heart of the health system: an activity convention, which regulates the State-doctor relationship, and a quality convention, which regulates the doctor-patient relationship.[5]

The literature on budgetary processes identifies a third convention, which is of particular importance when it comes to taking into account (as it does here) the budgetary environment: budgetary convention (Wildavsky 1964, 1975, 1988). This convention regulates the relationship between guardians and spenders of budgets within an organization by sharing responsibilities between them. The guardian looks after the budget as a whole to ensure that budgetary allocations conform to the rules of the organization, in particular those regarding deficits. By overseeing the budget, the guardian does not look after the services offered by his or her organization, because he or she knows that this is being looked after by the spender. Indeed, the spender is first and foremost concerned with the quality and quantity of services produced and offered under his or her watch, and he or she makes his budgetary requests accordingly, without any concern for the budget as a whole, since the guardian is looking after this.

Guardians have a number of reasons for limiting expenditures. If there is a deficit or mismanagement, they will be the first targets of criticism. Furthermore, their quest for power cannot be fulfilled by a growth in spending by their unit but by their control over other units' expenditures. Spenders have their own reasons to increase the quantity and quality of the services offered and therefore have reasons to increase their budget. It is easier to manage a growing budget than a shrinking budget, because it is easier to distribute additional resources to everyone than to have to choose who in your section will receive additional resources and who will not (or who will lose resources they already have). Furthermore, a section chief's prestige is tied in, lower down, with his or her ability to respond to the demands of his or her subordinates and, further up, with the share of the total budget he or she can obtain. Thus he or she will seek to increase the budget.

Trust is very important in the interaction between guardians and spenders. It is built on past decisions and, therefore, on learning. Without trust, guardians will impose strict controls, encouraging spenders to turn to other sources. Without trust, spenders will grossly overstate needs to ensure the minimum, encouraging guardians to impose stricter controls. Under the budgetary convention, then, responsibilities are shared between guardians and spenders for financial resources, control mechanisms, and sanctions aimed at dissuading potential abuses. As long as there is trust between guardians and spenders, the organization is saved the costs of non-cooperation, which are the costs of additional controls for guardians, lobbying, and searching for other funding sources for spenders.

Upon reflection, fiscal federalism in Canada can also be viewed as a budgetary convention regulating the relationship between Ottawa (guardian) and the provinces (spenders). As long as the actors share the responsibilities (the guardian looks after the budget as a whole and the spender looks after the quality and quantity of health care) and as long as there is trust between them, all of society is spared the costs of non-cooperation. From this vantage point, the agenda of the proponents of a stronger federal government risks breaking this convention and, as a result, adding to the costs of the health system the costs of non-cooperation. If fiscal federalism, as a convention, is not functioning properly, the provincial elite must devote a large portion of their resources (financial, organizational, and epistemic) to lobby the federal government or seek alternative sources of funding. When used in this manner, these resources are no longer available to develop reforms that can increase the quality and quantity of health services.

In addition, we should ask ourselves whether the five conditions provided for in the Canada Health Act (public administration, comprehensiveness, universality, portability, and accessibility) constitute a convention between the federal State and the Canadian taxpayers. Through this convention, the State identifies taxpayers' preferences (a health system that responds to these criteria) and the level of taxation they are prepared to assume. In exchange for compliance with the five principles of the act, taxpayers are prepared to pay the taxes growing out of their application. So long as there is trust between the federal State and the taxpayers on this question, the convention spares society the costs associated with the 'free-rider' risk, which would be generated by a lack of knowledge of the actual level of taxation that taxpayers are prepared to assume, and with the moral hazard to which taxpayers would have to expose themselves to learn the government's true intentions.

Taking into account the existence of these three conventions in the health system allows us to realize that contractual rules (which, for example, lead a doctor to reveal the information he or she possesses to the public authorities and patients or, in another example, tie a manager's salary to the attainment of budget objectives) and constraining rules (which introduce, for example, rationing that can bring spending under control) are effective to the extent that they do not threaten the conventions that exist in the health system. As pointed out by Béjean (1994), 'the conventions economy does not in an overall sense call into question the market economy nor the contractual coordination of individual decisions, but assumes that their effectiveness is dependent on these principles [conventions]' (296, our translation). The objective of expenditure or cost control must not be pursued to the detriment of the patient's, doctor's, or manager's interests. Or, put another way, financial capacity must not be strengthened to the detriment of organizational and epistemic capacities. The costs generated by a loss of trust between the actors in the health system could far surpass the savings that a series of rules imposed without regard to established conventions might yield.

Simplicity or Realism

Which theory should we choose? The standard, prevalent reply in economics is to choose the theory with the greatest predictive power (Friedman 1953). If we follow this logic, the unrealism of the behavioural assumptions is of little importance so long as the theory allows us to deduce hypotheses supported by systematic empirical observation. The greater the number of these hypotheses, the greater the theory's predictive power. This position is acceptable in the context of scientific research, but it is morally indefensible when it comes to applying public policy. Indeed, scientific research produces far more results that invalidate hypotheses than results that confirm them. For example, in their meta-analysis, Imbeau, Pétry, and Lamari (2001) showed that the 693 empirical results they analysed supported the hypothesis in only 20 per cent of the cases. And these findings deal only with results published in learned journals! Are we prepared to run the risk of this type of mistake in reforming the health system when we know full well that the basic assumptions of one theory are far less realistic than those of another? Applying the criterion of predictive power in choosing a theory with a view to informing public policy decisions is tantamount to experimenting on a population to validate the theory.

When the 'quasi-experiment' of the 'empirical test' (characteristic of social research) is replaced by an actual experiment on human subjects (characteristic of public policy), the criterion of the theory's predictive power must give way to that of realism when one must choose between theories that do not lead to the same recommendations. In the final analysis, it is not about choosing one theory and dismissing the others. Owing to the complexity of the social systems, we should make every effort to guard against this type of dogmatism, because the theories complement one another in that they each highlight a different aspect of the reality involved. If we limit ourselves to the conclusions of neo-classical theory, we risk overlooking an important aspect of the health system's capacity to respond to Canadians' health needs – its organizational and epistemic capacity.

Conclusion

Our examination of the sustainability of Canada's health system and the economic and political environment facing us today has led us to reformulate the question we began with, which has now become, How might the international context of fiscal discipline and the existence of two political agendas advanced by stakeholders in the discussions on reforming Canada's health system impact on the financial, organizational, and epistemic resources needed to respond satisfactorily to the health needs of today's and future generations? From the preceding discussion, five observations and five recommendations have emerged.

Observations

1 While necessary, sound management of the health system's financial resources is not enough to ensure its sustainability. Canada's fiscal situation over the past decade has led us to focus on financial resources. In doing so, we have often lost sight of the system's orga-

nizational and epistemic capacities. Only integrated management of all of the health system's capacities can shield us from pernicious, intolerable effects. Any change in financial management must be assessed on the basis of its impacts on the system's organisational and epistemic capacities.

2 Too much fiscal discipline can be counter-productive. When budget rules do need to be applied, they must emphasize as much as possible an incentive rather than a coercive approach. Coercive rules involve monitoring costs that are superfluous when agents have a personal stake in adopting the behaviour sought by the rule.

3 Trust is the cornerstone of the health system. Irrespective of the measures adopted to ameliorate the health system, the rules imposed to ensure improved efficiency must in no way undermine the trust that exists among the principal actors in the system: patients, physicians and other professionals, and managers; otherwise, monitoring costs will rise needlessly. The least costly and most efficient means of reforming the health system and ensuring its sustainability is to observe the conventions that link the system's main actors. Ignoring these conventions can only jeopardize the system's sustainability.

4 There are risks of disruption in budgetary convention in Canada, both within organizations and in federal-provincial relations. If we continue requiring budget spenders to play the role of guardians and to worry more about balanced budgets than quality of services, we run the risk of distancing them too much from their primary role, which is to improve the quality and quantity of care.

5 Because organizational and epistemic capacities are necessary to ensure the sustainability of the health system, it is essential to involve in the decision-making process specialists from fields other than economics and accounting (health specialists and social systems specialists). Increasingly, we are entrusting our accountants with the task of deciding the nature, quality and mix of services to offer, without asking ourselves if they are qualified to do so. With the best of intentions, they run the risk of weakening the system's organizational and epistemic capacities and thus setting it on the road to ruin. It would not be the first time that sorcerers' apprentices have created chaos while trying to put the house in order.

Recommendations

1 Ottawa must make it a priority to quickly restore its health funding

levels by earmarking budgetary surpluses for health before paying down the debt and cutting taxes. This will increase the system's capacity to respond to the health needs of the population.

2 We should unequivocally reaffirm the five fundamental principles of the Canadian health system (universality, accessibility, portability, comprehensiveness, and public administration) and continue to insist that the provinces meet these criteria as a sine qua non for federal funding. This will preserve public trust in our political institutions and in the health system.

3 The CHST should be the tool of choice for funding the health system, rather than the transfer of tax points. In this way, the federal government will maintain the leverage it needs to influence the evolution of the health system in the provinces.

4 We should encourage research on budgetary convention in health organizations with the aim of identifying the best ways of ensuring optimum allocation of financial resources without undermining organizational and epistemic capacities, and with the aim of increasing the trust of the managers and health stakeholders within these organizations.

5 We should support social research on the health system, in particular on the interaction among financial, organizational, and epistemic capacities.

NOTES

1 Recognizing this dual meaning, the Canadian Medical Association employs two different French translations of the term 'sustainability': 'En français, pour traduire "sustainable" dans le contexte du secteur de la santé, nous emploierons tantôt "durable" (santé durable), tantôt "viable" (système de santé viable). L'adjectif "viable" incorpore en effet les notions de durabilité et de développement' (2000, 1).

2 Bruce, Kneebone, and McKenzie (1997) published an interesting study on Alberta's experience of eliminating the deficit. For a description of the deficit elimination policy in Quebec, see Imbeau and Leclerc (2002). For a comparison of the experiences in Alberta, British Columbia, and Saskatchewan, see Imbeau (2000).

3 On the same theme, see Forest (2002).

4 Our discussion of the economic theories in this section is freely adapted from the writings of S. Béjean, whose insightful synthesis was of valuable assistance to us.

5 For a description of both conventions, see Béjean (1994), 272–85.

REFERENCES

Advisory Council on Intergovernmental Relations. 1987. *Fiscal Discipline in the Federal System: National Reform and the Experience of the States.* Washington, DC: Advisory Council on Intergovernmental Relations.
Béjean, S. 1994. *Économie du système de santé: Du marché à l'organisation.* Paris: Economica.
Bruce, C., R.D. Kneebone, and K.J. McKenzie, eds. 1997. *A Government Reinvented: A Study of Alberta's Deficit Elimination Program.* Toronto: Oxford University Press.
Canadian Medical Association. 2001. *In Search of Sustainability: Prospects for Canada's Health Care System.* Ottawa: Canadian Medical Association.
Commission sur le déséquilibre fiscal. 2001. 'Les programmes de transferts fédéraux aux provinces.' Montreal: Commission sur le déséquilibre fiscal. Background paper for public consultation.
Favereau, O. 1993. 'L'incomplétude n'est pas le problème c'est la solution.' Presentation to Cerisy Symposium, 'Limitation de la rationalité et constitution du collectif,' Cerisy, 5–12 June.
– 1989. 'Marchés internes, marchés externes.' *Revue Économique* 40(2): 273–328.
Forest, Pierre-Gerlier. 2002. 'Santé? La grande offensive des partisans de la privatisation.' In *Québec 2001 – Annuaire politique, social, économique et culturel,* ed. Roch Côté, 325–40. Montreal: Fides.
Friedman, M. 1953. 'The Methodology of Positive Economics.' In *Essays in Positive Economics,* ed. M. Friedman, 4–14. Chicago: University of Chicago Press.
Harrison, N.E. 2000. *Constructing Sustainable Development.* New York: State University of New York Press.
Imbeau, L.M. 2000. 'Guardians and Advocates in Deficit Elimination: Government Intervention in the Budgetary Process in Three Canadian Provinces.' In *Canada Observed: Perspectives from Abroad and from Within,* ed. J. Kleist and S. Huffman, 145–56. New York: Peter Lang.
Imbeau, L.M., and M. Leclerc. 2002. 'L'élimination du déficit budgétaire au Québec: Contexte et réalisation d'un engagement électoral.' In *Les engagements électoraux du Parti Québécois,* ed. F. Pétry, 67–81. Quebec City: Presses de l'Université Laval.
Imbeau, L.M., F. Pétry, and M. Lamari. 2001. 'Left Right Party Ideology and Public Policy: A Meta-analysis.' *European Journal of Political Research* 40: 1–29.

Millar, J. 1997. *The Effect of Budget Rules on Fiscal Performance and Macroeconomic Stabilization*. Ottawa: Bank of Canada.

Moreau, Y., M. Berthod-Wurmser, and Ch. Béchon. 1992. *Dépenses de santé; un regard international*. Paris: Ministère des affaires sociales et de l'intégration.

Ontario. Ministry of Health and Long-Term Care. 2000. *Public Information. Ministry Reports*. 'Understanding Canada's Health Care Costs. Final Report – Provincial and Territorial Ministers of Health, August 2000.' http://www.gov.on.ca:80//english/public/pub/ministry_reports/ptcd/ptcd_mn.html (January 2002).

Ort, D.L., and D.B. Perry. 1999. 'Provincial Budget Roundup.' *Canadian Tax Journal* 47(5): 1194–1213.

Perry, D.B. 1997. 'Provincial Budget Roundup.' *Canadian Tax Journal* 45(3): 451–72.

Richards, J. 2000. *Now That the Coat Fits the Cloth ... Spending Wisely in a Trimmed-Down Age*. Toronto: C.D. Howe Institute, No. 50.

Salais, R. 1989. 'L'analyse économique des conventions de travail.' *Economic Review* 40(2): 199–240.

Simon, H.A. 1978. 'Rationality as Process and as Product of Thought.' *American Economic Review* 68(2): 1–16.

Villedieu, Yannick. 2002. *Un jour la santé*. Montreal: Boréal.

Wildavsky, A. 1988. *The New Politics of the Budgetary Process*. New York: Harper-Collins Publishers.

– 1975. *Budgeting: A Comparative Theory of Budgetary Processes*. Toronto: Little, Brown and Company.

– 1964. *The Politics of the Budgetary Process*. Toronto: Little, Brown and Company.

PART III

THE SOCIAL AND LEGAL CONTEXT

8 Political Elites and Their Influence on Health Care Reform in Canada

JOHN N. LAVIS

There have been numerous and sustained calls for significant reform of health care in Canada. Commissions and task forces have recommended many changes, including service integration, user charges, primary care reform, and evidence-based practice (see, for example, for Alberta, Premier's Advisory Council on Health 2001; for Quebec, Commission d'étude sur les services de santé et les services sociaux 2001; and for Saskatchewan, Commission on Medicare 2001). The Canadian public began to call for large changes in the health care system in the early 1990s, which was significant given the many years of being generally satisfied with the system, unlike the citizens of many other countries (Donelan et al. 1999). But reform has been difficult to achieve (Lewis et al. 2001). In other countries, scholars and the media often identify political institutions – especially the many veto points at which opponents can kill reform efforts, coupled with powerful opponents to reform – as an important explanation for inertia (Immergut 1992; Marmor 2000; Morone 1992). In Canada, with our relative lack of veto points, scholars and the media are more likely to identify political elites as a reason for our lack of health care reform.

Who are these political elites, and how do they influence the prospects for change and for improved cooperation in bringing about change? The elites can include government officials at both the federal and provincial level who are engaged in constant finger pointing over health care, with federal government officials repeatedly saying to their provincial counterparts 'administer the system better,' and with provincial government officials responding 'give us the money we need to run the system properly.' Meaningful reform of any kind is difficult to achieve amidst such a dynamic, which some have called the 'politics of blame avoidance' (Weaver 1986; Pierson 1995). The elites can also include representatives from the dominant health care provider associations, especially physician and hospital associations (and more recently regional health authority associations), and representatives from biomedical industries and disease-based groups. Meaningful reform that involves these groups is perceived to be difficult to achieve without their support.

This chapter addresses the general question: How do political elites' interests and perspectives influence change in health care, either as barriers to or facilitators of change? More specifically, the chapter addresses the following four questions:

1 Which major reform efforts (both structural and substantive) have generally been supported by political elites, which have been opposed, and what explains these patterns of support and opposition?
2 Which major reform efforts (those in which change occurs and the nature of the change) have generally been most influenced by political elites, which have been least influenced, and what explains these patterns of influence or lack of influence?
3 How do political elites influence major reform efforts?
4` To what extent have regionalization and other approaches to integrating services altered whether and how political elites influence major reform efforts?

The chapter does not, however, assess the relative importance of political elites compared with other factors (such as public opinion, research knowledge, or political institutions) in their influence on health care reform; its goal is to shine a light on political elites as an important and often neglected factor in the dynamics of such reform.

Studying Political Elites

The influence of political elites on change in health care can vary dramatically according to the domain under discussion. For example, physician associations may be particularly influential when Canadian provincial governments are considering changes to physician remuneration mechanisms. Pharmaceutical companies may exert significant

leverage over changes to the Canadian federal government's prescription drug patent legislation. These political elites do not arise sponta-
neously, however, they are in large part created. Past reforms have
privileged some groups over others, and over long periods of time
groups acquire the knowledge, skills, and political resources to occupy
the position created for them (Pierson 1993, 2000). A physician association in a more market-driven health care system such as the United
States would exert little influence when health-maintenance organizations consider changing how they remunerate physicians. Similarly,
pharmaceutical companies would have little leverage in a country that
lacks a large research-based pharmaceutical industry.

This chapter focuses on the influence of political elites on possible
changes to the two core bargains that underpin medicare through the
Canada Health Act:

1 private practice for physicians with (first-dollar, one-tier) public (fee-
  for-service) payment (called the 'private practice, public payment'
  bargain by Naylor (1986)); and
2 private (not-for-profit) hospitals with (first-dollar, one-tier) public
  payment (the 'private ownership, public payment' bargain).

The payment features of the two core bargains are common to both
physician-provided and hospital-based services: cost-sharing is prohibited for insured services (which guarantees first-dollar coverage), as
is private insurance to cover these insured services (which supports a
one-tier system). Most Canadian physicians work in private practice
and are remunerated on a fee-for-service basis. Exceptions include
physicians working in organizations such as Quebec's Centres locaux
de services communautaires or Ontario's Health Service Organizations. Almost all Canadian hospitals operate as not-for-profit organizations owned by local communities or religious charities. Exceptions
include publicly owned facilities such as the now phased-out public
psychiatric hospitals and the for-profit cosmetic surgery facilities in
Ontario.

Studying the influence of political elites on real and proposed
changes to these two core bargains can provide a particularly illumi-
nating window into the politics of health care reform in Canada. These
bargains embody many of the core values that Canadians hold: an
aversion to people profiting from others' illness and an attachment to
allocating health care based on need, not ability and willingness to pay

(Mendelsohn 2002). These bargains also rule out some policy alternatives under discussion, such as user fees and a two-tier system for
insured hospital-based and physician-provided services, and the bargains would have to be re-opened before these policy alternatives
could be implemented. Moreover, these bargains influence the likelihood that seemingly unrelated policy alternatives will be adopted: service integration and major technology investments in primary care, for
example, are unlikely when many physicians continue to work as solo
practitioners in private practice.

This chapter adopts a case-survey approach to study the influence of
political elites on real and proposed changes to the two core bargains,
drawing conclusions from a survey of detailed case studies of particular policy decision-making processes that have been conducted by others (Gray 1991; Hacker 1998; Maioni 1995; Maioni 1998; Naylor 1986;
Taylor 1987; Tuohy 1999). The sampling from the pool of available
political analyses was conducted in two stages: (1) decisions in which a
core bargain was implicated were identified (for a total of six decisions); and (2) political elites that faced concentrated benefits or costs
in each decision (typically physician associations and hospital associations) were identified. Data about political elites' support for and
opposition to each of the six decisions, and their influence on each
decision, were then extracted from the political analyses. In doing so,
however, the chapter strives to recognize the dynamic nature of these
decision-making processes.

Two definitional issues arise from this approach. First: What constitutes a political elite when the analysis is focused on decisions involving the two core bargains? A group can comprise a political elite when
its voice is privileged in a debate about a change to one of the core bargains. Physician associations like the Canadian Medical Association
and their provincial counterparts clearly fall into this group (while provincial medical colleges, the profession's regulatory bodies, do not).
Hospital associations also fall into this group. But a group need not be
a stakeholder to be considered a political elite. The federal government
has responsibility as an overseer and partial source of finance: its voice
is clearly privileged in a debate about a change to one of the core bargains, so it too can be considered a political elite. For the purposes of
this chapter, provincial governments are not considered to be a political elite, however, because they constitute the final authority on physician and hospital services (as established by the Constitution Act,
1867). Provincial government officials are the decision-makers that

political elites try to influence. For both political elites and the provincial government officials that they are trying to influence, it is important to recognize that groups are not monolithic: physician and hospital associations and government officials, for example, are comprised of subgroups that may hold very different views than the dominant faction.

Second: What constitutes healthcare reform when the analysis is focused on decisions involving the two core bargains? For simplicity, the chapter uses the term health care reform to refer to changes to the two core bargains that underpin medicare (i.e., the core bargains with physicians and hospitals). Whether these changes constitute 'major' or 'meaningful' reform, a good outcome or a bad outcome, a likely possibility or a remote one, is left to the discretion of the reader. My colleagues and I have argued elsewhere, based on a historically grounded political analysis, that incremental changes probably offer more potential in the long-run for primary care reform given that such reform likely requires a revisiting of the core bargain with physicians (Hutchison, Abelson, and Lavis 2001) – a possibility that we considered unlikely at the time. But this chapter is about identifying insights based on an analysis with a longer time frame – a time frame that includes the decisions to create and entrench the two core bargains – and thus about identifying insights that can be used to inform whether and how to craft a new political bargain.

Political Elites' Support for and Opposition to Reforms That Implicate the Core Bargains

Five major decisions about Canada's provincial health care systems have implicated a core bargain (table 8.1). In three decisions that involved all provincial health care systems, federal government officials faced concentrated benefits (e.g., continued electoral office with a minority government in 1966) and concentrated costs (e.g., a substantial increase in financial obligations in 1945). In the three decisions that implicated the core bargain with physicians, the members of physician associations faced concentrated benefits (e.g., guaranteed payment for services provided by physicians in Saskatchewan in 1961 and across the country in 1966) and concentrated costs (e.g., lost income from extra-billing for physician services in 1984). Similarly, in the two decisions that implicated the core bargain with hospitals, the members of hospital associations faced concentrated benefits (e.g., guaranteed pay-

Table 8.1
Political elites' responses to major decisions and recommendations involving the core bargains with physicians and hospitals

Decisions[a]	Major elements	Response to Decision or Recommendation[b]		
		Federal government officials	Physician associations	Hospital associations
Health Insurance Proposal (1945)	• Failed attempt to introduce coverage for general practitioner-provided care, visiting nurse-provided care, and hospital-based care and (in later stages) medical specialist-provided care, other nurse-provided care, pharmaceuticals, laboratory services, and dental services	Weak support (relative to support in some provinces such as Saskatchewan)	Weak support	Weak support
Saskatchewan Hospital Services Plan (1946)	• Established (first-dollar, one-tier) public payment for hospital-based care • Enshrined the 'private ownership, public payment' bargain for hospitals	Neutral	Weak opposition	Weak opposition
National Hospital Plan (1957)	• Extended public health care regime to rest of Canada	Weak opposition then weak support (relative to support in some provinces such as Ontario)	Weak opposition	Weak opposition

Saskatchewan Medical Care Insurance Act (1961)	• Established (first-dollar, one-tier) public (fee-for-service) payment for physician-provided care • Enshrined the 'private practice, public payment' bargain for physicians	Neutral	Strong opposition (including a physicians' strike in 1962)	Not assessed
Medical Care Act (1966)	• Extended public health care regime to rest of Canada	Weak support (relative to support of coalition partner and to support in some provinces such as Saskatchewan)	Weak opposition in some provinces and strong opposition in Quebec (including a physicians' strike in 1971)	Not assessed
Canada Health Act (1984)	• Banned extra-billing by physicians (thereby reaffirming first-dollar coverage for physician provided care) • Entrenched the 'private practice, public payment' bargain for physicians	Strong support	Weak opposition in some provinces and strong opposition in Ontario (including a physicians' strike in 1986)	Not assessed

a Sources: Taylor (1987), Tuohy (1999).
b Sources: Gray (1991), Hacker (1998), Maioni (1995, 1998), Naylor (1986), Taylor (1987), Tuohy (1999).

ment for services provided by hospitals in Saskatchewan in 1946 and across the country in 1957) and concentrated costs (e.g., lost income from patients who could pay for a 'higher' level of care in 1957).

The one major proposal that was not acted upon would have generated additional bargains involving prescription drugs, home care, and dental care. Members of pharmaceutical company associations, nursing associations, and dental associations would have faced concentrated benefits and costs if this recommendation had been acted upon. Because these political elites did not face concentrated benefits and/or costs in subsequent decisions, however, the remainder of the discussion will focus on federal government officials, physician associations, and hospital associations.

Political elites' support for and opposition to reforms that implicate the core bargains have not remained constant over time. Federal government officials, for example, weakly opposed establishing the public payment bargain with hospitals *initially*, in large part because of concerns about its budgetary implications. But these officials came around to weakly support the bargain when Ontario's strong declaration of support brought to the fore electoral advantages that outweighed any financial concerns. Physician associations provided grudging support or at least muted opposition to the health insurance proposal in 1945 and yet they opposed all subsequent reforms that implicated the core bargains.

What explains the pattern in political elites' support for and opposition to reforms that implicate the core bargains? Political elites' positions appear always to have hinged on the circumstances surrounding these decisions. Certainly, any decision that would have (on balance) diminished the electoral or financial resources of a particular group, or threatened its autonomy, has typically been opposed by the group. The opposite also holds true: any decision that would have increased a group's electoral or financial resources or its autonomy has typically garnered their support. But a number of political analysts have concluded that political elites' positions are also influenced by other contextual factors, most notably by the strength of the forces supporting the core bargains (Hacker 1998; Maioni 1998; Taylor 1987; Tuohy 1999). Physician associations, for example, provided grudging support or at least muted opposition to one proposal that enjoyed widespread political and public support – the health insurance proposal in 1945. Given the limited opportunities for a veto in a parliamentary system with a party-government regime such as we have in Canada, once support builds for a particular decision it can become an exercise in frustration to oppose it formally (Hacker 1998; Maioni 1998).

A caveat: deducing political elites' support for and opposition to reforms that implicate the core bargains can be difficult for political analysts. The historical record can sometimes tell a very different story when groups like federal government officials and physician and hospital associations hold privileged positions in decision-making, as they do when the decisions implicate the core bargains. Federal government officials, for example, can convey their views informally through intergovernmental fora. Similarly, physician and hospital associations are often given the opportunity to participate in the decision-making process through 'joint management committees' in exchange for the information and expertise they can bring to the process and the compliance of their members once a decision has been made. This form of elite accommodation has been called a 'clientele pluralism' network (Coleman and Skogstad 1990).

Political Elites' Influence on Reforms That Implicate the Core Bargains

Despite the opposition to the introduction of the core bargains (and their entrenchment in the Canada Health Act) and the support in some quarters for these core bargains to be repealed, the 'private practice, public payment' bargain with physicians and the 'private ownership, public payment' bargain with hospitals remain intact. The majority of physicians continue to work in private practice and the vast majority of physicians have the option to do so. Almost all hospitals are private, not-for-profit facilities. Insured physician-provided and hospital-based services continue to be paid for by provincial health care insurance plans. Physicians and (to some degree) hospitals remain the fixed components of a system around which everything else is shuffled. By this I do not mean that the financial resources of physicians and the financial resources and autonomy of hospitals have not suffered over the last decade, but that the core bargains have proved remarkably resilient, in large part because of the influence of political elites.

Two groups of political elites appear to have most influenced both whether reform that implicates the core bargains occurs and the nature of the change (Gray 1991; Hacker 1998; Maioni 1998; Taylor 1987; Tuohy 1999). Federal government officials have been influential as a force for the entrenchment of the core bargains (e.g., maintenance of public payment for insured physician-provided and hospital-based services in the Canada Health Act of 1984) and as a force against proposed repeals of an element of the core bargains (e.g., introduction of user charges and thus a move away from first-dollar coverage of these insured services). Physician associations have also been influential as a force for the entrenchment of elements of the core bargains (e.g., maintenance of private practice and fee-for-service remuneration in the national Medical Care Act of 1966) and as a force against proposed repeals of an element of the core bargains (e.g., primary-care reform that involves a change in the physician-remuneration method from fee-for-service to capitation). Hospital associations have been far less influential, especially in recent times. Their influence was not even examined explicitly in political analyses of the Saskatchewan Medical Care Insurance Act (1961), the Medical Care Act (1966), or the Canada Health Act (1984).

What explains the pattern of political elites' influence on reforms that implicate the core bargains? Consider, for example, the changes recommended by recent commissions and task forces (table 8.2). Grouping the changes by policy category (following Lavis, Ross, Hurley et al. 2002) does not provide much illumination: 'big' policy changes such as regionalization were as likely to be implemented as smaller-scale policy changes such as revisions to scopes of practice. But identifying changes that implicate one of the two core bargains that have been studiously maintained for more than thirty years does provide illumination.

Federal government officials appear to have been most influential when the electoral resources that accrue from the 'public payment' elements of the core bargains were at stake. They have consistently rebuffed initiatives to increase the share of financing borne by individuals through out-of-pocket payments (i.e., user charges) or private insurance premiums and/or create a two-tier system for physician-provided and hospital-based care. Opinion polls clearly indicate that these initiatives would be unpopular with voters (Mendelsohn 2002). Not surprisingly, these officials have been least influential when the electoral advantages were not as clear-cut, such as with primary care reform that involves a change to physician-remuneration methods. While federal government officials created a transition fund to promote innovation in primary care delivery, provincial government officials have made the decisions about which models would be implemented and evaluated.

Physician associations appear to have been most influential when the professional autonomy that follows from the 'private practice' and 'fee-for-service' elements of the core bargain with physicians was at stake. For example, they have successfully opposed any primary care reform effort that would have changed physician-remuneration methods from fee-for-service to capitation (Hutchison, Abelson, and Lavis 2001). Indeed, the professional autonomy of physicians has suffered far more at the hands of private actors in the United States than at the hands of public actors in Canada (Grumbach and Bodenheimer 1990; Schlesinger 2002). Provincial government officials have been consistently unwilling to make decisions about reforms that might undermine the core bargain that governs their relationships with physicians. That said, these officials have certainly been willing to contain costs through a number of mechanisms that targeted physicians, which is likely the domain in which physician associations have had the least influence.

How Political Elites Influence Reforms That Implicate the Core Bargains

Political elites can draw on both their political resources and their financial resources to influence reforms. Federal government officials, for example, can speak directly to Canadians about the core bargains (a topic that many Canadians want to hear about), can control the agenda at Federal/Provincial/Territorial Conferences of ministers or deputy ministers at which the core bargains are discussed, and can take advantage of cleavages among their provincial counterparts on issues pertaining to the core bargains. Moreover, they can use the significant financial resources available to them to steer reforms that implicate the core bargains in the direction that suits them. Physician associations can also draw on a number of sources of influence. Their members, who are still viewed by many citizens as authoritative agents acting in their best interests, speak one-on-one with about 78 per cent of Canadians every year (Canadian Institute of Health Information 2002). Moreover, national and provincial physician associations have large annual budgets that can be used to pay for opinion polls and advertising campaigns. Hospital associations are in a relatively weaker position: their members have neither the professional autonomy nor direct patient contact that physicians enjoy and their budgets are a small fraction of physician associations' budgets.

Political elites can use their political and financial resources to influ-

Table 8.2
Changes recommended by recent commissions and task forces[a]

Policy category	Proposed policy change	Political bargain implicated?	If political bargain implicated, who could lose (gain) what?
Governance	Regionalization[b]	No unless hospital boards are replaced by regional boards	N/A
	Service integration[c]	Yes if it involves physicians or hospitals	Physicians and hospitals could lose autonomy
	Hospital restructuring[d]	Yes	Hospitals could lose financial resources and autonomy
Financial Arrangements	Change in public/private mix • Increase use of for-profit delivery (one type of privatisation)[e]	Yes if it involves hospitals	Hospitals could lose financial resources
	• Increase share of financing borne by individuals through out-of-pocket payments or private insurance premiums (another type of privatisation)[f]	Yes if it involves physicians or hospitals	Physicians and hospitals that treat poor (rich) patients could lose (gain) resources and federal government officials could lose electoral resources
	• Decrease share of financing borne by individuals through out-of-pocket payments or private insurance premia (e.g., pharmaceuticals and home care)[g]	No	N/A
	User charges[g-h]	Yes if it involves physicians or hospitals	Physicians and hospitals that treat poor (rich) patients could lose (gain) resources and federal government officials could lose electoral resources
	Two-tier[i-j]	Yes if it involves physicians or hospitals	Physicians and hospitals that treat poor (rich) patients could lose (gain) resources and federal government officials could lose electoral resources

Delivery Arrangements	Primary care reform with or without capitation payment for physicians[k]	Yes	Physicians could lose financial resources and autonomy N/A
	Revisions to scopes of practice[l]	No	N/A
Program Content	Evidence-based practice[m]	No	N/A
	More health promotion	No	N/A

a For reviews of the changes recommended by commissions and task forces in the more distant past, see Angus (1991) and Mhatre and Deber (1992).

b See, for example, Commission d'enquête sur les services de santé et les services sociaux (1988) on regionalization in Quebec; and Commission on Directions in Health Care (1990) on regionalization in Saskatchewan.

c See, for example, Commission on Medicare (2001) on service integration through primary care networks in Saskatchewan.

d See, for example, Commission on Directions in Health Care (1990) and Commission on Medicare (2001) on hospital restructuring in Saskatchewan, and Health Services Restructuring Commission (2000) on hospital restructuring in Ontario.

e See, for example, Standing Senate Committee on Social Affairs, Science and Technology (2001).

f See, for example, Premier's Advisory Council on Health (2001) on increasing the share of financing borne by individuals on physician-provided and hospital-based care through delisting services and charging variable premiums.

g See, for example, National Forum on Health (1997) on decreasing the share of financing borne by individuals on pharmaceuticals and home care through new national programs, and Commission d'étude sur les services de santé et les services sociaux (2001) on decreasing the share of financing borne by individuals on long-term care through a new long-term care insurance program.

h User charges are defined as any cost to the patient that varies directly with the amount of services used (the more services used, the more paid). Examples include a flat charge per service, co-insurance, deductibles, de-insurance, extra-billing, taxable benefits, and medical savings accounts.

i See, for example, Standing Senate Committee on Social Affairs, Science and Technology (2001) on two-tier options in Canada.

j A two-tier system is defined as a system that allows patients to pay extra for faster, higher quality or more comprehensive physician-provided or hospital-based care (i.e., more than just amenities).

k See, for example, Commission d'enquête sur les services de santé et les services sociaux (1988) on primary care reform involving alternative payment mechanisms in Quebec; Commission on Directions in Health Care (1990) and Commission on Medicare (2001) on primary care reform involving interdisciplinary teams in Saskatchewan; Commission d'étude sur les services de santé et les services sociaux (2001) on primary care reform involving family medicine groups in Quebec; and Premier's Advisory Council on Health (2001) on primary care reform involving alternative payment mechanisms in Alberta.

l See, for example, Health Professions Legislation Review (1989) on revising existing scopes of practice and establishing scopes of practice for new health professions in Ontario.

m See, for example, Commission on Medicare (2001) on the need for a Quality Council to facilitate evidence-based practice in Saskatchewan, and Premier's Advisory Council on Health (2001) on goal-setting to facilitate evidence-based practice in Alberta.

ence reforms in one of three ways. First, and least visibly, political elites exert their influence indirectly by engendering an anticipatory reaction (Lindblom 1982) on the part of provincial government officials (see, for example, Maioni 1998, 157). Political elites can be influential even when they do not formally oppose a reform proposal, and this constitutes an important and often overlooked type of political power (called 'the second dimension of power' by Gaventa 1980). Reform proposals may never make it past the consideration stage because provincial government officials anticipate opposition from political elites (called 'dominant structural interests' by Alford 1975) and do not feel they have the necessary political resources to take on this opposition. Second, and next most visibly, political elites exert their influence directly by voicing their opposition either publicly or behind closed doors. Third, and very rarely, political elites exert their influence by taking more extreme action: going out on strike. The latter two ways to exert influence have typically been the ones studied in political analyses, in large part because they lend themselves more readily to study.

Federal government officials have successfully drawn on their political and financial resources to help to create, entrench, and maintain the public payment element of the two core bargains. They have exerted their influence directly by voicing their opposition publicly as well as behind closed doors in, for example, Federal/Provincial/Territorial Conferences. But they have also reaped the benefits of these sources of influence in indirect ways: provinces are typically loath to propose a reform that implicates the public-payment element of the core bargains because they know that the reaction from the federal government will be hostile and the public will be generally supportive of this position. Exceptions to this general pattern do exist: Ontario and Alberta, for example, have sometimes acted under the impression that the electoral advantage to them of being seen to oppose the federal government outweighs the risk of engendering a hostile reaction.

Physician associations have also drawn on their political and financial resources, but in their case primarily to entrench the 'private practice' and 'fee-for-service payment' elements of their bargain with provincial governments. They too have exerted their influence directly by voicing their opposition publicly as well as behind closed doors in fora like the joint management committees that many provincial governments have established in conjunction with physician associations as part of their approach to elite accommodation. And they have also reaped the benefits of their political and financial resources in indirect ways: provinces have been hesitant to propose a reform that involves a move away from private practice and/or fee-for-service remuneration. Physician strikes have, however, been rare in Canada, with only one strike each in Saskatchewan, Quebec, and Ontario. These formal protests have never succeeded in reversing a provincial government decision and they have sometimes undermined Canadians' respect for physicians, and have thus risked physicians losing an important source of influence.

Service-Integration Efforts and Their Effects on Political Elites

Over the last decade a number of policy initiatives, many motivated in large part by a desire to integrate services, have had profound effects on hospitals. Most significantly, regionalization was accompanied in some provinces by the replacement of hospital boards with regional health authority boards. This change in governance altered a key element of the core bargain with hospitals: their autonomy as private institutions. In these provinces, hospitals remained publicly funded, not-for-profit facilities but hospital executives and managers now answer to boards that are accountable for the health of a geographically defined population, not to boards that are accountable for the role of a single facility in contributing to the health of a population from a (typically ambiguously defined) 'catchment area.' No comprehensive analyses have yet been conducted to establish whether this change in governance has led to different decisions about hospital services.

But even in provinces where regionalization was not accompanied by the replacement of hospital boards with regional health authority boards and in the one province where regionalization did not take place (Ontario), hospitals' autonomy was undermined. In Ontario, for example, a government-appointed Health Services Restructuring Commission made mock of many hospitals' autonomy through forced closures, conversions, and mergers. As well, the Ontario provincial government has appointed trustees to take over the administration of many hospitals, and has done so far more frequently than in past decades.

Unfortunately, no comprehensive political analyses of these hospital governance decisions have been conducted to determine whether hospital associations supported or opposed them. While hospital associations appear to have had little demonstrable impact on regionalization and the forms it took in different provinces, this would need to be confirmed through document reviews and interviews with political elites. Some hospital executives may well have supported a regionalization proposal given that it may have given them what they wanted: a larger remit (assuming that they were appointed to a comparable executive position in a new regional health authority). And while Ontario hospitals may have played a role in the Ontario provincial government's decision against regionalization, their autonomy was far from untouched at the end of the Health Services Restructuring Commission's mandate.

Similarly, no political analyses have been conducted on hospital associations' (or regional health authorities') influence on subsequent reform proposals that implicate the core bargains. Certainly, their purview does not include these domains. For example, hospital and regional health authority associations cannot consider new financing arrangements (e.g., user charges for hospital-based and physician-provided care) or new remuneration and delivery arrangements that involve physicians. And the hospital governance decisions over the last decade have, if anything, diminished further the potential influence of hospital associations on reforms that implicate the core bargains. While it appears that regional health authority representatives have emerged as a somewhat influential political elite in Quebec – where they have had several decades to acquire the knowledge, skills, and political resources to influence some aspects of the decision-making process – and the same is occurring in provinces that undertook regionalization more recently, the influence of regional health authority associations would also need to be confirmed through document reviews and interviews with political elites.

Over the last decade, a myriad of primary care reform pilot projects – many motivated in large part by a desire to integrate services – have been launched, albeit with little apparent effect on the core bargain with physicians (Hutchison, Abelson, and Lavis 2001). These projects have typically preserved physicians' autonomy by letting them choose whether and how they participate in a project and often by including a fee-for-service element in a blended remuneration method. Regionalization also had little apparent effect on the core bargain: physician services were excluded from regional funding envelopes in every Canadian province. Again, no political analyses of these regionalization decisions have been conducted to determine whether physician associations supported or opposed them, but the decisions were certainly consistent with physicians' desire for autonomy. Physicians, if not always hospitals, remain the fixed components in a system around which everything else is shuffled.

Physician associations' potential influence on subsequent reform proposals that implicate the core bargains appears little different after a decade of service-integration efforts. The primary care reform pilot projects and the regionalization decisions of the past decade have, if anything, confirmed the influence of physician associations on reforms that implicate the core bargain with physicians. The one change that may diminish this influence over time is physicians' work preferences, especially among female physicians who represent a growing proportion of physicians (Woodward, Ferrier, Cohen, and Brown 2001).

Caveats

This chapter addresses the influence of political elites that faced concentrated benefits or costs (i.e., federal government officials, physician associations, and hospital associations) in decisions in which the core bargains with physicians and hospitals were implicated. By design, it focused on what is a relatively 'closed' world (Berry 1989), albeit one that representatives from biomedical industries and disease-based groups can occasionally influence. Some groups, such as cardiovascular disease and cancer groups, may attempt to buy their way into this closed world by putting money into public-private partnerships. Other groups, such as HIV and breast cancer groups, may attempt to open it up so that they too can participate (called 'socializing conflict' by Schattschneider 1960). More often, these groups remain focused on other domains, most notably primary care (e.g., Hutchison, Abelson, and Lavis 2001), chronic care (e.g., Baranek, Deber, and Williams 1999), rehabilitation care (e.g., Gildiner 2001), and prescription drugs (e.g., Wiktorowicz and Deber 1997).

But the efforts of these political elites in other domains can have important spillover effects on the 'core' of our provincial health care systems. For example, recent research on the rehabilitation sector, a part of the health care system that has undergone a wholesale (and largely passive) privatization in provinces such as Ontario over the last fifteen years, has highlighted how a series of decisions made by a group of political elites – the insurers that provide automobile insurance, the employers that pay workers' compensation premiums, the for-profit rehabilitation companies that provide rehabilitation care, and the provincial governments and boards that regulate them – has created a second-tier of rehabilitation care (Gildiner 2001). This second tier is an option of last resort for individuals who did not sustain an injury either in an automobile accident or at work, and who cannot afford to pay the full cost of care (i.e., for many of the individuals who have been treated for acute injuries by physicians or in hospitals).

This chapter shines a light on political elites as an important and often neglected factor in the dynamics of health care reform. But their role can be overstated. Other factors, such as public opinion, research knowledge, and political institutions, also have a profound influence on health care reform. That said, we have a growing body of research knowledge about what works and doesn't work, and we have political institutions that offer at least the potential to minimize the capacity of narrowly focused groups to veto proposed changes. The question of how best to break out of our current patterns of engagement with political elites therefore warrants consideration even if these elites are not the sole influence on health care reform.

Implications

Based on this analysis, I propose three ways forward. The first way forward involves establishing a credible commitment between the federal and provincial governments about the public-payment element of the two core bargains. The most pressing concern for health care in Canada is the finger pointing between federal and provincial government officials that allows both to avoid accountability (and, when appropriate, blame). This finger pointing has existed for a long time but it has escalated in recent years with Ontario and Alberta provincial government officials' transition from problem-solvers to problem-makers within the federation. The result is the elevation of sectoral politics (where the focus of the entire policy community is on health care) to 'high' politics (where the focus turns to federal/provincial relations and health care is used as a political football). Meaningful reform of any kind is difficult to achieve when so much time is spent finger pointing.

A credible commitment between the federal and provincial governments should specify the 'public payment' elements of the two core bargains and any new bargains under consideration. For example, the commitment should specify whether (first-dollar, one-tier) public payment for physician-provided and hospital-based care will continue as specified in the two core bargains, whether public payment for prescription drugs and home care (as two possible examples) will be entrenched as new core bargains, the level or share of financing that the federal government will provide to provincial governments, and the nature of provincial governments' accountability for the performance of provincial health-care systems that federal government officials and the Canadian public can reasonably expect. Surely creative minds in federal and provincial departments of intergovernmental affairs can craft a commitment that ensures that the political benefits that accrue to both sides from a commitment are greater than the political costs to either side of withdrawing from or not supporting it. The time for blame avoidance is over.

The second way forward also involves establishing a credible commitment, this time between provincial governments and physician associations about the professional-autonomy element of the core bargain with physicians. After the finger pointing between federal and provincial government officials over health care, the next most pressing concern for health care in Canada is the inability of provincial government officials and physician associations to reconcile physicians' strong desire for professional autonomy (which does serve an important social purpose) and many groups' (including some physicians') strong desire for, say, organizational models that facilitate access to a comprehensive range of health care, funding mechanisms that provide incentives for team-based delivery models and evidence-based care, and technological innovations that will enhance the quality of drug prescribing. Meaningful primary care reform is difficult to achieve when the issue of professional autonomy is not given attention.

A credible commitment between provincial governments and physician associations should specify the proposed elements of a new core bargain with physicians. For example, the commitment should specify the organizational models within which physicians will work, the funding mechanisms through which they will be paid, the technology that they will have available to them, the working conditions that they can expect, the one-time transition costs that will be covered, and the nature of their accountability for the performance of the primary care system that provincial government officials and the Canadian public can reasonably expect. Surely creative minds in provincial health departments and in physician associations can craft a commitment that ensures that the political benefits that accrue to provincial governments match the professional and financial benefits that accrue to physicians.

The third way forward involves planning now to increase opportunities for and diminish constraints on the next round of health care reform by investing in training for new groups (e.g., nursing and home care associations) to acquire the knowledge, skills, and political resources to act as a countervailing influence on political elites privileged by past or current reforms. As physician associations have so well demonstrated over the last thirty years, groups can acquire the knowledge, skills, and political resources to occupy the position created for them. But given the long-standing lack of opportunities for other groups to contribute to discussions about reforms that involve the core bargains with physicians and hospitals, it will take proactive investments in training to help these groups catch up (Rachlis and Kushner 1994). Investments in nursing research and knowledge transfer funds, such as the one located at the Canadian Health Services Research Foundation, represent a step in the right direction.

Conclusion

Two political bargains, both in place for more than thirty years, have had a profound steering effect on Canada's health care system. Changes that would meaningfully alter the political bargain with physicians have not been successful. And changes that would meaningfully alter the political bargain with hospitals have for the most part been unsuccessful as well, even though hospital associations lost some of their already-limited potential to influence provincial government officials over this time period. With numerous and sustained calls for significant reform of health care in Canada, both from commissions and task forces and from the Canadian public, perhaps the time has come to act on what we've learned from past reform efforts. Doing so involves establishing credible commitments among the political elites who have much to lose (and potentially gain) by reopening the core bargains. To avoid such credible commitments will leave provincial governments where they've been for thirty years: reforming the 'periphery' of the system while leaving its 'core' (physician-provided and hospital-based services) largely untouched.

REFERENCES

Alford, Robert R. 1975. *Health Care Politics: Ideological and Interest Group Barriers to Reform*. Chicago: University of Chicago Press.
Angus, Douglas E. 1991. *Review of Significant Health Care Commissions and Task*

Forces in Canada Since 1983–84. Ottawa: Canadian Medical Association and Canadian Nurses Association.

Baranek, Patricia M., Raisa Deber, and Paul A. Williams. 1999. 'Policy Trade-Offs in "Home Care": The Ontario Example.' Canadian Public Administration 42: 69–92.

Berry, Jeffrey M. 1989. 'Subgovernments, Issue Networks, and Political Conflict.' In *Remaking American Politics*, ed. Richard A. Harris and Sidney M. Milkis, 239–60. Boulder, CO: Westview Press.

Canadian Institute for Health Information. 2002. *Health Care in Canada 2002.* Ottawa: Canadian Institute for Health Information.

Coleman, William G., and Grace Skogstad. 1990. *Policy Communities and Public Policy in Canada: A Structural Approach.* Toronto: Copp Clark Pitman.

Commission d'enquête sur les services de santé et les services sociaux. 1988. *Rapport de la Commission d'enquête sur les services de santé et les services sociaux.* Quebec City: Gouvernement du Québec.

Commission d'étude sur les services de santé et les services sociaux. 2001. *Emerging Solutions.* Quebec City: Gouvernement du Québec.

Commission on Directions in Health Care. 1990. *Future Directions for Health Care in Saskatchewan.* Regina: Government of Saskatchewan.

Commission on Medicare. 2001. *Care for Medicare: Sustaining a Quality System.* Regina: Government of Saskatchewan.

Donelan, Karen, Robert J. Blendon, Cathy Schoen, et al. 1999. 'The Cost of Health System Change: Public Discontent in Five Nations.' *Health Affairs* 18(3): 206–16.

Gaventa, John. 1980. *Power and Powerlessness: Quiescence and Rebellion in an Appalachian Valley.* Chicago: University of Illinois Press.

Gildiner, Alina. 2001. *What's Past Is Prologue: A Historical-Institutionalist Analysis of Public-Private Change in Ontario's Rehabilitation Health Sector, 1985–1999.* Toronto: University of Toronto Graduate Department of Health Administration.

Gray, Gwendolyn. 1991. *Federalism and Health Policy: The Development of Health Systems in Canada and Australia.* Toronto: University of Toronto Press.

Grumbach, Kevin, and Thomas Bodenheimer. 1990. 'Reins or Fences: A Physician's View of Cost Containment.' *Health Affairs* (Winter): 120–6.

Hacker, Jacob S. 1998. 'The Historical Logic of National Health Insurance: Structure and Sequence in the Development of British, Canadian, and U.S. Medical Policy.' *Studies in American Political Development* 12: 57–130.

Health Professions Legislation Review. 1989. *Striking a New Balance: A Blueprint for the Regulation of Ontario's Health Professions.* Toronto: Government of Ontario.

Health Services Restructuring Commission. 2000. *Looking Back, Looking For-ward: The Ontario Health Services Restructuring Commission (1996–2000) Legacy Report.* Toronto: Ontario Health Services Restructuring Commission.

Hutchison, Brian, Julia Abelson, and John N. Lavis. 2001. 'Primary Care in Canada: So Much Innovation, So Little Change.' *Health Affairs* 20 (3): 116–31.

Immergut, Ellen M. 1992. 'The Rules of the Game: The Logic of Health Policy-making in France, Switzerland, and Sweden.' In *Structuring Politics: Histori-cal Institutionalism in Comparative Analysis,* ed. Sven Steinmo, Kathleen Thelen, and Frank Longstreth, 57–89. Cambridge: Cambridge University Press.

Lavis, John N., Suzanne E. Ross, Jeremiah E. Hurley et al. 2002. 'Examining the Role of Health Services Research in Public Policymaking.' *Milbank Quarterly* 80(1): 125–54.

Lewis, Steven, Cam Donaldson, Craig Mitton, and Gillian Currie. 2001. 'The Future of Health Care in Canada.' *BMJ* 323: 926–9.

Lindblom, Charles E. 1982. 'The Market as Prison.' *Journal of Politics* 44: 324–36.

Maioni, Antonia. 1995. 'Nothing Succeeds Like the Right Kind of Failure: Post-war National Health Insurance Initiatives in Canada and the United States.' *Journal of Health Politics, Policy and Law* 20: 5–30.

– 1998. *Parting at the Cross Roads: The Emergence of Health Insurance in the United States and Canada.* Princeton: Princeton University Press.

Marmor, Theodore R. 2000. *The Politics of Medicare.* 2nd ed. New York: Aldine De Gruyter.

Mendelsohn, Matthew. 2002. *Canadians' Thoughts on Their Health Care System: Preserving the Canadian Model through Innovation.* Regina: Commission on the Future of Health Care in Canada.

Mhatre, Sharmila L., and Raisa B. Deber. 1992. 'From Equal Access to Health Care to Equitable Access to Health: A Review of Canadian Provincial Health Commissions and Reports.' *International Journal of Health Services* 22(4): 645–68.

Morone, James A. 1992. 'The Bias of American Politics: Rationing Health Care in a Weak State.' *University of Pennsylvania Law Review* 140(5): 1923–38.

National Forum on Health. 1997. *Canada Health Action: Building on the Legacy. The Final Report of the National Forum on Health.* Ottawa: Government of Can-ada.

Naylor, C. David. 1986. *Private Practice, Public Payment: Canadian Medicine and the Politics of Health Insurance 1911–1966.* Kingston: McGill-Queen's Univer-sity Press.

Pierson, Paul. 1993. 'When Effect Becomes Cause: Policy Feedback and Politi-cal Change.' *World Politics* 45: 595–628.

– 1995. 'Fragmented Welfare States: Federal Institutions and the Development of Social Policy.' *Governance: An International Journal of Policy and Administration* 8(4): 449–78

– 2000. 'Increasing Returns, Path Dependence, and the Study of Politics.' *American Political Science Review* 94(2): 251–67.

Premier's Advisory Council on Health. 2001. *A Framework for Reform: Report of the Premier's Advisory Council on Health.* Edmonton: Government of Alberta.

Rachlis, Michael, and Carol Kushner. 1994. 'Getting from Here to There: Strategies for Success.' *Strong Medicine: How to Save Canada's Health Care System.* Toronto: Harper Perennial.

Schattschneider, E.E. 1960. *The Semisovereign People: A Realist's View of Democracy in America.* Hinsdale: Dryden Press.

Schlesinger, Mark. 2002. 'A Loss of Faith: The Sources of Reduced Political Legitimacy for the American Medical Profession.' *Milbank Quarterly* 80: 185–235.

Standing Senate Committee on Social Affairs, Science and Technology. 2001. *The Health of Canadians: The Federal Role. Interim Report.* Volume 4: *Issues and Options.* Ottawa: Government of Canada.

Taylor, Malcolm G. 1987. *Health Insurance and Canadian Public Policy: The Seven Decisions That Created the Canadian Health Insurance System and Their Outcomes.* Kingston: McGill-Queen's University Press.

Tuohy, Carolyn J. 1999. *Accidental Logics: The Dynamics of Change in the Health Care Arena in the United States, Britain, and Canada.* New York: Oxford University Press.

Weaver, R. Kent. 1986. 'The Politics of Blame Avoidance.' *Journal of Public Policy* 6: 371–98.

Wiktorowicz, Mary, and Raisa Deber. 1997. 'Regulating Biotechnology: A Rational-Political Model of Policy Development.' *Health Policy* 40(2): 115–38.

Woodward Christel A., Barbara Ferrier, May Cohen, and Judy Brown. 2001. 'Professional Activity: How Is Family Physicians' Work Time Changing?' *Canadian Family Physician* 47: 1414–21.

9 Creating a More Democratic Health System: A Critical Review of Constraints and a New Approach to Health Restructuring

STEPHEN TOMBLIN

The twenty-first century opens with a fresh challenge for Canada's health care system. In response, academics and decision-makers are spending much effort and time conceptualizing and theorizing about two closely related issues: the benefits of public participation in the planning and implementation of health care services; and how we can go from 'here to there' to create a more open, democratic, and effective health system in an era when globalization, corporate concentration, and efficiency concerns are a high priority and the nation-state itself is being questioned from both above and below. These revolutionary changes that are taking place have posed a number of dilemmas for a country that has, in the past, relied upon health policy for the purposes of reinforcing a common sense of national identity and citizenship.

The dichotomous nature of the health restructuring debate and effort to balance competing objectives has made it difficult to advance new approaches. As one would expect, this has created problems as well as challenges for an already complex decision-making structure well known for its ideological diversity and territorial competitiveness. Four key issues need to be addressed in discussions over the future of health and health services in Canada. First, the advantages and disadvantages of public participation. Second, the different forms of public participation that have emerged. Third, the extent to which these forms of democratic engagement and accountability have made it possible for citizens to shape the values and direction of the health care system. Fourth, what can be done to sustain or encourage new levels of inclusion and participation.

The purpose of this chapter is to provoke discussion on the various constraints and contradictions that have worked against public involvement in health policymaking. The intent is to first provide a better understanding of why this has occurred and why this poses a problem for reformers hoping to achieve both health care reform and increased democratization. Emphasis is placed on exploring why public participation is important to the system, what has been accomplished, and what can be done to further enhance or encourage a more citizen-based approach to health policy.

Context

During this period of health care restructuring, old assumptions, visions, and organizations upon which our health governance system is based are being questioned and contested by critics. As a result of a broader understanding of the determinants of health, there has been growing pressure to change the Canadian health system. Even though reformers agree that new approaches are required, there are different models competing for power and public support. By nature, paradigm shifts are not smooth processes. Whether regime shifts occur depends on a number of factors, including the strength of the old Canadian policy regime and who controls the discourse.

A common challenge for reformers is the strength and autonomy of the old system of governance being contested. Changing citizen expectations or the behaviour of the policy actors is never easily accomplished so long as the old system remains institutionalized and rewards old patterns of behaviour. This essay is reflective and assumes that there is a need to understand the game we have built first before we can begin to assess the prospects for launching new health strategies. If we are committed to deal with a variety of new health challenges in a more participatory way, we should begin by analysing the policy context and the barriers to structural change. The traditional reliance that has been placed in the health system of governance upon market mechanisms as well as the medical pressure groups which have operated as 'agents of government' also need to be brought into the mix.

There are different views on whether the status quo is adequate, or whether there is a need for a different conceptualization of health, health delivery systems, scopes of practice, and ways to measure outcomes of interest. These debates involve value and political judgments and the system we have constructed has both systematic biases and means for defending itself. There are very different critiques and divergence of views on health issues and the kind of reforms required to address these.

For decades, health promotion advocates have presented a convincing argument that since social determinants of health matter more to the health of the population than biomedical services, it is only logical that new strategies and mechanisms replace outdated ones (Lalonde 1974). These efforts to establish a more 'people-centred,' community-based approach to health have been hampered by historical institutional arrangements and the competing elite (Raeburn and Rootman 1998). These researchers are highly critical of the monopoly of the medical profession and a health system that was never designed or intended to allow citizens and communities to directly participate in the creation of new forms of knowledge and dissemination required for addressing the social nature of disease. The population health approaches are concerned with social determinants of health and are aimed at planning health services based on the needs of the population. This is a more quantitative approach.

These various paradigms, which assume that direct public participation will improve the design and delivery of health services, have attracted much attention. They have played their part in legitimizing and mobilizing reform-seeking groups and politicians dedicated to their cause. However, competition between these approaches (despite various efforts to merge them) has complicated the quest of seeking a more participatory framework on determinants of health (Hayes 1999; Frohlich 1999; Beatie 1995; Federal, Provincial and Territorial Advisory Committee on Population Health 1994).

Furthermore, in other academic and political circles there is interest in reducing the role of the State, and particularly the national State. It is clear there are mixed motives and objectives in this fundamental struggle to control the future.

Currently in Canada there are divergent views on problem identification and the necessary changes required. In Alberta, British Columbia, and Ontario, for example, the provincial governments appear to be more concerned with fiscal realities and cost reduction than providing support for a failing public system. As a result, they are defining the crisis differently and have a more decentralized, market-oriented model in mind for restructuring. In Quebec, there would likely be less support than in Atlantic Canada for any approach calling for strengthening of the centre and increasing Ottawa's spending power. These ideological-territorial battles over redistribution through the Canadian welfare state are not new, but provide critical insights for understanding the different responses to the health crisis.

During the days of the Rowell-Sirois Commission and the Second National Policy, Ottawa assembled a group of experts who relied upon Keynesian assumptions about economic and social development to legitimize a push for a regime change that was supported by poor provinces but also 'threatened the economic and political powers of Alberta, Ontario, Quebec, and British Columbia' (Tomblin 1995, 34). The commission succeeded because it created a powerful national myth and then mobilized an influential coalition in support of a new common set of Canadian values and institutions. This was an important watershed in our history since it helped Canadians define themselves as different from Americans. This kind of vision has had less support in certain provinces and ideological circles. As a result, once in place, there was little political incentive to change it or open up Pandora's box, even when circumstances changed. Because the new approach became a symbol of national pride and not just a way to define and solve health problems, it later posed a dilemma for reformers.

The political right agrees with the assumptions of health-promotion reformers that there would be benefits associated with decentralizing power and making communities more responsible for health issues. Yet more attention is placed on the need to eliminate expensive State bureaucracies and cut costs. While both the political Left and Right see the value of these kinds of changes, the critiques presented to the public have been very different. Despite an apparent consensus on the merits of increased public participation, these deeply embedded historical divisions and dissimilar models of civic engagement have likely complicated the task of mobilizing the kind of public support required to effect change.

In this contest over ideas, public opinion can be an important catalyst for change. Yet, given the existing power and autonomy of the current system of governance with its well deserved reputation for elitism, behind the scenes approach to interest group politics, and concentrated executive-corporate power, it would be a mistake to assume that public opinion will necessarily determine the future direction of the health care system (Savoie 1999; Pross 1993). Plebiscitarianism and the concept of direct democracy is a popular idea for those who believe that the culture and health needs of Canadian society have changed, but even if this is true, our institutional system was never designed as a republic. Institutionally speaking, public opinion was never intended to determine policy and political outcomes in Canada. Consequently, there is a need for a more institutional or neo-institutional approach to the challenges of health restructuring.

Health reform cannot be viewed in isolation. Rather, it should be seen as part of a much larger ideological-territorial debate. Governments are being pressured from both above and below, and there are new voices calling for the weakening of the nation-state and the strengthening of continentalism and the role of subnational governments (Tomblin 1995). In provinces like Alberta, Quebec, Ontario, and British Columbia, alternative market-centred models and continental visions are now being conceptualized and debated in the health and other policy fields.

In Alberta, the Klein government hired Don Mazankowski to complete an analysis and a new health vision for the future (Alberta 2002). These reforms, which are the result of ideological-territorial struggle, will, when implemented, increase reliance placed on the private sector in the delivery of health services in that province but will also be used to pressure other provinces to adopt similar practices. The likelihood of this occurring depends on the capacity to develop new models or contest the ideas defended by the right. Real power comes from controlling public knowledge and forms of dissemination. The Alberta, Ontario, or more recent British Columbia visions of health naturally compete with more nation-centred, equity-focused approaches by the Atlantic provinces, Saskatchewan, and Manitoba. In the end, whether changes occur or not (and the direction these will eventually take) will ultimately depend on the sense that there is a policy crisis, the governance and decision-making processes involved, and the extent to which the general public is well informed. Much of this will also depend on the ideas that are presented and the way these debates are organized for public consumption. The public needs to be informed that there are a variety of options from which to choose, and not be bullied by right-wing critics, who may claim that there is no choice but the status quo and a private system, for example.

In the past, despite modernization theory and all the predictions about the inevitability of centralization, Canada continued to carve out a more decentralized path. In an era of globalization when there are predictions about the unsustainability and decline of the nation-state and associated policies, Canadians need to recognize that we can again make our own choices, but based on our own values, forms of public innovation, and evidenced-based knowledge.

Whether Canadian society buys into a new vision of public health will depend very much on the opportunities for a good debate. Despite much rhetoric about the need for civic engagement, Milner (2001) provides much evidence that civic literacy and political knowledge is not increasing in Canada. Understandably, democratic processes, forms of dissemination, and public institutions are important since they do play a critical role in deciding who participates and how issues are framed. Most citizens operate at the margin of politics and express themselves only occasionally, either through surveys or voting every few years.

Canada is not unique in feeling pressured to change. Jurisdictions and health systems around the world are being challenged both above and below. Globalization, new forms of communication dissemination, the rise of international organizations, and other factors have all played their role in supporting new conceptions of community and health. This has come in the form of new theories on social cohesion; external pressures for primary health care; grass-roots demands for increased control and participation in setting priorities for the health system, as well as new knowledge and evidence that social and economic conditions contribute more to our health status than medical care does (World Health Organization 1977, 1986). These democratizing pressures have both a domestic and international component (Commonwealth Foundation 1999; Wyman, Shulman, and Ham 2000).

In the current context, a number of Canadian citizens are not well-informed on contemporary health issues or new approaches. As a result, they continue to identify with the old regime. This naturally has created a number of dilemmas and contradictions for health reformers because some of the possible new remedies being proposed are considered to be unthinkable and unnegotiable.

Since various citizens accept the notion that the national Medicare system is what defines us as Canadians, it is little wonder that reforming the system has proven to be difficult. These kinds of issues have not received enough attention in the debate over health restructuring, and new calls for more direct public participation, which are popular with health reformers but also for the supporters of the Reform-Alliance Party, are being heard. They do, however, help explain the kind of political dilemmas that have been created and why bringing about a regime change has posed so many problems. These dilemmas also help us to better understand why the national government and others who benefit from the old regime would be motivated to perpetuate these old myths and refuse to give up control over the discourse, despite structural problems within the system.

Regime Changes

As illustrated by Peter Hall, the institutional-political context and rules and practices of the existing polity are important for understanding patterns of public opinion, institutionalized networks of policy innovation and learning, and also for determining whether new visions or theories are administratively and politically viable. Answering these kinds of questions requires knowing more about the structures, democratic practices, and dissemination processes that have been relied upon to define and solve problems and how these, in turn, have shaped political and policy outcomes, as well as reform processes (Hall 1989). Hence, assessing the extent to which there is likely to be increased public participation in the planning and/or delivery of programs in the near future (as advocated by various reformers) will ultimately depend on the strength of governance structures and decision-making practices.

As illustrated by Neil Bradford in Canada, our federal cabinet-parliamentary institutions and party/interest-group systems have not been effective catalysts for innovation. Nor have they been effective instruments for initiating new debates or mobilizing the kind of new coalitions required for institutionalizing new reforms. As a result, there has been a long history of relying on experts in Royal Commissions to fill this institutional gap (Bradford 1998). Therefore, whether a more people-centred health vision emerges in Canada or not will be greatly influenced by who controls the discourse and the strength of the old policy regime. Even though public opinion is important to any discussion on health reform, we also need to consider established political processes and traditions and the extent to which new models of civic engagement threaten or are compatible with these.

A major problem with the debate over revitalizing the health system is that it is dominated by various myths that have been politically constructed. For example, the idea of a publicly financed, integrated system where all Canadians have equal access to the same essential services at equal costs is largely a myth, but a convenient one. While various services are being privatized or delisted, many others like home care, dental, or pharmacare have never been fully covered by medicare or regulated by the Canada Health Act. Besides, depending on where you live in the country, the kinds of services available are not the same. Another powerful myth is the idea that biomedical services contribute most to our health status. These contradictions between 'myth' and 'reality' create public confusion and an opportunity and incentive for reformers to pressure for change. Despite this, these various myths do resonate with most Canadians and are a reflection of the old monopoly powers and institutions that we have relied upon to generate research and deliver programs. Under such circumstances, bringing about structural change has been difficult, despite much evidence that a more democratic, social-determinants approach would bring substantial health benefits.

The tendency has been for governments to respond to a difficult situation by 'blaming the other guy,' and defending the old monopolies and interests that they either inherited or relied upon to seize power in the first place. As in the past, our political institutions have proven incapable of advancing or championing new policy ideas on their own. This dangerous political game between Ottawa and the provinces has itself become a political problem and, as in the past, the solution has come in the form of a federal Royal Commission (Tomblin 1995, chap. 2; Bradford 1998, chap. 1). Predictably, the provinces have responded by having their own hired guns working on government-sponsored studies.

As a consequence of these developments, a number of Canadians have become increasingly cynical and frustrated with a system that provides little opportunity to take ownership of an issue that they care about. The only thing they can do is wait for the next government study, observe how the media responds, operate at the margins, and, if there is an opportunity, vote for or against the governing party.

Ironically, at a time when we are experiencing policy failure and there is a clear need for new approaches and more debate, the defenders of the old national paradigm appear to have little political incentive to frame these issues differently. Structural change does not always come easily (when circumstances change) because old, inherited, overlapping, societal and State traditions make it very difficult to change direction. According to the logic of neo-institutional thinking, our complex and divided federal system makes it possible for old identities, visions, and boundaries to survive and it limits what can be achieved, even when conditions change. This model offers critical insights for understanding the significance of inherited policy regimes and how these complicate any drive for structural change. According to Cairns (1995), 'We must learn to think in terms of politicized societies caught in webs of interdependencies with the state, and we must think of the latter as the embedded state tied down by multiple linkages with society, which restrains its manoeuverability' (33).

Public Attitudes

Canadians have often been characterized as more elitist, conservative, and less entrepreneurial than Americans (Lipset 1990). Such characterizations tend to play down the different regional subcultures and dialects that divide the nation or the recent impact of the Charter and other trends on Canadian culture (Cairns 1992). Even though there were always regional differences, historically speaking, most Canadians have come to identify with and support the concept of a publicly financed, socialized system of medicine.

With the democratization of various health services (beginning in Saskatchewan in the 1940s), the general public supported the notion of a public, universal system, despite the fact the system was never entirely public. The five principles specified in the Canada Health Act in the 1980s also struck a chord with voters and reflected the way most Canadians felt about health issues. Pierre Trudeau used this legislation to defend his pan-Canadian vision against continentalism, province-building, and Quebec nationalism.

In the past, despite the politically significant regional differences displayed by different provinces in the heated political battle that took place over the Second National Policy (1940s–70s) and pitted Ontario, Quebec, British Columbia, and Alberta against the central government and the have-not provinces, once the intense battle was over and the new policy regime was institutionalized, things did gradually settle down (Tomblin 1995, chap. 2). Naturally, there was little incentive to reopen the debate.

With the rise of free trade in the late 1980s (and the abandoning of the very idea of national policies during the days of the Macdonald Commission that helped spawn a new continental era) and the rise of more right-wing research institutes, there was a new opportunity for Ontario, Alberta, Quebec, and British Columbia to again defend a more decentralized, North American, neo-liberal vision. The strategy of aggressively pushing the health issue into the country's public discourse really only gained momentum in the late 1990s, a period of national crisis, public debt, neo-liberalism and increasing global-continental trade.

Health care became the dominant political issue during 1997 federal election (O'Reilly 2001, 18). As O'Reilly demonstrates, '[B]oth the federal and provincial/territorial governments were associated with grand vision statements during the second half of the 1990's' (21). The Ottawa-sponsored National Forum on Health provided another opportunity to make the case that principles and values associated with medicare still mattered.

There was a need for a new public discourse, and Ottawa had to respond to globalization and the fiscal imperative. Governments, in pursuing their goals, are often forced to deal with competing objectives and it has proved politically convenient to keep these debates in separate boxes. This helps to explain some of the ambiguity and slipperiness associated with public opinion, the aggressive style of federal-provincial sparring (shifting blame), and inconsistent, at times contradictory, government policies that have emerged. The federal government responded to this dilemma by supporting the principles of medicare, making cut-backs, and then blaming the provinces for mismanaging the system. With the provinces and political opposition divided, it proved to be an effective political strategy for the Liberal government, even if it did little to improve the overall health system. It also did much damage to federal-provincial relations. This intense, elite-dominated, insular, ideological-territorial competition has made it very difficult to bring Canadians together into the process of debating and reconstructing a national health vision.

The provinces responded by blaming Ottawa for cut-backs. Ironically, the increased salience of the health care issue may have made it more, not less, difficult to involve the public and reform the system. With the rise of a symbolic, high-stakes political game, health became an important intergovernmental issue. The governments responded in a predictable way, by seizing control of the issue. As a consequence, the public and other interests likely had fewer opportunities to control the health agenda or discourse.

There is much evidence to suggest that once health became the major intergovernmental issue, it was no longer possible to work through normal political processes. Rather, as evidenced by the recent

2002 premiers' meetings held in Vancouver to discuss the health policy crisis, coupled with the flurry of provincial-government-generated reports that have suddenly emerged, both levels of government have gone out of their way to try and gain control over what is discussed, the values and social interests that are most relevant to these discussions, and the course of actions being considered for reforming the system.

As in the past, Canadian citizens have taken on the role of spectators. Despite this, public opinion cannot and should not be considered unimportant to the changing politics of Canadian health policy. Quite the contrary, when effectively mobilized, public opinion can be a very powerful political weapon. Public opinion is a powerful political resource that governments and other powerful interests manipulate either to push forward a new approach or to defend the status quo. Since they play for different audiences and have competing interests, governmental and other interests who compete for power have a natural interest in shaping and mobilizing public opinion to serve their different territorial-ideological objectives. This helps explain why public opinion is by nature volatile and a slippery concept.

Public opinion has become highly volatile, full of contradictions, and difficult to predict (Milner 2001; O'Reilly 2001). Since political survival or pushing new ideas onto the public agenda depends on the ability to mobilize and shape public opinion, it is only logical that in this period of high-stakes politics and crisis that competing governments, medical organizations, or policy think-tanks would be motivated to shape public opinion, but based on competing territorial-ideological needs and objectives as many studies demonstrate (Rachlis et al. 2001; Fraser Institute 2001; Canadian Centre for Policy Alternatives 2000; *Canadian Perspectives* 2000; British Columbia Medical Association 2000; and Conference Board 2001). A major problem with many of these studies is that they are more prescriptive than concerned with advancing the public's understanding of new health issues. For the most part, even though there has been much more discussion and apparent interest in reforming the system and providing more opportunity for civic engagement, there is a lack of good comparative evaluation of the different reforms that have been tried provincially, and the 'best practices' associated with these. With the exception of a few good studies (Tuohy 1999; Adams 2001; and Bickerton 1999), there has been little analysis to inform those interested in this debate.

As a result of the walls that have been built by government and other key policy actors who have tended to dominate the discourse and agenda in this high-profile, symbolic debate, it has been very difficult for Canadians to come together, focus on common issues, or develop the kind of capacity that would be necessary for informed public participation and discussion. Citizens in Alberta tend to focus on the Mazankowski report (Alberta 2002), while in New Brunswick, most of the focus in the new millennium has been on their own government's vision (New Brunswick 2001). The same is true for other provinces. To a great extent, this competitive territorial-ideological debate has been organized to divide, not unite, the country on health issues.

Getting an accurate fix on public opinion is difficult given this context. In the early 1990s, Canadians were supportive and satisfied with their health care system. They felt their system was better than either the American or British systems of health governance (Blendon 1989; Tuohy 1999, 102; Gallop Canada 1991). More recently, there appears to have been a drop in public confidence (Angus Reid 2000). Even though there still remains strong support for the principles of a publicly funded, universal system, starting in the mid-1990s Canadians have become more concerned about the sustainability of the system (Tuohy 1999, 103). Canadians' values and attitudes appear to be changing, as has their sense of frustration over their inability to control the direction that the health system is taking. According to some, the growing sense of crisis has produced more openness to privatization and other, similar changes in service delivery (Conference Board of Canada 2001). Other polls demonstrate the opposite trend. A recent nationwide poll found that two-thirds of Canadians oppose the kinds of cost-cutting ideas being considered by governments in Alberta, British Columbia, and Ontario. Furthermore, the poll suggested that Canadians still have faith in and support the status quo. Most citizens think the solution is to improve rather than change medicare (*Globe and Mail*, 26 January 2002, 1).

As indicated by Hall (1989), since bringing about a change in regime requires first convincing others that the system has failed – and then mobilizing a coalition in support of a new approach – we should not be surprised that critics have acted this way. However, as was evident in the case of the Meech Lake Accord, the Charlottetown Accord, and various other examples, those critics seeking to change the regime are naturally motivated to convince others that the status quo is not an option – even when it may be. These things need to be taken into account as well.

Renewing Health Governance: Motivations and Barriers

We are living at a time when there appears to be much interest in searching for new values and democratic practices that better reflect new realities and contemporary thinking in the health field. Whether fundamental change occurs or not will greatly depend on the capacity of the old regime to adjust, and the power and resources available to the defenders of the status quo. The public health movement in Canada a century ago presented a different conception of health and evidence that public health measures mattered and did more to improve health status than medical services. Despite this, getting government financial and regulatory support was not easily achieved, and there was much opposition from those who had competing ideas or interests.

The biomedical model that gained prominence in the late nineteenth century and then exploded in the twentieth for various reasons, presented a different approach to analysing and treating health problems. It was argued that a clean environment was not enough to improve health status, what was required were new forms of diagnosis and medical care. New models of service delivery emerged and were debated in Canada. After the Depression and the experience of the war, there was much support for a universal system of coverage, especially as far as hospital and physician services were concerned. But there was never unanimous support for this approach. Ideological-territorial divisions coupled with the growth of powerful Canadian myths made it difficult to redefine health issues and to challenge the power of the medical profession or other established ideas, processes, or embedded institutions.

In the early 1970s, the health promotion and population health movements emerged to contest the ideas, processes, and institutions associated with the more hierarchical, expert-dominated, biomedical model. Reformers in their critiques argued there was little evidence that medical services improved the health of the population and, as a result, there was a growing need to better understand and address inequalities in health and especially social health determinants. As a result, there was increased pressure on and new interest in engaging the public more directly in defining the health problems and priorities. These clashed with traditional approaches.

Increasing the Role of the Public: Good or Bad Idea?

Since the Lalonde report (1974), various academic and government studies have highlighted the changing nature of health problems and the kind of new techniques and approaches required to address them. Public participation and community involvement in the planning and implementation is an important part of many of the new social determinant frameworks that have emerged. It is argued that there is a need for a redefinition of health in a way that would better recognize the importance of a clean environment, social cohesion, income, lifestyle behaviours, and other important determinants of health instead of focusing all of our energy on medical services.

Those interested in advancing public participation have done so by relying upon various methodologies and forms of analysis that seek very different objectives. Health promotion strategies, for example, have things in common with the defenders of new public management and defenders of globalized forms of governance (Barrows and Macdonald 2000). These various competing critiques aim to contest the State's top-down, hierarchal approach and replace it with one that devolves authority, improves efficiency, and strengthens the role of civil society. At the same time, strong ideological disagreements between the equity-centred health promotion perspective and the more market-centred new public management model have contributed to public confusion over the real objectives of a more community-based approach, which defenders of the old regime can and have used to defend the status quo.

Reformers have tended to assume that since the status quo is not an option, we have little choice but to adopt new solutions to address new problems. As a result, little attention has been placed on assessing the status of the social-determinants approach against the established paradigm or even new competitors. Nor has sufficient attention been focused on better understanding Canada's political cultural-institutional traditions that still endure today, and whether it makes sense to try and increase public participation within such a context without doing more preparatory work. There is also a need for further analysis of important changes that have occurred in an effort to increase civic engagement in the governance of the health system, and the impact these would have on priorities and power relations in the future. The rest of this chapter deals with democratic processes and practices of the Canadian public health system with the view that we need to better understand the obstacles to reform first before new strategies can be developed. As a result, as argued by Tuohy (1999), 'the organization and finance of health care delivery in Canada was much the same in the 1990s as it was in the 1970s' (90). However, there have been many attempts to reform the system.

Benefits of Public Participation

Since health involves much more than medical services, it is imperative that there are increased opportunities for public participation and community-determined priorities and mandates. These are required so new frameworks and approaches can be developed in light of new evidence that population health needs are influenced by various socio-economic determinants. We need to recognize the value of more evidence-based, community-centred, integrated structures and systems that are more interdisciplinary in approach and more capable of reinforcing the kind of collective willingness required for the public to take ownership of health issues, while avoiding the competitive turf wars fought among the competing elite across disciplines and communities that have characterized these debates in the past. Since democracy comes in different forms, there are dissimilar models for encouraging or increasing public participation in the governance of the health system. In order to understand which forms of public participation might be best for Canada, we need to take into account cultural and institutional traditions and the kinds of reforms being proposed.

As indicated by Tuohy (1999), there are three institutions that have been relied upon in our health decision-making system. None of these were specifically designed to facilitate direct public involvement. These mechanisms include the market, the State, and a collegial system. In the case of the latter, for example, members of the medical profession have historically performed an important role as 'agents of government.' These organizations that were created to carry out these kinds of functions were never very open or democratic. As Pross (1975) has demonstrated, Canada's institutionalized pressure groups had a good understanding of how a cabinet-parliamentary government operates, and preferred working behind the scenes, outside of the public view (10). In the process, they have played an important role in both designing and implementing various public policies and have enjoyed much autonomy. As Tuohy (1999) points out, in describing this kind of arrangement, '[w]ithin broad budgetary parameters established by provincial governments, physicians have been central to decision-making systems at various levels from central joint profession-government "management" committees at the provincial level, to the level of autonomously constituted hospital medical staffs, to the level of independent individual practices' (30).

Even though this mix of institutions and policy traditions served us well in the past, they also likely made it difficult to implement new reforms, including the notion of empowering communities and allowing them to take more control over health issues. In practice, from the start, there were various components of our health system that were never intended to be controlled by public institutions. For example, the medical profession is paid, for the most part, on a fee-for-service basis. Other professions such as physiotherapy, dentistry, the pharmaceutical industry, chiropractics, home care professionals, massage therapy, and optometry do not receive the same level of public recognition or financial support. There is evidence that a number of these professions would have preferred operating within the public- rather than private-market system, but they were never given much chance to do so, in part because of opposition from the medical profession (O'Reilly 2001, 28–9). The medical profession has attained a special status within the Canadian society, which is further reinforced by its historical domination over medical research and education. There is little question that the dominant status and legitimacy of the bioscientific medical profession has been greatly enhanced by its control over what is taught and the kind of issues and themes that are researched at medical schools.

Over 30 per cent of health expenditures are private and not covered by provincial public programs, and the same services are not covered in every province (O'Reilly 2001, 40). As with any institution, the market mechanism has both strengths and weaknesses. However, it was never designed for the purposes of direct community empowerment or civic engagement. Even though the pharmaceutical drug industry in Canada would be concerned about public relations, for example, there has been little incentive for this industry to build the kind of mechanisms that would be required to allow citizens more effective control over company decisions. When we consider the economic power and interest that drug companies have in promoting and defending the old biomedical model – coupled with their close links with government, the medical profession, and medical research – this poses yet another big challenge for those seeking a more determinants, community-centred, population approach to health (Lexchin 2002).

A third mechanism that has been involved in establishing general principles and controlling the direction of health policy is the State. The nature of our political institutions and the way they are structured are important for understanding where we have been and where we are likely going on this issue. It is also important for addressing the issue of Canadians' sense of ownership and control, or lack of, over the health system.

As we have seen, even though there has been much national debate on the future direction of the Canadian health care system, it is for the most part a provincially based system. Federalism is about diversity and what we really have is a series of provincial health care systems that both compete and cooperate. Recently, it has become clear that federal-provincial competition has made it difficult for Canadians to work together on health issues and to feel part of a common project.

The federal government, through its spending power, Royal Commissions, research institutes, intergovernmental bargaining, and legislation, has tried to influence and create a national political discourse only with limited national processes and institutions. It has also played its part in promoting and building political coalitions, shaping common values, and turning issues to its own advantage. All of this has complicated the reform of the health system because, while the public has come to identify with the idea of a national health system, there have been few institutional opportunities for them to actually engage on a national basis, unless Ottawa decides to mobilize a coalition. As indicated by Banting (1987), Ottawa has a long history of exploiting the welfare state and its spending power primarily for purposes of legitimizing the power of the centre (176). In the past, provincial governments have responded by asserting and defending their own jurisdictional powers and territorial interests against outside attacks.

Reform and Restructuring Projects: Are They Making a Difference?

Recently, there have been various attempts to restructure and reform both the intergovernmental and health system. This is evident in the 1984 Canada Health Act and various intergovernmental agreements, including the Social Union Framework Agreement (Adams 2001). Much of this was in reaction to growing public cynicism and frustration. However, as far as some critics are concerned, these kinds of reforms did little to address underlying structural problems, encourage significant public participation, or push the system in a direction that would address data requirements and other limitations or reflect the variety of new practices and models that are available for addressing health problems. For instance, a number of critics have expressed concerns about the fact that while the Canada Health Act deals with older established areas of health policy (such as hospital and physician services), it provides little support or guidance for a number of other essential services such as pharmacare, health promotion, or home care. Adams (2001) argues that for the most part the Canada Health Act does not 'speak to the contemporary concerns of the quality of health, relevance, responsiveness, and acceptability of services to the public, the efficiency, effectiveness or affordability of the services, the public accountability for the services provided and their outcomes, or the manner in which the services are delivered to and accepted by the public' (65). Nor was it designed to go very far in encouraging the development of new models and tools required for adequately addressing non-medical determinants of health.

Despite these limitations, we do need to draw attention to the fact that there seems to be growing recognition and increasing opportunities for contesting old approaches in a way that could, if it continues to be supported, strengthen public participation and improve our ability to address new health problems based on evidence, while generating better outcomes. The focus will now shift to discuss some of these reform ideas and initiatives, taking into account both sides of the issue and paying attention to some of the constraints involved, in an attempt to better inform the commission's discussions and final recommendations.

There are various challenges in assessing the Canadian experience of public participation in terms of governance of the health system. Part of the problem is that there are different criteria and objectives that could be assessed, depending on the values, interests, processes, or assumptions informing the analysis. For most economists, and certain interests, keeping costs down would likely be a top priority. For others, health outcomes, social cohesion, or dealing with health inequalities is considered to be more important than economic efficiencies. There is not a universal approach for assessing various new experiments in stakeholder-community participation and how these have worked in coming to terms with a variety of health challenges.

As noted by Howlett (2000), there is much Canadian material on the 'role played by private- or public-sector patrons in aiding the formation' and 'tools related to group creation and manipulation' required for legitimizing old power structures and approaches (419). Effecting internal changes and replacing embedded societal and State institutions (and corresponding interests and values) is easer said than done, even in a period of crisis. The fact that change is never neutral and there are winners and losers makes it difficult to build support for any new model, particularly if the old regime remains strong, underlying structural conditions do not change, and there is little opportunity to contest established monopolies and old sources of knowledge, innovation, or popular myths that have been politically constructed and institutionalized.

The fact that there are various experiments, commissioned studies, and planning processes taking place and organized by competing stakeholders, and ideological-territorial interests is a reflection of our diverse, democratic system that is trying to adjust to a policy crisis and to new sources of competition. This is something we should be proud of but we also need to make sure that the competition is fair and balanced, or within the 'public interest.' As discussed above, the public has always been part of the health system, but because of our institutional structure and cultural traditions, the tendency has been to view society as a resource to be manipulated and organized by the competing elite.

Understandably, unless conditions change and there is both incentive and opportunity to properly assess the pros and cons of public participation on the governance of the health system (whether we are dealing with dissimilar models of regionalization, new forms of direct democracy, fee-for-service, new human-health-needs-based forecasting models, privatization, or other restructuring ideas), it is unlikely that we can go very far in judging these experiments and their impacts on reducing costs or on improving the health needs of the population – unless certain things continue to happen.

Judging Recent Restructuring Experiments in Public Participation

Health care reform and the need to improve health, reduce costs, and deal with a series of policy crises has become a popular national preoccupation in Canada, as it has in other countries. Much of the restructuring has been designed for the purposes of:

- shutting down hospitals, removing duplication and other expensive forms of infrastructure (especially in rural communities);

- eliminating full-time nurses and administration;
- institutionalizing, where possible, and promoting through public rhetoric a more non-institutional, community-based, determinants health model;
- regionalizing health services within provinces (subprovincial restructuring has occurred everywhere except Ontario); and
- finding new ways to promote policy learning and coordinate services across provinces (cross-provincial regionalism).

As a result of globalization, increasing costs, changes in fiscal federalism, rural depopulation, and rise of new social movements, there is growing pressure to reform or replace the current health system and the kind of policy instruments associated with it. Yet there are a number of powerful countervailing forces that should not be underestimated, nor should we assume that some of the new reforms and mechanisms that have emerged are necessarily within the public interest or even intended to push the system in a new direction. In the end, whether or not new forms of public participation and health models replace old approaches will greatly depend on the extent to which current processes, forms of knowledge, and structures are considered creditable by policy actors, and whether there is sufficient public trust or legitimacy associated with the old system. If not, there will be little choice but to consider new approaches and policy instruments more capable of mobilizing a new coalition in support of a new regime. Otherwise, other political competitors will take on this role.

Subprovincial regionalization is a very popular health restructuring strategy that, in theory at least, attempts to reduce costs and avoid duplication, while also providing increased opportunities for citizens and communities to participate more directly in health decision-making. Regionalization as an approach to restructuring has much to offer, but a major problem with evaluating this concept is that it has various meanings in different policy settings and can be used to defend very different, even competing objectives, which may be politically controversial. For example, in the field of economic development, regionalization tends to be associated more with addressing efficiency issues than dealing with equity concerns. It has been used to justify cutting services or downloading blame. Cross-border regionalism (for example, recent efforts of the Atlantic premiers to coordinate and integrate health policies) and subprovincial regionalism logically work at cross-purposes since the more power is devolved at the community level and the more policy diversity that exists, the more difficult it will be to integrate or coordinate policies at the executive level across provinces (Tomblin 2002; Council of Atlantic Premiers 2001). Understandably, this could complicate future nation-centred campaigns seeking to coordinate cross-jurisdictional health policy integration and collaboration across the country. Hence, there may be a need to coordinate these different regional experiments or at least take into account their impacts on other planning experiments.

It is too early to say anything substantive at this stage about the nature or impact of this restructuring approach on patterns of public participation in the governance of the health system until more comparative research is available. At the cross-provincial level, since these discussions take place at the executive level and behind closed doors, there has been limited opportunity to promote direct public input.

Subprovincial regionalization involves both devolution as well as centralization of power. In practice, regionalization may involve the elimination of local community structures and hospitals that people identified with, may have influenced, and depended upon. Whether newly appointed, integrated boards are more democratic and accountable is still open to debate, but the majority of provinces have so far avoided establishing even partially elected boards. Likewise, devolution of power depends on having sufficient resources and capacity to make independent decisions at the community level. Since provincial governments continue to maintain ultimate control over these kinds of experiments (as evidenced in recent massive changes in British Columbia that were imposed from above), it is still open to question whether community-based forms of subprovincialism have the kind of autonomy and capacity that would be necessary to gain control over the principles and future direction of the health system. Moreover, since these new regional structures never had a direct impact on doctor salaries or the economic market-practices of drug companies (Lomas 2001), the jury is still out on whether regionalization, by itself, can, at least as currently structured, ever hope to generate the type of knowledge or even mobilize the kind of public enthusiasm and support required for addressing certain problems or for moving the health system in a new direction. In the case of Nova Scotia, for example, the 1996 provincial government campaign to erect community regional governance structures that appeared to strike a chord with the public was completely stymied by the decision of the new regional hospitals to 'remain outside of the regional structure.' In the end, this kind of power and

defensive strategy 'effectively undermin[ed] the province's restructuring effort and depriv[ed] the regional and community health boards of
institutional support' (Redden 1999, 1373). Unless or until these power
differentials and institutional deficiencies are addressed, regionalization remains a limited option.

The question of which forms of public participation are most useful
for the effective operation of the health system has received some
attention in the literature, as has the issue of how different forms of citizen participation influence problem definitions and policy solutions.
But, here too, there is a need for further research. The results of one
study based on a survey of members of health boards in Saskatchewan
suggest that regionalization has improved the system, resulted in better decisions, and enhanced local control (Lewis et al. 2001). However,
there was some confusion among board members on what kind of
powers the boards actually had, and much criticism of provincial government restrictions and lack of board autonomy. There was also evidence that there were few differences in preferences of appointed
versus elected members, or between health providers and board members without a health background. The research provided no evidence
that appointed or elected members perceived health problems differently, which refutes the claims of some critics that these kinds of institutions are bound to be dominated by special interests and hence
incapable of defending or promoting the public interest. It should be
noted, however, that 'there were no objective measures or survey items
to verify the regional health authorities have in fact developed locally
sensitive mechanisms for improving effectiveness and efficiency'
(Lomas 2001, 344). While there was clear support among board members for the need to reform the system based on a wellness as opposed
to a biomedical model, there was also a majority perception that the
kind of vision or plan that would be required to build public support
and implement this new paradigm never materialized.

There were other problems identified by this study. A major problem
was the lack of public interest in voting for board members. Since only
10 per cent of citizens even bothered to vote, this does not bode well
for those who would like to build support for a more legitimate and
democratic health system. If this lack of public support is a result of
mistrust, these legitimization problems may need to be better understood and then addressed. Another problem identified by the study
was the problem of deficits, especially in Regina. In fact, in 2000, the
decision was made to eliminate the practice of partially elected boards

and appoint a commissioner to investigate this problem and experiment. For the time being at least, it does not appear that this experiment in democratization is operating efficiently or is in a position to become more fully institutionalized; in fact, it has been temporarily abandoned. Regionalization experiments in other parts of the country also seem to be in a constant state of restructuring, which indicates their lack of legitimacy, autonomy, or capacity to deal with new health challenges, especially those related to costs. In addition, it seems logical that these authorities have never been in a good position to mobilize the kind of coalition necessary to defend themselves against outside competitors, adjacent ideas, processes, and expectations.

There are different perspectives on which forms of public participation would be best suited for the efficient functioning of our health care system. Much of this depends on the values or priorities that are being promoted or defended. On the political Right, the idea of decentralization, civic engagement, and making communities more aware of the costs and responsibilities for delivering services is im-portant to this system of analysis. The same could be said for various advocates of private-public partnerships, even though the jury is still out on whether private medicine is more efficient than public services (Canadian Health Services Research Foundation 2002; Wilson 2001).

Within the United States, such critiques are a clear reflection of cultural, institutional, and policy traditions and have likely contributed to a tradition of not relying upon the State to deal with problems of disparity, including health disparities. Various critics suggest that too much localization and, democratization may create a situation where there is less willingness or opportunity for redistributing resources to those most in need or unable to defend themselves. This has certainly been evident in conflicts between have and have-not provinces, but also between urban and rural communities within Canadian provinces. Traditionally, Canadian cultural, institutional, and policy traditions have been more collectivist in orientation and, as a result, more focused on equity issues and problems of need.

There is always a danger that too much decentralization, democratization, or privatization could create a very different political dynamic in the country and make it much more difficult to deal with disparity problems or build a coalition in support of a needs-based health system, which has always reflected Canadian collectivist traditions as opposed to American values of individualism. In Oregon, for example, experiments with more direct participatory forms of governance seemed to have worked to the disadvantage of certain groups, and especially those with low socio-economic status (Redden 1999). Hence, there is still some question whether a more participatory model would foster a better health system for everyone. In fact, it could very well add further to health and income disparities, but this does help explain why such an approach is more popular on the Right.

A patient's charter is another instrument for reforming the health system and linking the public to it. It has received a fair bit of attention in various restructuring debates. In the United Kingdom, for example, the idea first emerged in 1991 under the Thatcher government (Tuohy 1999). It was revised in 1995 and later abandoned. It has been the centre of much controversy and debate ever since. Some of the problems with the idea of a patient's charter have included the fact that it was a top-down creation; people and stakeholders did not identify with it and were threatened by it; the charter was designed to promote a consumerist culture or approach rather than a needs-based one; it encouraged competition and not the sharing of best practices across health units; the emphasis was more on process, rather than outcomes; the focus was more national than community-based; it 'encouraged people to cheat'; reinforced a 'blame culture'; and 'it muddled the concept of rights and aspirations giving patients rights but no effective redress when these rights were not delivered' (Dyke 1998).

Another problem with the idea of a patient's charter is that it creates a discourse focused on rights and this makes it far more difficult for politicians to make changes that require, by definition, compromising rights. As well, in the United States, the concept of a patient's charter has been justified as a means for guaranteeing a certain level of service. A major problem with this approach is that it would further complicate health processes and the mechanisms required for protecting patients' rights, which would add further costs for an already very expensive system. There would also be a new incentive to do more medical tests, which, in practice, would further drive up medical costs. Since there have been various problems associated with implementing this concept in other jurisdictions, it seems logical that we should adopt a cautious, more incremental approach. In Britain, for example, there was not the kind of policy capacity or support required to implement these new measures, and there were various negative political and policy outcomes as a result (Tuohy 1999, 182–3).

Where Do We Go from Here?

By exploring the symbolic myths and institutional realities of the health system in Canada, this chapter has shed light on the various obstacles that inhibit public control of the principles and direction of the health care system. The intent has been to confront some of these myths and provoke discussion, but in a way that allows us to better understand the processes and mechanisms that have produced and sustained them. The hope is that by providing more details on the health policy system, public discussion will be stimulated and understanding of a complex policy field enhanced.

The question needs to be raised about the kind of democracy we have or the kind we would like to have. The purpose of much of this chapter has been to reflect on how difficult it has been to increase public ownership and control over market mechanisms, executive-dominated intergovernmental relations, or collegial arrangements. These are the structures and processes that we have relied upon but were never intended to provide many opportunities for increasing direct public participation in the health system. Canada's more collectivist cultural traditions are reflected in the public institutions that we have built, and we need to consider both the advantages as well as disadvantages of these. Despite much rhetoric from the Right, however, democracy is not just about numbers. In fact, direct forms of democracy, as evident in the Oregon case study discussed above, do pose problems for those individuals or communities who may not have the resources or skills required to defend their interests satisfactorily in a more pluralistic, competitive system.

Canadian representative forms of democracy have always had built within them ways of ensuring that these kinds of interests were not ignored. It has always been understood that effective policy development requires identifying both winners and losers of policy change and then finding ways for compensating or assisting those who have been hurt, but in a way that benefits everyone. As a result, these kinds of policy lessons should not be ignored in the pursuit of a more democratic health care system. If we were to ignore them, the political and policy outcomes could be very negative. We need to better understand what we have created, what has worked, and what can be done to refine and improve the system, and we need to do so based on evidence and new partnerships, and forms of dissemination that will appeal to Canadians, address their concerns, and reflect their values.

A realistic transformation of the health system is necessary, but it must be based on first understanding and acknowledging what we have created together as a country. It must avoid mechanisms, processes, or approaches that will force provinces, communities, and citizens away from turning inward and adopting ill-conceived competitive territorial-ideological strategies that will likely have a very negative impact on the health of individuals and communities in the long run. It also requires identifying and conceptualizing both the barriers and facilitators of reform, and then developing new strategies carefully designed to build public support for new reforms and include communities in both the research and implementation process, but without undermining or threatening traditions of collective responsibility that have been so important to Canadian values.

We have created a situation where the State's task of managing health issues and renewing the consensus of who we are as a people and what values count most has posed as much of a challenge as managing a complex health system. What is now required is a new determination to find ways of moving the system forward and facilitating new innovative strategies, different kinds of knowledge and partnerships that are better designed for gradually breaking down some of the old boxes and replacing them with new ideas, processes, and institutions. This will require a better understanding of the connections between new and old health strategies for individual and community health and discovering new innovative ways for connecting and encouraging different, integrated forms of knowledge (biomedical, social-determinants approaches, local community traditions), and finding ways for integrating these in a way that will help us produce better health strategies without creating unnecessary and unproductive political divisions or abandoning what has worked in the past.

Relying upon commissioned studies and new forms of research and dissemination has a long tradition in Canada. We should continue to develop and expand this tradition by continuing to foster the growth of diverse, high-quality, evidence-based research that is more capable of challenging and contesting the dominance of a well-entrenched, province-centred, top-down, market-biased, biomedical policy regime. In this period of policy crisis, there is much pressure to reconceptualize health issues, bring in a more community-based research-policy agenda and push the system in a new direction. In the end, this form of public involvement, which has a long history in Canada, will likely have more impact and be more useful to the longevity and efficient functioning of the health system than many of the reforms (which Canadians have not been very enthusiastic about) in more right-wing critiques.

Recently, there have been many attempts to change the way we investigate and conceptualize human needs in Canada. There is much more interest and emphasis placed on promoting interdisciplinary approaches and finding new creative ways for directly linking researchers, decision-makers, citizens, and communities together in an effort to better understand the impact of old and new strategies on human, community, and environmental health, which have always been closely related but analysed in separate boxes (Lavis et al. 2002; Lavis 2002). This is reflected in various research initiatives, which include the Coasts Under Stress Project; Canadian Health Services Research Foundation; Canadian Institutes of Health Research; Canadian Population Health Initiative; Canadian Regionalization Research Centre; and Policy Research Initiative.

At the provincial level, there has also been much interest in creating public access points and data sets required to bring communities and citizens more directly into the research and policy process. In Newfoundland and Labrador, for example, the rise of the Strategic Social Plan and the development of community accounts that provide useful information on non-medical health determinants for the public, have been very positive and progressive experiments. Similar experiments exist in other provinces. These kinds of initiatives should continue to be supported, but the federal government needs to also play a role in establishing and maintaining the kind of information infrastructure and research links across provinces that will enable Canadians everywhere to support, shape, and compare best practices from a national perspective. The idea of involving citizens on any new structures designed to overview the Canada Health Act, for example, would be an improvement. But given the fact that the act is limited in scope, there is an even greater need for other reforms, especially those that would ensure that policymakers in non-health policy sectors are forced to consider health outcomes. New ways need to be found to ensure this kind of information is available and used to pressure governments to take into account the health effects of their actions. This idea will not be popular with established interests, but it will be embraced by the general public.

Given the massive disparities between the province-centred, biomedical model, and other approaches to health, it is critical that we further develop support mechanisms required for institutionalizing a more community, social determinants, evidence-based paradigm. It is critical that there be a balanced approach to knowledge creation and dissemination, and if we continue to build new data sets and research-policy traditions that are more open, transparent, and inclusive, it will be much easier for the public to feel empowered and in control of health issues. Even if the costs are high, the costs and consequences of allowing others to have a monopoly over these kinds of activities are likely much higher and also pose a threat to national cohesion and traditions of inclusion. From this perspective, it would also make sense to reduce the influence of drug companies on research and training of doctors, and reduce or even eliminate their advertising activities. There should also be appropriate steps taken to ensure that doctors are encouraged to promote new health practices (especially wellness), and this might involve new forms of resource allocation or moving away from a fee-for-service payment system. It is time for Canadians to take back control over their health system in a way that will strengthen and improve it.

Whether in the area of primary care, regionalization, community and home care programs, and health promotion, there is much interest in developing new alternatives and strengthening public ownership and control over the system. Unfortunately, these new innovations and movements, which pose a threat to the expertise and dominance of the old biomedical model and associated interests, tend to be isolated and lack the kind of political resources and autonomy required to effectively challenge the medical world view. To meet these new challenges and to provide ample opportunity to engage Canadians in a debate that is less divisive and does not simply reflect the ideological-territorial interests of the established regime, there is a need to provide a clearer direction, shift the balance, and mobilize frameworks and new forms of knowledge for the progressive democratization of the health system. In terms of increasing Canadians' sense of control over health restructuring, the best approach would be to provide more opportunities for alternative models of health to integrate research on a national basis, promote common values, and build the kind of support required to bring about fundamental change.

The best way to increase public ownership and control over the general principles and direction of the health system is to ensure that old monopolies are challenged, and new ideas and options like regionalization and population health approaches are considered. This will require new effective national mechanisms for comparing best practices and integrating research across jurisdictions, while providing Canadians with more opportunity to engage in an open and honest dialogue. We need to continue to support and look for ways that will challenge the power of old monopolies, improve the design of alternatives, and make it easier for Canadians to debate and consider alternative approaches beyond the rather narrow range of options presented by defenders of the old regime. This could come in the form of support for interdisciplinary, cross-provincial research, and a permanent national commission that would be responsible for providing a clear direction, identifying best practices, and reporting on reform initiatives across the country. As mentioned, in Canada, commissions have played this role in the past and we could go further in creating a permanent structure. New ways also need to be found to ensure that all governments and stakeholders in the health system provide the kind of information required to integrate research and make it possible to evaluate the outcomes achieved by new community models and approaches. Such a commission could also ensure that policymakers and the public are well informed on how decisions in other policy fields influence health outcomes. If these things were done, Canadians would develop a greater sense of control over their health system, and they would have more options from which to choose.

NOTES

I have benefited from participating in various research programs involving regionalization over the years. The support of the Social Sciences and Humanities Research Council (SSRHC)–sponsored Challenges and Opportunities of the Knowledge-based Economy in Newfoundland and Labrador Project; SSHRC and Natural Science and Engineering (NSERC)–sponsored Coastal Communities Under Stress Project; and the Canadian Health Services Research Foundation Career Renewal Award are greatly acknowledged and appreciated.

I also wish to acknowledge several people who provided advice on the discussion paper. They include Jim Feehan, Doreen Neville, Michael Wallack, Gail Tomblin-Murphy, Chris Page, Peter Boswell, Jeff Jackson, Dwight Nelson, Stephen Bornstein, Renee Lyons, and Lesley Tomblin.

REFERENCES

Adams, Duane, ed. 2001. *Federalism, Democracy and Health Policy in Canada.* Montreal: McGill-Queen's University Press.

Alberta. 2002. *A Framework for Reform: Report of the Premier's Council on Health.* Commissioned by the Government of Alberta. http://www2.gov.ab.ca/ home/health_first/ documents_maz_report.cfm.

Barrows, David, and H. Ian Macdonald, eds. 2000. *The New Public Management: International Developments.* Toronto: Captus Press.

Beatie A. 1995. 'Evaluation in Community Development for Health: An Opportunity for Dialogue.' *Health Education Journal* 54: 465–71.

Bickerton, James. 1999. 'Reforming Health Care Governance: The Case of Nova Scotia.' *Journal of Canadian Studies* 34(2): 159–90.

Blendon, Robert. 1989. 'Three Systems: A Comparative Survey.' *Health Management Quarterly* 11(1): 2–10.

Bradford, Neil. 1998. *Commissioning Ideas: Canadian National Policy Innovation in Comparative Perspective.* Toronto: Oxford University Press.

British Columbia Medical Association. 2000. *A New Course for Health Care* (July).

Cairns, Alan. 1995. *Reconfiguration: Canadian Constitutional Citizenship and Constitutional Change.* Toronto: McClelland and Stewart.

– 1992. *Charter versus Federalism.* Montreal: McGill-Queen's University Press.

Canadian Centre for Policy Alternatives, with the British Columbia Government and Services Employees' Union. 2000. *Without Foundation: How Medicare Undermined by Gaps and Privatization in Community and Continuing Care* (November). http://www.policyalternatives.ca/bc/withoutfoundation. html.

Canadian Health Services Research Foundation. 2002. *Myth: For-profit Ownership of Facilities Would Lead to a More Efficient Healthcare System.* http:// www.chsrf.ca/docs/resource/myth6_e.pdf.

Canadian Perspectives. 2000. 'The Medicare Crisis: A Citizens' Guide to a Real Crisis in Medicare' (Spring): 8–11.

Commonwealth Foundation. 1999. 'Citizens and Governance: Civil Society in the New Millennium.' A report prepared by the Commonwealth Foundation. http://commonwealthfoundation.com.

Conference Board of Canada. 2001. *Canadians' Values and Attitudes on Canada's Health Care System: A Synthesis of Survey Results.* Ottawa: Conference Board of Canada (January).

Council of Atlantic Premiers. 2001. *Working Together for Atlantic Canada: An Action Plan for Regional Co-operation.* Halifax: Council of Atlantic Premiers.

Federal, Provincial, and Territorial Advisory Committee on Population Health. 1994. *Strategies for Population Health: Investing in the Health of Canadians*. Prepared for the Meetings of the Ministers of Health, Halifax, Nova Scotia, 14–15 September.

Fraser Institute. 2001. *Moving Beyond the Status Quo: Alberta's 'Working' Prescription for Health Care Reform*. http://www.fraserinstitute.ca/publications.pps/49/section_01.html.

Frohlich, Katherine. 1999. 'Collective Lifestyles as the Target of Health Promotion.' *Canadian Journal of Public Health* (November-December): S11–S13.

Gallop Canada. 1991. *The Gallop Report*. Toronto (August).

Globe and Mail. 2002. 'Majority Rejects Health Changes,' 26 January, A1.

Hall, Peter. 1989. *The Political Power of Ideas*. Princeton: Princeton University Press.

Hayes, Michael. 1999. 'Population Health Promotion: Responsible Sharing of Future Directions.' *Canadian Journal of Public Health* (November-December): S15–S17.

Howlett, M. 2000. 'Managing the "Hollow state": Procedural Policy Instruments and Modern Governance.' *Canadian Public Administration* 43(4): 412–31.

Lalonde, M. 1974. *A New Perspective on the Health of Canadians*. Ottawa: Information Canada.

Lavis, John N. 2002. 'Ideas at the Margin or Marginalized Ideas? Nonmedical Determinants of Health in Canada: Policymakers Outside Canada's Health Sector Have Not Made Much Use of What Is Known About Health Effects of Their Policies.' *Health Affairs* (March/April): 107–12.

Lavis, John N., et al. 2002. 'Examining the Role of Health Services Research on Public Policy-making.' *The Milbank Quarterly* 80(1): 125–54.

Lewis, Stephen et al. 2001. 'Devolution to Democratic Health Authorities in Saskatchewan: An Interim Report.' *CMAJ* 164(3): 343–7.

Lexchin, Joel. 2002. 'Profits First: The Pharmaceutical Industry in Canada.' In *Health, Illness, and Health Care in Canada*, ed. B. Singh Bolaria and Harley Dickinson, 700–21. Toronto: Nelson Press.

Lipset, Seymour Martin. 1990. *Continental Divide*. New York: Routledge.

Lomas, J. 2001. 'Past Concerns and Future Roles for Regional Health Boards.' *CMAJ* 164(3), 356–7.

Milner, Henry. 2001. *Civic Literacy: How Informed Citizens Make Democracy Work*. Hanover, NH: University Press of New England.

New Brunswick. 2001. *Renewing Health Care for New Brunswickers: Regional Health Authorities, A New Direction for the 21st Century*. Fredericton: Government of New Brunswick.

O'Reilly, Patricia. 2001. 'The Canadian Health System Landscape.' In *Federalism, Democracy and Health Policy in Canada*, ed. Duane Adams. Montreal: McGill-Queen's University Press.

Pross, A. Paul. 1993. *Group Politics and Public Policy.* 2nd ed. Toronto: Oxford University Press.

– 1975. *Pressure Group Behaviour in Canadian Politics*. Toronto: McGraw-Hill Ryerson.

Rachlis, Michael, et al. 2001. 'Revitalizing Medicare: Shared Problems, Public Solutions.' Study Prepared for the Tommy Douglas Research Institute (January). http://www.tommydouglas.ca.

Raeburn, John, and Irving Rootman. 1998. *People-Centred Health Promotion*. Toronto: John Wiley and Sons.

Redden, J. Candace. 1999. 'Rationing Care in the Community: Engaging Citizens in Health Care Decision Making.' *Journal of Health Politics, Policy and Law* 24(6): 1364–89.

Savoie, D.J. 1999. *Governing from the Centre: The Concentration of Power in Canadian Politics*. Toronto: University of Toronto Press.

Tomblin, Stephen. 2002. 'Regionalization: Does It Really Matter?' Paper presented at the Health Institute, Dalhousie Law School, March.

– 1995. *Ottawa and the Outer Provinces*. Toronto: Lorimer.

Tuohy, Carolyn. 1999. *Accidental Logics: The Dynamics of Change in Health Care Arena in the United States, Britain and Canada*. New York: Oxford University Press.

Wilson, Donna. 2001. 'Public and Private Health Care-systems: What the Literatures Says.' *Canadian Public Administration* 44(2): 204–31.

World Health Organization. 1997. *New Players for a New Era*. Fourth International Conference on Health Promotion, Jakarta, Indonesia, 21–25 July. Conference Report. World Health Organization, Geneva/Minister of Health, Indonesia.

– 1986. *Ottawa Charter for Health Promotion*. Geneva: WHO.

Wyman, Miriam, D. Shulman, and L. Ham. 2000. 'Learning to Engage: Experiences with Civic Engagement in Canada.' Ottawa: Canadian Policy Research Networks.

10 Could New Regulatory Mechanisms Be Designed after a Critical Review of Health Technology Innovations?

PASCALE LEHOUX

This chapter was prepared at the request of the Commission on the Future of Health Care in Canada. The following question was submitted to the author: How will diagnostic and therapeutic technologies and procedures drive costs in the foreseeable future? The Commission also submitted a series of specific questions aimed at identifying technologies that may have an influence on health care and costs, the extent to which the cost of these technologies would be offset by a reduction in required services, and how expenditures could be controlled.

Researchers who have attempted to address the issues raised by the Commission have encountered daunting conceptual and empirical difficulties (Chernew et al. 1998; Ahrens 1998; Boldy and Lewis 2000; Bryan, Buxton, and Brenna 2000; Rettig 1994). First, the word 'technology' refers to many very different things, from implants to medical imaging to surgical technology. Next, while it is possible to demonstrate that a particular technology can, under specific conditions, generate cost-savings, it is still extremely risky to generalize from such conclusions to other organizational contexts and other technologies. Finally, the time frame in which the costs and benefits of a technology are measured has a considerable impact on the findings. In other words, because the nature, role, operation, and effects differ greatly from one technology to another, it is impossible to measure their overall impact on costs. Only a comparative empirical approach could identify relatively robust dynamics, analysing them within a typology of economic impacts. To my knowledge, this exercise has been attempted at least twice (Mohr et al. 2001; AHQ 1989). Such an exercise can give us a better understanding of the ways in which technologies reduce or increase certain costs (days of hospitalization, emergency visits), but does not allow us to propose new ways of regulating access to these technologies. Furthermore, it was not possible to conduct empirical analyses in the context of this study.

Therefore, in order to develop a rigorous and useful analysis of the issues raised by the Commission's questions, I first decided to reformulate them from a broader perspective: Could the design of new regulatory instruments benefit from a critical assessment of the value of innovative technologies and processes? Then, to enrich the discussion, I chose to tap a body of multidisciplinary literature, including the analytical frameworks from the field of sociology of innovation (Akrich 1994), and emphasize the importance of R&D activities that generally take place 'upstream' from clinical adoption of technologies. My decisions are supported by three observations that are both personal and empirical.

Three Aspects of the Technology Issue

First, in the course of my research, it has become clear that the value of technology is often defined from a narrow utilitarian perspective that measures costs and clinical outcomes only (survival, objective measurement of functional capacities, diagnostic precision), assuming in principle that those outcomes are beneficial or desirable. Such a perspective is in contradiction with sociological analyses which indicate that the population as well as affected patient groups are more interested in the practical consequences of treatments (quality of life, autonomy, after-effects) and their ethical significance (e.g., why screen or diagnose if treatment is not possible?) (Blume 1997; St-Arnaud 1996, 1999; Heitman 1998). Hence the importance of expanding the discussion on the value of technologies beyond their clinical and economic outcomes (Giacomini et al. 2000).

Second, the growing complexity of 'technological systems' is very often underestimated, causing us to ignore their 'real cost,' to mismanage their use and replacement, and to not exploit their full potential (Casey 1998; Patton 2001). This latter observation is closely related to my training in industrial design, which prompts taking a closer look at how technologies are understood, managed, and used in the real world. It is critical that we rid ourselves of an idealized conception of technologies, which holds that acquiring them is all that is necessary to be able to benefit from them. Technology historians insist on the major changes that have occurred over the last twenty years (Tenner 1996; Rip, Schot, and Misa 1995). They say that we are no longer mere manipulators of tools whose immediate results can be observed and controlled, but managers of 'portions' of technological networks whose ramifications and scope far exceed the skills of a single occupation or profession. The result is a situation of great interdependence where a series of distinct, specialized skills are required to introduce, maintain, and utilize technologies (Casey 1998). The latest report of the Auditor General of Quebec (Le Vérificateur général du Québec 2001) refers to this systemic complexity when it confirms that existing radiology equipment has not been appropriately managed, that many pieces of equipment are obsolete or not used for lack of human or financial resources to operate them, and that public health is being compromised as a result.

Third, while efforts have been made towards a more rational adoption of technologies, including by means of health technology assessment, that approach nonetheless leads to some difficult choices. What proportion of our collective resources are we prepared to invest in increasingly specialized and costly services? Is judicious funding and regulation of technology use possible? How can we ensure that access to these services remains equitable and fair? These questions cannot be resolved solely by evaluating the effectiveness, safety, and cost of technologies; they also require an examination of the ethical and sociopolitical aspects that accompany technological change (Cookson and Maynard 2000; Lehoux and Blume 2000). In this chapter, I therefore stress the need to renew regulatory mechanisms by expanding forums for public deliberation, since the issue of the proper use of technology has to be discussed in the public arena and not just within expert groups – which are and will be increasingly subject to pressure from such stakeholders as medical professional bodies and the biomedical equipment industry (Jasanoff 1990; Cozzens and Woodhouse 1995; Giacomini 1999; Faulkner 1997).

Study Design

In attempting to clarify and articulate these three observations, the study develops the idea that a new way of regulating the design, management, and use of technologies must be adopted, and proposes a new role for the federal government. The objective of the first section of the chapter is to analyse the tensions between the market value of technologies (i.e., their return once they are introduced on the market), their clinical value (what they allow clinicians to know and do), and their social value (the positive and negative changes they can bring). The second part stresses the importance for the federal government of creating new 'upstream' regulatory instruments that can influence R&D processes and the adoption of innovations, in order to promote the marketing and utilization of technologies that more clearly contribute to the collective well-being. The chapter concludes with a series of recommendations aimed at promoting innovative activities within a joint cross-sectoral approach, with the objective of reconciling the market, clinical, and social values of technology

Redefining the Value of Technology

From a commercial standpoint, technologies generate revenue for professionals, manufacturers, and distributors. This largely explains the pressure exerted for their adoption and utilization (Gelijns and Rosenberg 1994; Cookson and Maynard 2000). From a clinical standpoint, they give physicians greater capacity for action by generating knowledge (diagnostic capacity), and permitting intervention on the human body and its physiological functions (therapeutic capacity) which influences the health or quality of life of patients. It is relatively rare for a new technology to produce clinical outcomes that are not considered 'promising' by the clinicians concerned (McKinley 1981; Goodman and Gelijns 1996; Rothman 1997). From a societal standpoint, technology affects the redistribution of costs and benefits among various social groups and transforms expectations about health care systems.

It is argued in the following pages that, while assessment allows to determine more precisely the clinical value of innovations, it very often obscures their market value and hardly provides an analysis of their social value. It is important to better define these last two aspects in order to consolidate the role of assessment in decision-making and develop effective regulatory instruments.

Transforming the Human Body and the Health Care System

Health technologies are attracting media attention and prompting numerous controversies. There have been major breakthroughs in many fields, transforming the relationship with the human body and the health care system. Imaging technologies now make it possible to intervene at earlier stages. Genetic testing can predict disease development at the fetal stage. Tissue engineering can reconstruct the human body from hybrid materials (half -human/animal and half-artificial) (Hogle 2000). Some of these innovations make certain practices technically possible although they remain socially and ethically questionable (cloning, 'patenting life forms,' use of stem cells in research, heterografts). Indeed, the turn of the millennium has very clearly been characterized by major technological developments concurrent with the need to introduce ethical guidelines and legal rules to prevent things from getting out of hand (Daniels 1993; Callahan 1990). It is in a context of tension between 'innovation' and 'regulation' (Rip, Misa, and Schot 1995) that most medical technologies are being developed and adopted.

In more concrete terms, there are six major sectors where rapid and important developments are noted in the literature. (1) With the advent of informatics and the development of by-products from defence technologies (such as ultrasonography), there has been an increase in medical imaging possibilities (Blume 1992). Because they use different imaging processes, magnetic resonance, positron-emission tomography, and axial tomography yield different information. As a result, they cannot easily be substituted for one another. (2) More and more telehealth projects using videoconferencing or digital data transmission by Internet, telephone line, optical cable, or satellite are being introduced in different health care sectors, including home care. In addition, information systems are transforming the management and storage of administrative clinical data and information sharing among facilities. (3) The biotechnology sector, which encompasses various classes of innovations, is in full expansion. The best-known applications are: Apligraf,™ an artificial skin cultivated from the patient's cells, whose uses include the treatment of major burn victims and was authorized in 1999 by the FDA; and Carcitel,™ a cartilage which prevents or reduces the effects of bone ageing and improves the healing of fractures (Hogle 2000). (4) Vaccines have helped to eradicate many infectious diseases, but research in the field is continuing, aimed at diseases thus far considered chronic (such as Parkinson's). (5) Research on new materials and micro-electronics has made it possible to design implants such as ventricular aids for heart disease patients, or cochlear implants which restores certain auditory functions in deaf persons. (6) Finally, medications are administered by increasingly varied and enhanced devices, such as patches, programmable pumps and inhalators, with more refined pharmacological action.

All of these innovations are being used in an organizational context that is becoming ever more diverse. Hence the necessity, in the assessment field, of introducing the concept of modes of intervention or treatment. Not only are the new technologies means of treatment but they also lead to new care delivery models, as in the case with nonintrusive surgical techniques. Some of these enable surgeons to operate using local anaesthetics in out-patient clinics, while others reduce patient convalescence time. The home care sector is booming thanks to devices that are lighter, more compact, and more mobile, not to mention easier to use, to the point that patients are becoming their primary users (mechanical infusion devices to administer antibiotics, oxygen concentrators, remote monitoring systems for diabetes, heart disease, or high-risk pregnancies). For a growing number of congenital diseases or defects, several prenatal tests are available, including genetic screening. This is controversial, since the 'treatment' generally proposed to pregnant women is abortion. A great future in being predicted for gene therapy, which is said to make possible early intervention in utero, although significant results have yet to be seen. Finally, while organ grafts have been a reality for some time now, there is controversy over the possibility of procuring organs in economically disadvantaged countries and of using animals for this purpose.

In summary, the last twenty years have seen numerous clinical and organizational innovations in the health care sector. They are transforming not only the nature of care, the ways it is provided and the flows of private and public spending, but also the expectations of the population (Bastian 1998).

Putting a Figure on Health Spending

Since the late 1970s, the impact of technologies on health expenditures has generated a fair amount of literature (Chernew et al. 1998; Ahrens 1998; Boldy and Lewis 2000; Bryan, Buxton, and Brenna 2000; Rettig 1994). It is difficult to quickly summarize this material since authors adopt different analytical perspectives and do not measure economic impacts in the same way. Should we focus solely on the cost of new technology and assume *substitution* effects? In other words, should we postulate that use of this technology renders previous forms of patient management obsolete? Should we include the cost of *complementary* services generated by the use of technology? This applies particularly to the medical follow-up, testing, and treatment required by patients who have been treated by means of new technology but not necessarily cured. What about technologies used in the context of a new *model* of service organization? For example, the measurement of costs associated with technologies used in out-patient and/or home care services raises certain methodological challenges: (1) we must ensure that the costs of all components of the intervention are captured (pre- and post-operative, telephone follow-up, information management, costs borne by patients); and (2) to be able to generalize from the outcomes, we must next ensure that these models are fully implemented (personnel training, monitoring tools, care protocols, patient selection) (Coyle, Davies, and Drummond 1998; Jonsson and Husberg 2000; Arno, Bonuck, and Padgug 1995).

Furthermore, it is often found that increasing recourse to the out-patient method, while potentially reducing the unit cost of interventions, increases the intensity and volume of hospital services, and consequently total expenditures (Chernew et al. 1998). Gelijns and Rosenberg (1994, 42) identify three main mechanisms by which costs are affected by technology use: (1) increased intensity of interventions (the 'technological imperative'); (2) introduction of new technologies and adaptation of existing technologies for other purposes; and (3) expansion of therapeutic and diagnostic information.

Generally speaking, the literature supports the idea that technology is one of the main factors behind rising health expenditures. Chernew et al. (1998) recently reviewed this literature as well as studies of the impact of managed care on the adoption of new technologies in the United States. Each of the eleven studies they identified pertaining to the cost impacts of technology concludes that technology has contributed to a substantial increase in expenditures. For example, Newhouse (1992, 1993), adopting a 'residual' approach that determines the total increase in health spending while neutralizing the effects of non-technological factors such as inflation, the ageing of the population, and increases in personal income, has concluded that technology was the main growth factor in the period following the Second World War. Peden and Freeland (1995) have estimated that, since the 1960s, 70 per cent of the increase in spending has been attributable to the development and distribution of medical technologies, which they claim were largely induced by the deployment of health insurance (on this subject, see Danzon and Pauly 2001). The studies listed by Chernew et al. that have adopted an 'affirmative' approach – focusing on the economic impact of a technology used for a specific health problem – have come to similar conclusions (Legorretta et al. 1993; Cutler and McClellan 1996; Lu-Yao et al. 1993).

Since they associate technology with increased spending, these studies tend to support the view that tighter control over the adoption and use of technology is necessary. However, the review by Chernew et al. (1998) indicates that, even though managed care seems to succeed in containing spending increases, the effects observed may only be transitional, in that the adoption of new technologies has been delayed but not avoided. It is also clear that the choice of technology in an 'affirmative' study will have a determining effect on its results. Weisbrod (1991) suggests that, for some pathologies, technology has been able to reduce costs substantially (e.g., the polio vaccine). In a recent issue of *Health Affairs* (September/October 2001), a number of authors go so far as to say that the overall cost of technology development yields health gains that are significant enough to justify an increase in spending. For example, Cutler and McClellan (2001) have observed that in four out of five clinical cases, interventions have yielded benefits outweighing their costs (heart attacks, treatment of underweight babies, depression, and cataracts); only one showed costs equivalent to the benefits generated (breast cancer). To calculate these benefits, the authors estimate that a year of good health is valued at US$100,000 (so if expenditures do not exceed that figure, the intervention is considered 'cost-effective'). They also argue that people whose lives have been saved or whose health has been restored will make an economic contribution to society by (re-)entering the labour market and spending income. While they recognize the importance of reducing the use of technologies that yield marginal benefits, the authors fear that policies of technology cost-containment, including managed care, will be detrimental to the productivity of health care systems over the long term by limiting innovation.

However, nothing indicates that the main issue for health policy is to determine the degree to which technology is responsible for increased spending. The solution probably does not lie in adopting fewer new technologies. It is more important to get a better understanding of the relationship between the nature of the technologies and expenditures, as well as the incentives for the development and use of innovations. Gelijns and Rosenberg (1994) emphasize the need to take a critical look at technological development: 'Empirical analyses that *unpack* the forces underlying technological change and its relationship to health care costs are urgently needed to strengthen the basis for future policy making' (94). Some authors say that the current context is driving manufacturers to develop technologies that help reduce costs (Goodman and Gelijns 1996; Arno, Bonuck, and Padgug 1995). However, if such technologies are deployed in an environment where physicians are given financial incentives to use them, not only is it possible that total expenditures may rise, but there may also be unnecessary and potentially risky treatments. Table 10.1 summarizes the impacts that broad technology categories are likely to have on health care spending.

In summary, the clinical value of medical innovations is often difficult to determine, and their contribution to society remains open to debate. On one hand, sceptics underscore how much innovations cost. On the other, enthusiasts emphasize their intrinsic value in pushing back the frontiers of medicine. Health technology assessment (HTA) has been a product of this type of confrontation in virtually all industrialized countries.

The Challenge of Assessment: Estimating the Value of Technologies

Since the late 1980s, Canada has enjoyed an excellent international reputation in the field of HTA. Directly contributing to this reputation has been the work of agencies established since the end of that decade in various provinces (BCOHTA, HSURC, AHFMR-HTA Unit, ICES, AETMIS) and at the national level (CCOHTA). HTA is a field of applied, interdisciplinary research oriented towards policy development. It examines the clinical, economic, ethical, legal and social dimensions of the introduction, use and dissemination of technologies and new methods of providing health care (Banta and Perry 1997; Battista et al. 1994). HTA aims to encourage clinicians, managers, and planners to become more rational in their decisions, practices, and policies.

Nonetheless, the challenge is a formidable one. On the one hand, the number of technologies that can be submitted for assessment far outstrips the current capacity of these agencies (Battista, Lance et al. 1999; Goodman 1992). On the other, the receptivity of health care decisionmakers to using this evidence has to be increased and supported by appropriate structures and incentives (Garber 1994; Roberts 1999; Lehoux, Battista, and Lance 2000). In other words, there are now tangible achievements in HTA, but they have to be consolidated. That consolidation should rest on two main initiatives.

Table 10.1
Potential effects of broad categories of technologies on expenditures and health

Categories	Effects on health	Increased expenditures	Expenditures avoided
Prevention (healthy workplaces and neighbourhoods)	– Reduction of risk factors / trauma – Quality of life	– Costs of establishing and monitoring a program	– Reduction of mortality/morbidity
Screening	– Less uncertainty – Timely management	– Acquisition costs – Costs of establishing and monitoring a program – False positives, false negatives	– Early treatment likely to reduce mortality/morbidity
Diagnosis	– Less uncertainty – Timely management	– Acquisition costs – Low substitution	– Timely treatment likely to reduce mortality/morbidity
Non-intrusive surgery	– Faster healing/ convalescence – Quality of life	– Acquisition costs – Increased volume of services – Complications	– Reduction of mortality/morbidity – Reduced lengths of stay
Chronic treatment	– Reduction of pain, symptoms and disability – Quality of life	– Recurring costs	– Control of mortality/morbidity
Palliative treatment	– Reduced suffering	– Increased intensity of services	– Less aggressive therapy
Technical aids	– Minimization of disability status	– Recurring costs	– Social integration
Drugs (for preventive, curative or palliative purposes)	– Healing/control of pain and symptoms – Quality of life	– Recurring costs if problem is chronic	– Control of mortality/morbidity
Home/community care (for preventive, curative or palliative purposes)	– Non-institutionalized convalescence – Reduction of pain, symptoms – Quality of life	– Private expenses – Recurring costs if problem is chronic	– Reduced lengths of stay – Institutionalization deferred

322   Pascale Lehoux

Figure 10.1
Traditional conception of technology development

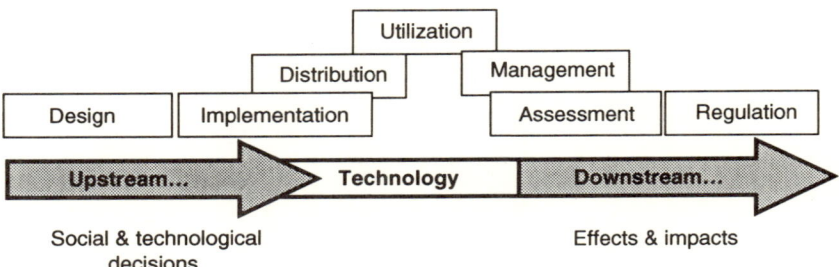

Source: Lehoux 2002.

First, a better conceptualization of health technologies is required (Giacomini 1999; Lehoux and Blume 2000). Figure 10.1 illustrates a linear model where a technology is developed through successive, incremental phases. Within this model, the assessment cannot really generate rigorous data unless it focuses on the clinical use of the technology, because that is when its effects can best be measured in random clinical trials (Goodman 1992). However, major works in the sociology of technology have clearly demonstrated that formative decisions are made well upstream from this clinical phase (Koch 1995; Rip, Schot, and Misa 1995; Latour 1989). The cost of technologies is largely determined by decisions that involve both technical choices (material, functionalities, energy, performance) and social choices (level of competencies required, clinical information, context of use) (Callon 1989; Williams and Edge 1996). A more elaborate conceptualization of health technologies should recognize that assessment of R&D activities is just as important, since the time has come to make changes and encourage the development of less expensive technologies (this idea is developed in the second section of this chapter; see Shine 1997; Coile 2000). A more elaborate conceptualization should also encourage the use of qualitative HTA research, including case studies that offer more refined organizational analyses and interviews or focus groups that clarify the views of users of technologies (professionals and patients) (Giacomini et al. 2000).

Second, dissemination of HTA projects has to be improved and should target broader groups (Cookson and Maynard 2000; Koch 1995). Patient groups and the general population in particular are still poorly informed about the effectiveness, safety, and cost of technologies. The public's main sources of information are the health columns in the popular press, which usually vaunt the promises of medical research or doggedly pursue the funding problems of public health care systems (Rabeharisoa and Callon 1998). The result is an ambiguous situation where the argument of the 'demand' for new technologies is used by promoters of technology and clinicians to justify higher spending – and even recourse to private funding – when the distribution of more balanced information on technology might strengthen the role of patients in clinical decisions (Domenighetti, Grilli, and Liberatti 1998; Bastian 1998).

What do we mean by more balanced information? For instance, when AETMIS assessed the benefits and risks of using antigens to screen for prostate cancer, at a time when this practice was spreading rapidly, a special section was developed to clarify the potential effects on men (impotence, incontinence) and the likelihood of their occurrence (CETS 1995). In addition, the report clearly explained the important epidemiological concept of overscreening to make clear to readers that instead of dying *of* this cancer, the large majority of men afflicted by it will die *with* this condition. This sort of knowledge allows for a more critical estimate of the social value of a technology.

In short, HTA can play an important role in rationalizing the use of technology. However, it will be necessary both to refine its analytical framework and to increase the dissemination of its results. The objective is to develop a general culture that is more critical of technology promises.

Wanting Innovation, Underestimating the Risks, and Demanding Perfection

Why should we adopt such a critical attitude? Is it not a disguised way of supporting certain forms of rationing? Even of trying to curb innovation? A review of the initial objectives of HTA and a brief analysis of the current situation should clarify this call for a culture of questioning.

When the Office of Technology Assessment (OTA) was created in the United States in the early 1970s, technology assessment was deemed relevant because of the need to know the risks for patients of certain forms of treatments (also for healthy individuals, for screening tests). It must be remembered that the introduction of X-rays in the early twentieth century – before the risks of radiation exposure were known – generated rather high mortality and morbidity (Blume 1992). Not until the 1980s did the notion of effectiveness truly begin to take shape and the methodology of randomized clinical trials became grounded in medical research (Koch 1995). During this period, studies on regional variations in practices fuelled the idea that clinical decisions were not based on explicit effectiveness criteria. In the 1990s, the advocates of HTA promoted it as one of the best ways to prevent ineffective, unnecessary and harmful technologies from entering health care systems (Marmor and Blustein 1994; Johri and Lehoux 2003). The cost concept was gradually introduced, along with various tools that were supposed to make it easier to compare different therapeutic options for a given disease (cost-effectiveness) or different health programs (QALY, DALY) (Coyle, Davies, and Drummond 1998). Finally, at that time, there was a proliferation of initiatives relating to evidence-based clinical practices.

Technological scepticism is thus a feature of a relatively recent historical trend, but one which tends to focus on scientific assessment of the effectiveness, safety, and cost of technology. So, during that same period, what was happening on the R&D side? Are ineffective, unnecessary, and harmful technologies being put on the market today? A prudent response would be to say not many (excluding drugs and medical devices available over the counter). It is probably impossible to provide empirical support for this observation. However, it is becoming increasingly clear from the findings of HTA agencies that current and future medical technology issues cannot be boiled down to a simple, black-and-white choice between adopting and not adopting. The decisions that are required today are much more sophisticated and must be based on varied and ingenious regulatory instruments.

For a growing number of technologies, it is a matter of determining in which clinical and organizational contexts, for which patients, and with what level of professional supervision can their use be beneficial. Regulation of this type of practice has to be based on clear guidelines, explicit selection criteria, proven care protocols, and appropriate care infrastructures. The complexity of certain technologies demands not only the presence of specialized personnel (such as biomedical engineers, laboratory technicians, genetics consultants, or computer specialists), but also adapted infrastructures and effective monitoring programs (for example, a breast cancer screening program requires both equipment that is perfectly maintained and quality assurance mechanisms). Deployment of specialized technologies in the absence of these types of organizational conditions is tantamount to tacit acceptance of high public-health risks.

Furthermore, in many cases, restricting access to patient groups for whom a treatment has been deemed effective raises ethical issues (Nord 1999; Giacomini et al. 2000; St-Arnaud 1999). Can treatment be denied because the health status, age, or social environment of the individuals concerned do not meet the ideal conditions for success? How do we respond to patient groups that are demanding faster access to innovations (Barbot 1998)? Finally, some practices, such as assisted reproduction techniques, genetic screening, home telemonitoring, and routine testing, seem to be capitalizing on recent social transformations that reveal a close connection between increasing medicalization and the fear of disease together with a quest for the perfect body (Heitman 1998). The more the notion of technological infallibility is reinforced, the higher the expectations of clinical practices. This in a context where the 'demand' for technology is not only based on laudatory information sources but is also rather easily manipulated by the proponents of new technologies (Blume 1997).

This brief analysis of the current situation identifies three types of concerns. First, the development of health technologies is greatly encouraged by the fact that they are intrinsically perceived as highly desirable and vehicles of progress. Second, the risks associated with their use are probably more difficult to estimate than was believed at the time that HTA was developed, given that the decision to use them is more complex and requires the establishment of sophisticated regulatory and control structures. Third, it seems paradoxical that public expectations of technology are so high, given the publication of scientific studies and HTA results that show the limits to the effectiveness of technology and that highlight the probabilities of success and side-effects.

Before concluding this first section, it is important to return to the initial question: How can the value of technologies be defined? The links between three dimensions of their contribution seem particularly relevant to this study (see fig. 10.2). From the federal government's standpoint, the market value of technologies cannot be concealed. The health technology market has major development potential (Zinner 2001; MIC 1987; CST 1993). It would be naïve to try to regulate access to medical technologies in health care systems (downstream) without examining the incentives for their development (upstream). So there is

Figure 10.2
Reconciling the three components of value of technologies

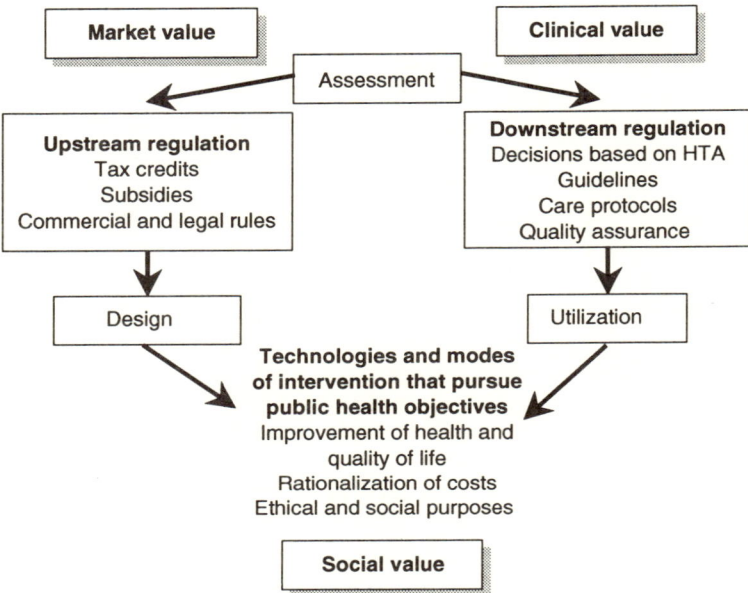

reason to ask whether medical technology R&D activities supported by the federal government are coordinated with the concerns of provincial and territorial health care systems. In other words, is there any coherence between innovative industrial activities and the goals of health care systems?

Next, the tensions observed between 'innovation' and 'regulation' seem significant enough to examine, much more closely than has been done thus far, the ways in which the economic and clinical contributions of technologies are consistent with their social value. Do technological developments that are increasing the diagnostic and therapeutic capacities of clinicians correspond to specific health needs? Do we know exactly what the population and patients want? Are those desires reasonable and legitimate in light of the distribution of collective resources and social transformations that they imply? How can these issues be democratically debated? To date, HTA has concentrated on evaluating the clinical effects of technologies and, to some extent, on analysing their costs, but the social, ethical and legal dimensions have received only ad hoc or superficial treatment (Lehoux and Blume 2000). In years to come, the role of HTA will be increasingly important. It will not be possible to fully assume that role unless analysts succeed in estimating the 'real cost' of the technologies – including the costs of setting up genuine maintenance and quality assurance programs and systematic strategies for the training and skills maintenance of care-giver teams – and unless they can enrich and clarify a critical social debate, especially about the notions of ethics and fairness (Cookson and Maynard 2000).

Rethinking the Instruments of Technology Regulation

Why should we want to link the market, clinical, and social values of technologies? First, because the processes for designing and marketing medical innovations have changed dramatically over the years and directly affect the nature, cost, usefulness, and relevance of these tech-nologies. Next, because the issue of containing the costs associated with technology has special significance when formulated so as to grasp the commercial and financial dynamics underlying all the phases of technological development (from upstream to downstream). Finally, because it appears increasingly urgent to coordinate federal and provincial technology development policies with those designed to rationalize health services. This second section of the study thus suggests some avenues for the federal government to coordinate R&D support activities with technology regulation instruments. The objec-tive is to promote the marketing of technologies that more clearly con-tribute to the collective well-being.

Are Our Technology Policies Schizophrenic?

In Canada, the balance of trade for biomedical equipment is generally negative (CST 1993). This means that we import more technologies than we export. This 'shortfall' has been and remains a recurring argu-ment in federal and provincial science and technology policies for con-solidating the industrial fabric and R&D activities of this sector (CST 1993; MIC 1989). More concretely, at the federal level, three types of policies directly affect health technologies. First, commercial policies can influence the financing and creation of firms primarily involved in the medical equipment field (tax credits, entrepreneurship subsidies, international import and export agreements) (Zinner 2001). Second, policies that aim to support R&D generally can promote the development of specific technology niches that will have the medium- and long-term effect of transforming health care services (biotechnologies, telecommunications, micro-electronics). Third, health policies have a more direct impact on the supply of health care, particularly those that regulate the entry onto the Canadian market of equipment and drugs (approval, formularies, improvement of technical capacities). To date, however, there seems to be relatively little effort towards harmonizing the effects of these various policies. There is even reason to ask whether some of them are not 'schizophrenic.' On the one hand, the government feels obliged to consolidate a profitable and growing industry. On the other, it imposes rigorous measures to control health spending.

How do we go about harmonizing policies that pursue apparently divergent ends (profitability versus efficiency)? Is it possible to promote the development of lucrative firms while limiting their revenues? Does this not amount to squaring the circle (Brown and Brown 2001; Goldstein 2001; Johnson 2000; Levin-Scherz 2001; Smith 2000)? The profit motive is indeed a powerful driver in the design and marketing of medical technologies. The potential number of patients likely to benefit from a technology is naturally an important factor in the decision to innovate in a given technological niche, as is the magnitude of the barriers limiting access to those patients (approvals, patents, competition, reimbursement policies). We are now seeing developments in the home care sector which, because it is not clearly covered in the Canada Health Act, are designed to short-circuit health structures so as to access patients directly. Furthermore, the biomedical equipment industry is clearly more fragmented than the drug industry (Zinner 2001). It contains big as well as small players. Their medium- and long-term capacity to amortize R&D expenditures, outstrip the competition and win the trust of buyers is highly variable. Equally variable are the human and financial resources they require to bring innovative projects to completion. For this reason, it is conceivable that some firms would be interested in committing to specific R&D projects if the government, in return, would agree to provide them with financial, organizational, and commercial support.

The prospect of intervening at the technology design phase is clearly attractive once we accept that it is during that phase that critical decisions to the efficiency of the heath care system are made. For example, Christensen, Bohmer, and Kenagy (2000) explain why it is helpful to promote the entry on the market of what they call 'disruptive technologies': those that disrupt private preserves in the medical technology market by simplifying both the organizational contexts in which technologies are used and the level of skills required to use them. One obvious example is the development of personal computers. Users do not have to master esoteric programming languages, prices are now more accessible, and they are relatively simple to use. An example in the medical field is the development of low-intensity mobile radiology units. They are inexpensive (10 per cent of conventional radiology equipment) and can be used by non-specialized care providers. According to Christensen, Bohmer, and Kenagy, this sort of project meets with immense resistance from the giants of medical imaging and clashes with corporate mentalities.

Another example deserving of more detailed examination is the technological evolution of the management of diabetics. A series of innovations (injection devices, blood glucose monitors, automated monitoring of physiological parameters) has made it possible to expand the role of patients while simplifying and reducing the procedures and material required. It is entirely possible (if the professional corporations agree to revise certain rules governing reserved procedures) that primary care may become an important locus for the development of 'disruptive technologies' that could be used in Canada and exported abroad (including to developing countries).

All the same, how would it be possible, in practical terms, for R&D support policies to be linked to public health objectives so as to produce more efficient technologies that contribute to the collective well-being? Three arguments can be made. First, health economists have made it clear that the dynamics of the health care market do not adhere to conventional postulates of markets regulated by the free play of supply and demand (Evans 1984; Contandriopoulos et al. 1993). 'Consumption' of care is very often not a matter of choice. Patients generally do not play an informed role because they largely depend on information transmitted by those who prescribe the services or make the equipment. It therefore seems legitimate for the government to intervene, through public policies, to ensure that manufacturers and distributors of biomedical equipment develop technologies that satisfy more explicit health objectives, as opposed to simply regulating access to those technologies entering the market after being developed.

Second, the dynamics that lead to the production of new technological knowledge and innovation have evolved over the past twenty years. Gibbons et al. (1994) stress the new attributes of what they refer to as Mode 2. This is a process of knowledge production that involves closer interaction between universities, government, and the private sector. In this context, the creation of new knowledge is clearly oriented towards solving concrete problems, taking various forms such as the search for market outlets for new processes and emerging technologies, or the development of more efficient social programs. Development of such knowledge would require the formation of heterogeneous and relatively short-lived teams, capable of sharing and integrating a variety of expertise for specific projects. Such focusing of research activities around concrete objectives would legitimize the contribution of non-academic players to assessing the quality and relevance of research work, which would no longer be judged solely by the traditional disciplinary yardstick (originality in terms of advancement of knowledge, methodological rigour, general applicability of results). Under Mode 2, the fact that knowledge is cross-disciplinary and 'contextualized' takes on particular importance and tends to erase the traditional boundary between fundamental research (generally in a single discipline) and applied research. Finally, under Mode 2, knowledge is disseminated through more informal channels, outside of scientific institutions (prestigious journals, conferences for informed publics).

If this Mode 2 is as prevalent as Gibbons et al. suggest, it would seem not only relevant but necessary for the government to help define the 'concrete problems' of our health care systems and to offer objectives to be achieved for the development of new medical technologies. For example, a greater role for the government in piloting projects under a Mode 2 knowledge production would have the advantage of encouraging the development and distribution of 'disruptive technologies' capable of generating savings and responding to certain health needs.

Third, it is clear enough that some health innovations – genetics and tissue engineering being the most visible – will raise major ethical and social issues over the next twenty years. The government's responsibilities with respect to those issues will be of two kinds: limiting the amount of social drift, and defining public access to certain technologies, whether or not they are included in the basket of insured services (Daniels 1993; Callahan 1990). Although moratoriums have been imposed in various industrialized countries (on cloning, for example), public and private research centres are clearly engaged in a fierce competition to be the first to make major breakthroughs and secure associated royalties (Hogle 2000). Furthermore, national borders are proving easily permeable, since science in these sectors is developing solely by means of networks of international co-operation (Guston 1999). What lessons can be drawn from this? The dynamics that underlie the development of socially ambivalent technologies are at once powerful and complex. It would be naïve to think it is possible to control them totally. These research centres will succeed in obtaining the financial resources required, sometimes outside of control mechanisms. It is also probable that patient groups will become increasingly demanding (with or without direct encouragement from the technology promoters; see Blume 1997; Barbot 1998) in a context where they are presented with solutions to their health problems or where the legitimacy of the government as a third-party payer is compromised. The cost argument cannot be the sole reason used to deny access to technology. The State will have to stand as a credible interlocutor, capable of representing the interests of each of its current and future citizens.

In summary, this analysis identifies three reasons the federal government must revise (if not reinvent) its role in technology regulation: (1) the negative effects of market incentives on the supply of care; (2) the advisability of intervening in innovation processes so as to orient the nature of technologies and their impact on costs; and (3) the social and ethical issues raised by the scope of modern techno-scientific breakthroughs which demand that a collective position be taken. These reasons should convince us of the relevance of government intervention both 'upstream' and 'downstream' of technology development, but one important question remains: How can the federal government give concrete direction and support for specific R&D projects in the medical field and promote the appropriate use of technology?

New Policy Instruments for Regulating Innovation

I mentioned earlier that the main issue for technology and health spending is not to control the adoption of the technologies but to more finely regulate the patients for whom and the organizational clinical conditions under which the technologies should be used. To clarify this change of perspective, I first summarize the current instruments for 'downstream' regulation and then define the forms that new 'upstream' regulatory mechanisms might take.

'Downstream' Regulation

The usual mechanisms for regulating technology use are largely based on professional colleges, specialists' associations, hospital administrations, payer agencies (physician reimbursement, specific insurers such as occupational health and safety, automobile insurance, offices for disabled persons) and provincial and territorial health departments (including other administrative levels such as regional boards or councils) (Davies 1999). Table 10.2 indicates the principal existing mechanisms and offers examples of technologies which, by virtue of their nature and cost level, are candidates for regulation through these mechanisms (Battista et al. 1999). Very often, to better manage the use of a technology, more than one mechanism has to be applied. Table 10.2 also indicates the main players likely to influence decisions and contribute to policy implementation. At each of these decision-making levels, there are effectiveness, cost, and ethical criteria (accessibility, fairness, principles of beneficence and non-maleficence, informed consent) in play. The overall objective is to guarantee that technologies are used to provide health status gains to those persons who can benefit from them through competent professionals, within appropriate infrastructures, and at an acceptable cost.

As stated earlier, fine regulation of the use of technologies and of the introduction of new modes of treatment will be necessary. This type of regulation assumes that training, guidelines, and health protocols, will play a more important role. In the home care sector, for instance, intravenous antibiotic therapy can be administered by different means (programmable pump, elastomeric or mechanical devices, gravity). Very often, however, nurses do not have access to protocols issued by professional organizations and mainly resort to 'in-house' protocols which vary from one physician or hospital to another and are not systematically updated (Lehoux et al. 2001). In addition, the number of devices available makes it more complicated for nurses to use them (increasing the risk of error), since each one has features that are slightly different (alarms, programming, tube insertion, and so on).

'Upstream' Regulation

This study suggests that new instruments or mechanisms have to be devised to guide the development of technology and modes of treatment. Such a proposal requires substantial reflection and analysis, which is not possible within the scope of this study. However, the following avenues might be explored. First, in a context of Mode 2 knowledge production, the State's role should be redefined to ensure that current R&D initiatives support not only the sectors that have commercial opportunities, but above all those that are likely to yield public

Table 10.2
Instruments of 'downstream' regulation

Decision-making levels	Instruments	Examples
Macro: Provincial departments		
Interlocutors: Specialists' associations and institutions	Procurement policy	Distribution of radiology equipment (TEP, magnetic resonance, etc.)
Interlocutors: College of physicians, specialists'/GPs' associations	Public health policy	Prostate cancer screening program
Interlocutors: Specialists' associations and institutions	Policy on the organization of specialized care	Organ transplant centres
Meso: Institutions		
Interlocutors: Specialists	Routine examination policy	Pre-operative chest X-rays
Interlocutors: Hospital programs and patient groups	Reimbursement of equipment Mused at home	Use of portable oxygen therapy cylinders
Interlocutors: Specialists	Resource utilization policy	Reuse of biomedical instruments (catheters, pacemakers, etc.)
Micro: Clinical practice		
Interlocutors: Specialists' associations and patient groups	Reimbursement of medical interventions	Laparoscopic cholecystectomy
Interlocutors: College of physicians, specialists' associations and patient groups	Guidelines	Breast cancer screening
Interlocutors: Specialists in private practice and patients	None (apart from public information)	Laser vision correction

health and efficiency gains. In telemedicine, for example, there must be currently almost a hundred pilot projects across Canada to which various governments are making financial contributions. Is it possible to better target the distance services that can be offered and the regions where such services are desirable? How can we ensure that these projects are accompanied by evaluative research that allows us to improve technology decisions and know the conditions under which use of these technologies will be beneficial? A complete analysis of the benefits of projects funded through the Health Transition Fund (HTA), which have featured some of the elements suggested above, should help to identify success factors for this type of initiatives.

Second, the market logics that preside over the development of medical technologies impose certain constraints that are detrimental to or limit the marketing of 'disruptive technologies.' Indeed, why would firms agree to commit to the production of technologies likely to reduce the market share of other products they manufacture? Why would small and medium-sized businesses take the risk of developing a technology that generates little profit and whose sales are expected to be low? If our society is relying on innovation to such an extent to resolve health problems while being reluctant to spend more, is it not necessary in turn for it to call into question some of the forces driving that innovation? In other words, it may be that the development of technologies which more clearly contribute to the collective well-being has to be supported by incentives other than just profit. For example, guaranteed markets, tax credits, and special subsidies (SME-oriented R&D support) could be granted in order to reduce commercial constraints that now stand in the way of these initiatives. The federal government seems particularly well positioned to design and introduce such instruments, which should necessarily proceed from joint efforts of the business and health sectors.

In summary, the second section of the study has tried to demonstrate that the issue of technology's impact on costs can only be resolved by agreeing to examine all the factors that influence both the 'supply' of and the 'demand' for technologies. This perspective forces us to acknowledge the 'schizophrenic' character of public policies which, on the one hand, encourage R&D likely to lead to commercial applications and, on the other, impose a rationalization of health spending. Given that the health 'market' is imperfect, a general policy of laissez-faire would be a dangerous proposition; I feel it is important to point out that the State and civil society must intervene 'upstream' of technological development in order to facilitate the design and use of technologies as well as the modes of intervention, which are beneficial to health and socially legitimate. This latter point implies the establishment of cross-sectoral regulatory instruments and mechanisms of public consultation (Bohman 1996).

Recommendations

This final section contains a series of recommendations that promote innovative activities within a cross-sectoral approach whose objective it is to reconcile the market, clinical, and social values of technologies. Three sets of recommendations are offered. The first is to support the 'upstream' regulation of technology by developing an environment conducive to the design of efficient technologies. These recommendations imply an analysis of current trade and commerce legislation. The second is to harmonize and consolidate 'downstream' regulatory instruments so as to refine our capacity to manage the use of technologies. The third is to promote a culture that is critical of technology by expanding the public target of HTA and creating expanded forums for public debate.

Beyond these three sets of recommendations, and given that the study suggests a new role for the federal government in the technology sector, it would also be helpful to assess the advisability of creating an independent cross-sectoral agency at the national level with the mandate to:

- examine all commercial and health policies that impact on the design and marketing of health technologies;
- identify the public health and efficiency objectives to which medical technologies introduced and used in Canada should contribute;
- work closely with divisions at Health Canada responsible for the approval of biomedical equipment and the introduction of drugs on the Canadian market; and
- develop commercial and legal strategies and incentives for private firms and multidisciplinary teams to design and market technologies that contribute to the efficiency of health care systems.

Recommendation 1: Encourage Innovation Where It Matters for the Canadian Population

This study postulates that national and provincial departments of health can play a greater role in R&D activities in order to target sectors where there are few or no therapeutic options and where more cost-effective technologies and modes of treatment could be developed. This assumes that the government can hire specialist resources that are competent to identify and prioritize promising projects.

Research

- Support research that documents and clarifies the views of patients and the population on the usefulness and relevance of medical innovations.
- Inform the population and clinicians of the results of this research.
- Encourage the development of results measurement that takes better account of the practical consequences of treatments on patients' lives.
- Support the use of such results measurement in clinical, administrative and policy decisions.

Trade and Health

- Support firms that are interested in developing technologies that can better meet the expectations of the population and patients.
- Reward innovations, including new modes of intervention, that meet public health objectives and serve to minimize costs by granting their manufacturers special subsidies.
- Provide forms of tax credits to compensate manufacturers who select technological niches where the profit margin is limited but health needs are high.
- Identify collective purchasing strategies to increase bargaining power in order to reduce the costs of acquiring technologies.

Recommendation 2: Manage the Complexity of Technological Systems

This study has stressed that the technological developments we are now witnessing are of unprecedented nature and scope. The medical imaging sector aptly illustrates the need to review the ways in which we acquire, finance, manage, and use health technologies. The following recommendations are therefore intended to suggest an organizational framework that includes all of the elements for offering safe, effective, and quality care.

Training (support for provincial initiatives)

- Consolidate all training programs (including continuing education) in the health sector and strengthen the human capital required for the appropriate use of technologies (physicians, nurses, biomedical engineers, managers).
- Increase the number of biomedical engineers and ensure that sufficient trained technology maintenance staff is available to guarantee the equipment's technical compliance.
- Ensure that nurses have access to provincially proven and standardized care protocols.

Technology Funding Policies

- Harmonize terms and conditions for the funding (combination of federal, provincial, and private sources) of very expensive equipment such as that used in medical imaging.
- At the time of acquisition, provide for funding of the replacement of technologies and of their careful and regular maintenance.

Technology Distribution Policies

- Develop specific distribution plans for specialized technologies that take account of the needs of the population and the availability of human resources and necessary infrastructures.
- Encourage the concentration of specialized technologies in major centres.
- Make managers and clinicians accountable for the proper operation and compliance with safety rules of technologies they adopt and use.
- Penalize establishments that adopt technologies without making use of protocols and guidelines validated by professional organizations and without maintaining strict quality standards.

Recommendation 3: Enhance the Process of Rational Assessment by Organizing Structures for Public Deliberation

The final set of recommendations is based on the idea that a culture that takes a critical stance towards technology can contribute to better use of technologies by clinicians and patients and to better public policies. Moreover, the social and ethical issues surrounding new technologies require that structures for public deliberation be put in place.

Research

- Consolidate HTA capacity at the national, provincial and local levels (particularly in university hospitals).
- Strengthen interdisciplinary efforts in HTA activities.
- Develop analyses that encompass the notion of fairness in technology assessment.

Training (support for provincial initiatives)

- Introduce HTA concepts in medical, nursing, and biomedical engineering teaching curricula.
- Encourage specialized training programs in HTA.
- Strengthen the capacity of planners and managers to use HTA results and develop incentives that can strengthen the role of assessment in administrative and clinical policies and decisions.

Communication and Consultation

- Increase the dissemination of HTA results to decision-makers.
- Support adapted dissemination of HTA results to the population and patient groups.
- Set up structures for public consultation and deliberation.
- Release to the media the results of these consultation proceedings.

Conclusion

This chapter sought to offer a rigorous and useful analysis of technological issues that the Commission was mandated to scrutinize, by addressing the following question: Could the design of new regulatory instruments benefit from a critical assessment of the value of innovative technologies and processes? To enrich the discussion, I tapped a body of multidisciplinary literature, including work on the sociology of innovation. A major emphasis was also placed on R&D activities that generally take place 'upstream' from clinical adoption of technologies. Finally, three sets of recommendations were developed.

The issue of the cost impact of technologies may well remain on the agenda of provincial and federal governments for decades to come. Nothing indicates that our health care systems have reached a state of balance with respect to structural and technological change. One might even be tempted to venture the opposite, in view of the strength of innovative activities and the growing pressure from budget constraints. Many are taking advantage of this period of tension to suggest greater privatization of the supply and funding of health care. In this study, I have deliberately avoided a discussion of this issue. The private sector is behind every technological innovation: without a for-profit market, there would simply be no manufacturing firms and no technologies. With regard to medical technologies, however, the question as we see it is not to determine whether increasing to role of the private sector is likely to improve the performance of our health care systems, but rather to examine how public health concerns can be harmonized with the constraints and interests of the technology market.

This chapter proposes a new role for the federal government, that is, to pilot the development of technologies that are more efficient and more socially legitimate. It also suggests some innovative and, indeed, surprising actions. However, it seems useful to give closer consideration to the financial, legal, and commercial instruments that would allow manufacturers and distributors to benefit from producing technologies which, instead of magnifying the negative effects of budget constraints, could more clearly contribute to the collective well-being. Obviously, this will require a transformation of the commercial culture of manufacturing firms. In this turbulent era, therefore, we will have to introduce new ways of regulating technologies, while re-examining the incentives and constraints that structure the ways they are designed, purchased, managed, and used.

NOTE

The author wishes to thank those who generously agreed and comment on preliminary versions of this study: Renaldo N. Battista, Agence d'évaluation des technologies et des modes d'intervention en santé (AETMS), Department of Epidemiology and Biostatistics, McGill University; André-Pierre Contandriopoulos, Department of Health Administration (DASUM), Groupe de recherche interdisciplinaire en santé (GRIS), University of Montreal; Jean-Louis Denis, DASUM, GRIS, University of Montreal; Mira Johri, DASUM, GRIS, University of Montreal; Paul Lamarache, DASUM, GRIS, University of Montreal; Jean-Marie Lance, Agence d'évaluation des technologies et des modes d'intervention en santé (AETMIS); Marie Rachelle Narcisse, Public Health doctoral candidate, University of Montreal; Raynald Pineault, Department of Social and Preventive Medicine, GRIS, University of Montreal.

REFERENCES

Ahrens, T. 1998. 'Impact of Technology on Costs and Patient Outcome.' *Critical Care Nursing Clinical North American* 10: 117–25.

Akrich, Madeleine. 1994. 'Comment sortir de la dichotomie technique/société? Présentation des diverses sociologies de la technique.' In *De la préhistoire aux missiles balistiques. De l'intelligence sociale des techniques*, ed. B. Latour and P. Lemonnier, 105–31. Paris: Éditions La Découverte.

Arno, P.S., K. Bonuck, and R. Padgug. 1995. 'The Economic Impact of High-tech Home Care.' In *Bringing the Hospital Home: Ethical and Social Implications of High-tech Home Care*, ed. J.D. Arras, W.H. Porterfield, and L.O. Porterfield, 220–34. Baltimore: Johns Hopkins University Press.

Association des hôpitaux du Québec (AHQ). 1989. *L'impact économique de l'évolution technologique médicale dans les centres hospitaliers. Projet coût de système.* Montreal: AHQ.

Banta, David, and Sean Perry. 1997. 'A History of ISTAHC: A Personal Perspective on Its First 10 Years.' *International Journal of Technology Assessment in Health Care* 13: 430–53.

Barbot, Janine 1998. 'Science, marché et compassion. L'intervention des associations de lutte contre le sida dans la circulation des nouvelles molécules.' *Sciences sociales et santé* 16: 67–93.

Bastian, Hilda. 1998. 'Speaking Up for Ourselves: The Evolution of Consumer Advocacy in Health Care.' *International Journal of Technology Assessment in Health Care* 14: 3–23.

Battista, Renaldo et al. 1994. 'Lessons from Eight Countries.' *Health Policy* 30: 397–421.

– 1999. 'Health Technology Assessment and the Regulation of Medical Devices and Procedures in Quebec: Synergy, Collusion or Collision?' *International Journal of Technology Assessment in Health Care* 15(3): 593–601.

Blume, Stuart. 1992. *Insight and Industry: On the Dynamics of Technological Change in Medicine.* Cambridge, MA: MIT Press.

– 1997. 'The Rhetoric and Counter-Rhetoric of a "Bionic technology."' *Science Technology and Human Values* 22: 31–56.

Bohman, James. 1996. *Public Deliberation: Pluralism, Complexity, and Democracy*. Cambridge, MA: MIT Press.

Boldy, D., and J. Lewis. 2000. 'Controlling Health Care Costs Whilst Improving Population Health: What Are the Issues and Can It Be Done in Hong Kong?' *Asia Pacific Journal of Public Health* 12, Supplement S71–3.

Brown, M.M., and G.C.Brown. 2001. 'Will Disruptive Innovations Cure Health Care?' *Harvard Business Review* 79(2): 151.

Bryan, S.M. Buxton, and E. Brenna. 2000. 'Estimating the Impact of a Diffuse Technology on the Running Costs of a Hospital: A Case Study of a Picture Archiving and Communication System.' *International Journal of Technology Assessment in Health Care* 16(3): 787–98.

Callahan, Daniel. 1990. *What Kind of Life: The Limits of Medical Progress*. Washington, DC: Georgetown University Press.

Callon, Michel. 1989. 'Society in the Making: The Study of Technology as a Tool for Sociological Analysis.' In *The Social Construction of Technological Systems*, ed. W.E. Bijker, T.P. Hughes, and T.J. Pinch, 83–106. Cambridge, MA: MIT Press.

Casey, Steven 1998. *Set Phasers on Stun, and Other True Tales of Design, Technology and Human Error*. 2nd ed. Santa Barbara: Aegean Publishing Company.

Chernew, M.E. et al. 1998. 'Managed Care, Medical Technology, and Health Care Cost Growth: A Review of the Evidence.' *Medical Care Research Review* 55: 259–88.

Christensen, C.M., R. Bohmer, and J. Kenagy. 2000. 'Will Disruptive Innovations Cure Health Care?' *Harvard Business Review* 78(5): 102–12, 199.

Coile, R.C. Jr. 2000. 'The Innovator's Dilemma: Disruptive Technologies.' *Russ Coiles Health Trends* 12(12): 2–4.

Conseil de la science et de la technologie (CST). 1993. *Urgence technologie. Pour un Québec audacieux, compétitif et prospère*. Quebec: Publications officielles du Québec.

Conseil d'évaluation des technologies de la santé du Québec (CETS). 1995. *Screening for Cancer of the Prostate: An Evaluation of Benefits, Unwanted Health Effects and Costs*. Montreal: CETS.

Contandriopoulos, André-Pierre et al. 1993. *Regulatory Mechanisms in the Health-Care Systems of Canada and Other Industrialized Countries: Description and Assessment: Final Report*. Montreal: University of Montreal, Groupe de recherche interdisciplinaire en santé (GRIS).

Cookson, Richard, and Alan Maynard. 2000. 'Health Technology Assessment in Europe: Improving Clarity and Performance.' *International Journal of Technology Assessment in Health Care* 16(2): 639–50.

Coyle, D., L. Davies, and M.F. Drummond. 1998. 'Trials and Tribulations:

Emerging Issues in Designing Economic Evaluations Alongside Clinical Trials.' *International Journal of Technology Assessment in Health Care* 14: 135–44.

Cozzens, Suzan, and Edward Woodhouse. 1995. 'Science, Governments, and the Politics of Knowledge.' In *Handbook of Science and Technology Studies*, ed. S. Jasanoff, G.E. Markle, J.C. Petersen, and T. Pinch, 533–53. Thousand Oaks, CA: Sage Publications.

Cutler, D.M., and M. McClellan. 1996. *The Determinants of Technological Change in Heart Attack Treatment.* Cambridge, MA: NBER Working Paper No. 5751.

– 2001. 'Is Technological Change in Medicine Worth It?' *Health Affairs* 20(5): 11–29.

Daniels, N. 1993. 'Rationing Fairly: Programmatic Considerations.' *Bioethics* 7: 224–33.

Danzon, P.M., and M.V. Pauly. 2001. 'Insurance and New Technology: From Hospital to Drugstore.' *Health Affairs* 20(5): 86–100.

Davies, B.J. 1999. 'Cost Containment Mechanisms in Canada.' *Croa Medical Journal* 40(2): 287–93.

Domenigehtti, G., R. Grilli, and A. Liberati. 1998. 'Promoting Consumers' Demand for Evidence-Based Medicine.' *International Journal of Technology Assessment in Health Care* 14: 97–105.

Evans, Robert. 1984. *Strained Mercy – The Economics of Canadian Health Care.* Toronto: Butterworths.

Faulkner, A. 1997. 'Strange Bedfellows' in the Laboratory of the NHS? An Analysis of the New Science of Health Technology Assessment in the United Kingdom.' In *The Sociology of Medical Science and Technology*, ed. M.A. Elston, 183–207. Oxford: Blackwell.

Garber, A.M. 1994. 'Can Technology Assessment Control Health Spending?' *Health Affairs* 13: 115–26.

Gelijns, Annetine, and Nathan Rosenberg. 1994. 'The Dynamics of Technological Change in Medicine.' *Health Affairs* 13(3): 28–45.

Giacomini, Mita. 1999. 'The Which-Hunt: Assembling Health Technologies for Assessment and Rationing.' *Journal of Health Politics, Policy, and Law* 24: 715–58.

Giacomini, Mita et al. 2000. 'Using Practice Guidelines to Allocate Medical Technologies: An Ethics Framework.' *International Journal of Technology Assessment in Health Care* 16: 987–1002.

Gibbons, Michael et al. 1994. 'Introduction.' In *The New Production of Knowledge: the Dynamics of Science and Research in Contemporary Societies*, M. Gibbons et al., 1–16. London: Sage Publications Ltd.

Goldstein, D. 2001. 'Disruptive Innovations Threaten Revenues and Profits.' *Management Care Interface* 14(4): 50–2.

Goodman, Clifford. 1992. 'It's Time to Rethink Health Care Technology Assessment.' *International Journal of Technology Assessment in Health Care* 8: 335–58.

Goodman, Clifford, and Annetine Gelijns. 1996. 'The Changing Environment for Technological Innovation in Health Care.' *Baxter Health Policy Review* 2: 267–315.

Guston, David. 1999. 'Stabilizing the Boundary between US Politics and Science.' *Social Studies of Science* 29: 87–112.

Heitman, Elizabeth. 1998. 'Ethical Issues in Technology Assessment: Conceptual Categories and Procedural Considerations.' *International Journal of Technology Assessment in Health Care* 14(3): 544–66.

Hogle, L.F. 2000. 'Réglementer les innovations utilisant des tissus humains: hybrides et gouvernance.' *Sciences Sociales et Santé* 18(4): 53–73.

Jasanoff, Sheila. 1990. *The Fifth Branch: Science Advisers as Policymakers.* Cambridge, MA: Harvard University Press.

Johnson, D.E. 2000. 'Will Disruptive Innovations Cure Health Care?' *Harvard Business Review* 78(6): 197–8.

Johri, Mira, and Pascale Lehoux. 2003. 'The Great Escape? Health Technology Assessment as a Means of Cost Control.' *International Journal of Technology Assessment of Health Care* 19: 179–93.

Kleinke, J.D. 1997. 'The Industrialization of Health Care.' *Journal of the American Medical Association* 278(17): 1456–7.

Koch, E.B. 1995. 'Why the Development Process Should Be Part of Medical Technology Assessment: Examples from the Development of Medical Ultrasound.' In *Managing Technology in Society: The Approach of Contractive Technology Assessment,* ed. A. Rip, T.J. Misa, and J. Schot, 231–60. London: Pinter Publishers.

Latour, Bruno. 1989. *Science in Action: How to Follow Scientists and Engineers through Society.* Cambridge, MA: Harvard University Press.

Le Vérificateur général du Québec. 2001. *Rapport à l'Assemblée nationale pour l'année 2000–2001.* Quebec: Publications officielles du Québec.

Legorreta, A.P. et al. 1993. 'Increased Cholecystectomy Rate After the Introduction of Laparoscopic Cholecystectomy.' *JAMA* 270: 1429–32.

Lehoux, Pascale. 2002. 'Nouvelles Technologies en santé: valuation et conflits de perspectives.' *Santé et systemique* 6: 251–67.

Lehoux, Pascale, and Stuart Blume. 2000. 'Technology Assessment and the Sociopolitics of Health Technologies.' *Journal of Health Politics, Policy, and Law* 25(6): 1083–120.

Lehoux, Pascale, Renaldo Battista, and Jean-Marie Lance. 2000. 'Monitoring Health Technology Assessment Agencies.' *Canadian Journal of Program Evaluation* 15(2): 1–33.

Lehoux Pascale, Charland Carole, Pineault Raynald, Richard Lucie, and Joce-lyne St-Arnaud. 2001. *Convivialité et cadre organisationnel des technologies uti-lisées à domicile. Rapport 1 : Résultats de l'enquête par questionnaire auprès des gestionnaires des programmes de soins à domicile des CLSC.* Montreal: University of Montreal, GRIS.

Levin-Scherz, J. 2001. 'Will Disruptive Innovations Cure Health Care?' *Harvard Business Review* 79(2): 150–1.

Lu-Yao, G.L. et al. 1993. 'The Prostate Patient Outcomes Research Team: An Assessment of Radical Prostatectomy.' *Journal of the American Medical Associa-tion* 269: 2633–6.

Marmor, T.R., and J. Blustein. 1994. 'Cutting Waste By Making Rules: Promises, Pitfalls and Realistic Prospects.' In *Understanding Health Care Reform*, ed. T.R. Marmor, 8–106. New Haven: Yale University Press.

McKinlay, John. 1981. 'From Promising Report to Standard Procedure: Seven Stages in the Career of a Medical Innovation.' In *Technology and the Future of Health Care*, ed. J.B. McKinlay, 233–69. New York: Milbank Memorial Quarterly.

Ministère de l'Industrie et du Commerce (MIC). 1987. *L'industrie du matériel médical au Québec.* Quebec: Publications officielles du Québec.

Mohr, P.E. et al. 2001. *The Impact of Medical Technology on Future Health Care Costs.* Project HOPE, Final report. Bethesda: Center for Health Affairs.

Newhouse, J.P. 1992. 'Medical Care Costs: How Much Welfare Loss?' *Journal of Economic Perspectives* 6: 3–21.

– 1993. 'An Iconoclastic View of Health Cost Containment.' *Health Affairs* 15: 152–71.

Nord, Eric. 1999. *Cost-Value Analysis in Health Care: Making Sense out of QALYs.* Cambridge: Cambridge University Press.

Patton, G.A. 2001. 'The Two-edged Sword: How Technology Shapes Medical Practice.' *Physician Exec.* 27: 42–9.

Peden, E.A., and M.S. Freeland. 1995. 'A Historical Analysis of Medical Spend-ing Growth, 1960–1963.' *Health Affairs* 14: 235–47.

Rabeharisoa, V., and M. Callon. 1998. 'L'implication des malades dans les activités de recherche soutenues par l'Association française contre les myopathies.' *Sciences sociales et santé* 16(3): 41–65.

Rettig, R. 1994. 'Medical Innovations Duels Cost Containment.' *Health Affairs* 13: 7–27.

Rip, Arie, T.J. Misa, and J. Schot, eds. 1995. *Managing Technology in Society: The Approach of Constructive Technology Assessment.* London: Pinter Publisher.

Roberts, Janet. 1999. 'Coalition Building and Public Opinion: New Reproduc-tive Technologies and Canadian Civil Society.' *International Journal of Technol-ogy Assessment in Health Care* 15: 15–21.

Rothman, David. 1997. *Beginnings Count: The Technological Imperative in American Health Care*. New York: Oxford University Press.

St-Arnaud, Jocelyne. 1996. 'Réanimation et transplantation; la mort reconceptualisée.' *Sociologie et Sociétés* 28(2): 93–108.

– 1999. *Enjeux éthiques et technologies biomédicales*. Montreal: Presses de l'Université de Montréal.

Shine, K.I. 1997. 'Low-cost Technologies and Public Policy.' *International Journal of Technology Assessment in Health Care* 13(4): 562–71.

Smith, J.T. 2000. 'Will Disruptive Innovations Cure Health Care?' *Harvard Business Review* 78(6): 197–8.

Tenner, E. 1996. *Why Things Bite Back? Technology and the Revenge of Unintended Consequences*. New York: Vintage Books.

Weisbrod, B.A. 1991. 'The Health Care Quadrilemma: An Essay on Technological Change, Insurance, Quality of Care, and Cost Containment.' *Journal of Economic Literature* 29: 523–52.

Williams, Robert, and David Edge. 1996. 'The Social Shaping of Technology.' *Research Policy* 25: 865–99.

Zinner, D.E. 2001. 'Medical R&D at the Turn of the Millennium.' *Health Affairs* 20(5): 202–9.

11 Strengthening the Foundations: Modernizing the Canada Health Act

COLLEEN M. FLOOD AND SUJIT CHOUDHRY

The Canada Health Act (CHA) states that its purpose is to 'establish criteria and conditions in respect of insured health services and extended health care services provided under provincial law that must be met before a full cash contribution may be made' (CHA 1985, sec. 4). But to view the CHA as simply a dry and dusty spending statute, whereby the federal government transfers funds to provinces that comply with certain conditions, belies the importance of the CHA in the hearts and minds of Canadians. For most Canadians, the CHA has become a document of near constitutional status, emblematic of Canadian values and a guarantee for all Canadians of the security of health insurance. The link between the CHA and Canadian identity is reinforced by the sharp contrast between the universal scope of Canada's Medicare program and the partial scope of health insurance in the United States (Naylor 1999, 24), where 16.3 per cent of the population (OECD 2001, table 146) is left without the day-to-day security of even the most basic health insurance coverage (Reed and Tu 2002).

In this chapter, we explore how to modernize the CHA so that the values Canadians cherish in the distribution of health care will continue to be realized in the twenty-first century. We propose a number of significant reforms to the CHA. Our vision is ambitious, and the reforms proposed are sweeping in nature. We have two caveats for readers. First, we do not have space in this chapter to work through in detail each proposed reform or the mechanisms for their implementation, the latter being particularly critical. Second, we wish to stress that none of our proposals detract from a publicly funded health care system in which all Canadians are assured of access to the care they need. But notwithstanding our commitment to this fundamental principle, we do think that the means whereby this principle is achieved require change, which in turn, requires amendments to the CHA itself. The need for reform is particularly pressing because the prospects for enforcing the act in its current form have been greatly diminished by federal-provincial conflict over the stability and level of financing. The CHA needs to be strengthened so it becomes a beacon for innovative reform and continual improvement as opposed to a lightning rod for dissent.

In the first half of the chapter, we discuss the five criteria of the CHA (public administration, comprehensiveness, universality, portability, and accessibility) and whether or not these criteria satisfy the values and needs of contemporary Canada. We make several recommendations for clarifying and embellishing the five criteria. We also discuss the CHA's explicit prohibitions on extra-billing and user charges. As well, we discuss the enforcement of the CHA to date. Our most important recommendation arises from the difficulty that the federal government has had in enforcing compliance with the five criteria, some of which are described in very broad terms – for example, what does it mean to require that provincial insurance plans be 'comprehensive'? We argue that accountability should focus primarily on the *processes* that provincial governments have in place to meet the five criteria. Different provinces will employ different means to achieve the values represented by the five criteria.

We also discuss the extent to which the CHA restricts the potential for innovative health care reform. We conclude that the CHA does not impede reform of the *delivery* of health care but does exclude experimentation with private financing. Moreover, we note that there is no evidence that increased private financing would solve any of the problems that medicare is currently experiencing.

Although we consider our recommendations regarding the five criteria to be critical, our most sweeping ones fall in the second half of the chapter. These recommendations pertain to enforcing the CHA and respond to the dysfunctional relationship that has developed between the federal and provincial governments over the governance of health care. We propose the creation of a permanent, independent tribunal for resolving disputes as well as an independent, national commission that would reward provinces for engaging in innovative reform.

We also recommend creating separate legislation to provide national standards for insuring pharmacare and home care and discuss a number of constitutional methods for moving forward to create those standards. In particular, we recommend creating a new companion legislation similar to the CHA.

Assessing the CHA: Does It Satisfy the Values and Needs of Contemporary Society?

The CHA ensures full public funding for a range of hospital and medical services. The act does so by requiring provinces to cover 'insured health services,' which it defines as all 'medically necessary' hospital services, 'medically required' physician services, and surgical-dental services that need to be performed in a hospital. To obtain federal funding contributions, each provincial insurance plan must meet the five criteria: public administration, comprehensiveness, universality, portability, and accessibility. The CHA also expressly prohibits extra-billing and user charges for insured health services, and requires the federal government to withhold one dollar of federal funds for every dollar paid if provinces allow these practices. The five criteria and prohibitions *do not* apply to 'extended health care services.'[1]

For Canadians, these criteria and prohibitions have evolved into the touchstones of a just and fair health care system. We discuss below the relative importance of each and consider the extent to which they need to be clarified or amended to reflect contemporary needs. We first discuss universality, portability, and public administration – perhaps the least controversial of the five criteria. We then move on to (and spend considerably more time on) the far more difficult criteria of comprehensiveness, issues of accessibility, extra-billing and user charges, and finally, problems of enforcement.

Universality

The criterion of 'universality,' under section 9 of the act, requires a provincial plan to entitle 100 per cent of qualified provincial residents to receive 'medically necessary' hospital services and 'medically required' physician services on uniform terms and conditions. Universality is a *fundamental* value that ensures a national plan for all Canadians. That said, the Canadian model (a universal plan funded by general taxation revenues) is not the only model that can provide the security of health insurance to all citizens. The Netherlands, for example, manages to achieve near universal coverage through compulsory *social insurance* for the poorer 65 per cent of the population, while leaving the remaining 35 per cent to purchase private insurance. Social insurance is funded *progressively* (i.e., according to people's means) by employer and employee contributions, which are a percentage of annual income. And through extensive regulation, the Dutch manage to ensure functional equivalence between the coverage provided by social and private insurance (Flood 2000a, chap. 3).

However, the Dutch system is not clearly so much more efficient than the Canadian one that we should abandon our principle of universality when it comes to core services such as hospitals and physicians. Nor is it clear that reforming the Canadian system along the lines of the Dutch system (with its mixture of private and social insurance) is feasible, given the historical development of Canada's health care system. Canada has neither a long history of sickness funds and social insurance nor a commitment to what the Dutch call 'social solidarity,' a value that enables them to harness both the private and quasi-public sphere in pursuit of the public interest. Thus, we would recommend that a modernized CHA retain its core commitment to universal coverage for hospital and physician services while increasing financial flexibility.

A commitment to universality does not necessarily mean a commitment to funding universal coverage from general taxation revenues. Indeed, the CHA does not require this, although most provinces have opted to fund health insurance in this way. International experience demonstrates that it is possible to achieve universal coverage through a variety of means – public financing through general taxation revenues, social insurance (i.e., funding through compulsory premiums), and the regulation of private insurance. Within Canada, the provinces are already experimenting with different mechanisms for providing universal coverage for services and goods outside the rubric of the CHA. For example, Quebec has put in place a pharmacare plan that ensures coverage for all citizens by regulating private insurance schemes and requiring contributions by employers and employees as a fixed percentage of annual income. We think there could be future benefits if Canada were to experiment with *different* methods of achieving universal coverage.

Below we argue for new federal legislation that would provide national standards for the insurance of pharmacare and home care. Like the CHA, such legislation would not require health care to be funded from general taxation revenues. But unlike the CHA, it should explicitly permit provincial insurance plans to be funded progressively through employer and employee contributions, as long as coverage is universal. Indeed, there may be a significant benefit to moving to premiums, because separating funds for health care from general taxation revenues would assist in ensuring the stability of funding. It would also reduce the tension between the drive to increase public spending on health and the desire to cut taxation rates. Moreover, as private insurers already have a significant presence in the market for insuring prescription drugs and, increasingly, home care services, requiring them by law to achieve universal access is unlikely to raise the expropriation provisions under NAFTA, whereas nationalizing them clearly would (Epps and Flood 2002).

Recommendations

• The criterion of universality be maintained for hospital and physician services.
• As we develop national standards for insurance programs covering pharmacare and home care, that there be a requirement for universality and for progressive funding, but not necessarily from general taxation revenues.

Portability

Section 11 of the CHA requires a province's plan to insure all residents within three months of arrival in the province. In terms of interprovincial portability, plans must pay for the cost of services used by residents who travel to other Canadian provinces at the rate approved by the plan of the province in which the services are provided or by agreement otherwise. In terms of Canadians visiting foreign countries, provincial plans must reimburse at least the amount that would have been paid for similar services rendered in the province. Sections 11(2) and (3) provide that the portability criterion is not contravened by a requirement that a patient obtain consent from the provincial plan before receiving non-emergency care when in another province or country.

Quebec breaches the portability criterion by refusing to compensate for health care services that its residents receive in other provinces. Five other provinces breach the requirement that they reimburse the cost of services provided outside of Canada at a rate similar to the one paid for services rendered in the province (Office of the Auditor General 1999, chap. 29). Eliminating the requirement for out-of-country coverage would not offend, in our opinion, the core principle of fairness that underlies the CHA, as it is reasonable to assume that Canadians who can afford to travel to foreign jurisdictions can also afford to purchase travel insurance. Moreover, we think the coverage currently provided is likely to cover only a small percentage of the total costs incurred by cross-border travellers, for example, to the United States. The existence of even some coverage by provincial plans may provide a false sense of security to Canadian travellers and deter them from purchasing full private travel insurance. Other countries such as the United Kingdom, New Zealand, and Australia, do not provide out-of-country coverage for emergency services unless they have negotiated reciprocal agreements with the country in question and are able to ensure that their citizens are *fully* covered for the costs.[2] For these reasons, we believe the requirement for provinces to insure out-of-country treatments should be deleted from the portability requirement. Of course, the elimination of this requirement from the CHA would not prevent any province from electing to provide out-of-country coverage as an additional benefit for its citizens.

Recommendation

• The criterion of portability be amended to eliminate the requirement that provinces pay for out-of-country treatment.

Public Administration

The CHA has become an icon of Canadian values, yet its actual content is poorly understood. This is most true of the requirement of 'public administration.' This criterion requires that the plan be 'administered and operated on a non-profit basis by a public authority appointed or designated by the government of the province' (sec. 8(1)(a)). Notably, it does *not* require that all *providers* be either non-profit or public. Thus the public administration criterion does not prevent a province from contracting out the delivery of publicly funded services to private, for-profit providers. In fact, for-profit providers such as physicians have long been central to the system. To be sure, some have argued that allowing physicians to operate on a for-profit basis is significantly different from contracting out to for-profit firms responsible to shareholders (Evans et al. 2000). However, there is nothing in the CHA to prevent private, for-profit providers from participating in the publicly funded system, whether they are physicians or firms. Moreover, we would submit, the participation of private, for-profit firms (e.g., for-profit hospitals or laboratories) does not contravene the underlying values of the CHA, provided the services delivered are *fully publicly funded*.

Notwithstanding the permissibility of contracting out to private, for-profit entities under the CHA, interest groups continue to oppose these sorts of reforms by arguing that they contravene the act. These objections attract support because no crisp distinction is made in public discourse between financing (which the CHA appropriately safeguards as public) and delivery (which has historically always been a mixture of public, not-for-profit and private, for-profit providers). The unspoken concern behind the opposition to private, for-profit firms may be that by condoning the participation of for-profit providers, we are on a slippery slope towards more private financing in the system. We do not doubt there would be significant regulatory challenges if there were a significant increase in the number of private, for-profit firms operating in the health care sector, particularly in acute care. But given the evidence that for-profit hospitals in the United States are associated with higher mortality rates than not-for-profit hospitals, most provinces are unlikely to facilitate the introduction of a large for-profit hospital sector (Devereaux et al. 2002). Moreover, a strong commitment to full public funding, along with rigorous enforcement of the prohibitions on extra-billing and user charges, should be sufficient to keep a check on for-profit firms trying to circumvent the restrictions of public financing or trying to create de facto a two-tier system. If we are not correct in this prediction, then the CHA may have to be revisited. For the time being, there seems to be sufficient evidence both for and against for-profit delivery in different spheres that this matter is best left to each province's discretion.

We also question whether 'public *administration*' is as fundamental to Canadian values as 'public *governance*.' The act currently allows provinces to 'designate any agency to receive ... any amounts payable ... and to carry out on its behalf any responsibility in connection with the receipt or payment of accounts rendered for insured health services' (sec. 8(2)(a) and (b)). The public administration criterion, as it is currently configured, *implies* a *passive* insurance model, where governments simply administer and process claims made by physicians and hospitals for services provided. The assumption underlying this language is that all care prescribed and provided by physicians must be 'medically necessary' and therefore should be publicly funded. This kind of language is at odds with the contemporary practice of health care systems. In response to ever-increasing costs in health care, insurers around the globe, whether public or private, increasingly use a variety of techniques (sometimes called managed care) to try to influence the allocation decisions made by physicians (Flood 2000a). Thus, to speak of public *administration* belies the significant *governance and management* roles.

Also, the criterion of public administration, as it is presently worded, could be interpreted as reducing the flexibility that provinces need to experiment with different management models. Should provinces be prevented from contracting with private, for-profit organizations to manage publicly funded health insurance plans? Would it contravene the criterion of public administration if provinces were to devolve budgets to groups of doctors (who are private, for-profit providers) and require those groups to manage these funds? Although we do not think the current wording of the CHA would prevent this kind of managerial innovation, ongoing disputes over these kinds of questions could be avoided if the criterion of public administration were updated by amending it to 'public governance.'

There are other reasons to prefer the word 'governance' over 'administration.' When we speak of governance, we begin to get to the heart of what has been lacking in the Canadian system and what is required to ensure sustainability. In our opinion, the most significant problem is a failure to commit to strong governance and accountability for decision-making (Choudhry 2000; Flood 2000a, chap. 4; Institute for Research in Public Policy 2000; Flood 2000b). Here, we do not mean accountability solely for dollars spent, but accountability to citizens for how the system is governed and for the delivery of timely and high-quality health care. We are thinking of democratic accountability: how to ensure that the State, and decision-makers empowered by it, take responsibility for the decisions they make, and are accountable in a fair and more direct and timely manner than is possible through elections every four or five years. This could take a variety of forms and will differ from province to province. For example, provinces might choose to devolve and decentralize decision-making closer to affected communities, make consultation mandatory, elect regional health authorities, ask citizens to choose primary care groups, establish patients' bills of rights, or create patient ombudspersons (Flood 2000a, chap. 4; Institute for Research in Public Policy 2000; and Flood 2000b).

The federal government could take a lead here by amending the CHA to include a richer definition of public administration, namely, 'public governance and democratic accountability.' Some might argue that our logic is circular here, for if 'public administration' is not clear, then neither is 'public governance and accountability.' However, as we discuss below, the primary mechanism for enforcing public governance and democratic accountability should be asking the provinces to account for the *processes* they have instituted to improve public governance and democratic accountability. Thus, the provinces themselves will flesh out the meaning of the criterion through governing their respective plans. They will, in effect, bind themselves through this process.

To further the accountability of federal and provincial governments, we also recommend that the federal government be held to account for the total sums transferred to the provinces for health, and the provinces for the spending of all federal transfers. To facilitate this, it is vital that health care transfers be decoupled from transfers for social assistance and postsecondary education under the Canada Health and Social Transfer (CHST). In its stead, there should be a separate federal transfer, which we would call the 'Canada Health Transfer.' Whatever benefits there are from the flexibility of consolidating federal funds are overwhelmed, in our view, by the loss of accountability for expenditures on health.

Recommendations

- The federal government monitor the growth of health care delivery by for-profit firms but acknowledge that the CHA does not preclude their participation, *provided services are fully publicly funded.*
- The criterion of public administration be recast as 'public governance and democratic accountability.'
- The CHA require provinces to account for the processes they have in place to further improve public governance and democratic accountability within their systems.
- Federal transfers for health be separated from other transfers to ensure clear lines of accountability on the part of federal and provincial governments.

Comprehensiveness

If a health insurance plan fails to cover what society considers necessary care, it will ultimately lose legitimacy in the eyes of the public. Failure to ensure comprehensive coverage will also diminish the incentive of wealthy Canadians to support the plan politically and their wish to remain in it (Hirschman 1970; Flood 2000a). We approach the difficult issue of comprehensiveness in the following stages:

1 How provinces determine which hospital and physician services are publicly funded.
2 The accountability of provinces for their processes to decide which hospital and physician services are publicly funded.
3 What the CHA could do to make *effective* health care services the priority for public funding.
4 How the CHA fails to cover important health care services such as prescription drugs and home care.
5 How to ensure the integration of funding and delivery of care for a broader range of services than those protected by the CHA.

How Provinces Determine Which Hospital and Physician Services Are Publicly Funded

Which hospital and physician services are publicly funded turns on the interpretation of the phrases 'medically necessary' and 'medically required.' However, these key phrases are not defined in the CHA and have also not been defined operationally in provincial legislation (Canada Royal Commission on New Reproductive Technologies 1993, 80). In practice, provincial governments and medical associations negotiate which services are to be publicly funded in the process of determining the fees that physicians will receive in exchange for providing services. This method attributes a great deal of power to physicians and reflects the accord reached between physicians and governments at the time the foundations of medicare were established, that is, that physicians would accept public insurance provided that public insurers did not interfere with their clinical autonomy (Tuohy 1999). The decision process has been primarily a one-way highway, with new services being added to and few removed from the list that is publicly funded. More recently, there has been some movement in the opposite direction. Increasingly, provincial governments are 'delisting' certain services on the grounds they are not 'medically necessary' or 'medically required.' As with the decision to publicly fund a service, the decision to delist is made jointly by provincial governments and medical associations. In Ontario, for example, a 'Physician Services Committee,' composed of representatives of the Ministry of Health and Long-Term Care and the Ontario Medical Association, makes delisting decisions.

Accountability of Provincial Decision-Making Regarding
What Services to Publicly Fund

Presently both the process of deciding which services to fund and the process of delisting rely on provincial governments to represent public values and on physicians to apply technical expertise.[3] However, there are strong arguments that this is an impossible task because, at present, the process for determining what is 'medically necessary' is too intimately connected to the process for determining compensation rates for physicians.

Should we amend the CHA to include a substantive definition of 'medically necessary'? The difficulty is that what goods and services are 'medically necessary' change over time as technology, resources, and values change (Caulfield 1996). Rather than trying to nail down a definition, which will inevitably be superceded, it is more important to develop better *processes* for determining what is or is not 'medically necessary.'

A recent report commissioned by Premier Klein of Alberta (the Mazankowski report) has called for the establishment of a permanent, expert, and independent panel to determine which services are or are not 'medically necessary' and, therefore, publicly funded (Klein 2001). If implemented and made truly transparent, this initiative would be a significant improvement over the existing system where these decisions are made behind closed doors by provincial governments and medical associations. We advocate that the CHA be amended to require all provinces to establish transparent, democratic, and accountable processes to determine on an ongoing basis what should be covered in the public system.[4]

An important issue is whether or not the decision-making process for determining what is 'medically necessary' could be used as a method to whittle away the core of publicly funded services. Except for services such as cosmetic surgery and infertility treatments, the custom has been to publicly fund in full hospital and physician services if 'medically necessary.' Moreover, it has traditionally been thought that services that are not 'medically necessary' and hence not publicly funded would not be provided by the *private sector*, because there would be no demand for medically unnecessary services. However, while services may not be beneficial enough to warrant public funding, there is increasing recognition that patients may still benefit from them enough to wish to buy them. This approach raises concerns about creating a two-tier system, an issue we discuss further under extra-billing. It also raises potential conflicts of interest for physicians who work in both the public and private systems and, who, at least in the absence of sophisticated regulation, would have a financial incentive to shift patients into a privately financed system for their services. This is particularly a concern if, as the Alberta government is planning, the intention is to encourage supplementary private insurance to help provide coverage for services that are not 'medically necessary' but still considered sufficiently beneficial to be privately provided.

Concerns that the process of deciding what is 'medically necessary' is being used to whittle away at the scope of publicly funded services suggests we may need to redouble our efforts to find a substantive definition of 'medically necessary.' On balance, however, we think that by requiring provinces to establish transparent, democratic, and accountable processes, the core of Medicare will be protected. With such processes in place, the experience both domestically and internationally is that there is no political will to significantly reduce the range of publicly funded hospital and physician services (Flood, Stabile, and Tuohy 2002; Jacobs, Marmor, and Oberlander 1999). Once the prospect of rationing services is made explicit and transparent, citizens will not be prepared to exclude patients from getting the health care services they need. Also, at the limit, the federal government can claim that a province is delisting services that are 'medically necessary' and withhold federal transfers. As we argue below, the reasonableness of the federal government's interpretation could be reviewed by an independent dispute resolution tribunal.

What the CHA Could Do to Make Effective *Health Care Services the Priority for Public Funding*
Whatever process is used to determine which services are publicly funded, it must be noticeably generous in its inclusion from the start. Why is this? On the one hand, we may conclude that a certain kind of procedure or test is not 'medically necessary' for a population. However, it will always be the case that for certain patients in certain circumstances a particular kind of procedure or test will be by far the most cost-effective and appropriate treatment. Thus, being too utilitarian in our calculations will lead both to inequity and frustration with the system on the part of physicians and their patients.

On the other hand, our present system, which gives physicians complete control over allocating public funding to a very broad range of services, results in the provision of some services for which there is little or no evidence of effectiveness. Estimates of the cost of inappropriate use generated by physicians vary but are sometimes as large as 30 to 40 per cent of the cost of all services (Stoddart et al. 1993, 6). For ordinary Canadians, this may be hard to understand given the difficulties many have in accessing care, but variations in the number of health services supplied in communities without different health needs support this contention (Roos and Roos 1994; Canada National Forum on Health 1997, 20). For example, there are significant variations in the number of hysterectomies performed in Ontario, with no underlying objective clinical reason why there should be such wide variations and with no apparent difference in patient outcomes (Coutts 1998). The goal of the publicly funded system should be to encourage the delivery of health care for which there is *evidence of effectiveness*. While the CHA states this goal implicitly by requiring provinces to determine what is 'medically necessary,' it needs to be more explicit so that the process is disentangled from the one to determine remuneration for physicians.

The CHA's Failure to Cover Prescription Drugs and Home Care
The CHA does not protect what have become very important health care services: prescription drugs, medical equipment, or diagnostic services used outside of hospitals; ambulance services; dental care; and home care services. By giving primacy to 'medically necessary' hospital services and 'medically required' physician services, the act skews public financing towards those services. The systemic impact is that hospital and physician services receive high rates of public funding (91.1 per cent and just under 99.0 per cent, respectively), while prescription drugs, for example, are funded at a rate of just 36 per cent (Canadian Institute for Health Information 2001). Canada may seem to be a model for ensuring fair access to physician and hospital services, but, among developed OECD countries, it stands in the odd company of Mexico, the United States, and Turkey in not ensuring universal access to prescription drugs (Jacobzone 2000; Willison et al. 2001).

The principles of the CHA, laid down in the 1950s and 1960s, have served Canadians extremely well over the decades. Now, however, advances in technology and changes in demographics have revealed the system's inflexibility. There is now less need for health care services to be delivered in hospitals and much greater need for prescription drugs and home care services outside the hospital, neither of which is consistently publicly funded. The core value that lies behind the criterion of comprehensiveness is that people should have access to needed

services. Most Canadians would probably agree that it is more important for people with diabetes to get insulin than an annual general
checkup, but the CHA does not currently reflect that value because it
requires full public funding of the latter (if medically required) but not
the former. Moreover, those people who have private insurance for
prescription drugs are more likely (all other things being equal) to use
more publicly funded physician services (Stabile 2001).

To ensure that Canada's health care system is comprehensive, we
believe it is essential to create national standards for insuring prescriptions drugs and home care. The most feasible way to do so, in our
opinion, is to create companion legislation to the CHA, which would
be enforced through conditional federal transfers. This companion legislation would allow provinces more flexibility to experiment with the
mix of public and private financing (including user charges) than the
CHA allows. At the same time, companion legislation (which we
might call the 'Canada Pharmacare and Home Care Act') would have
to contain minimum standards regarding access for example, the
income level below which user charges are unacceptable. We discuss
our reasoning more fully below.

In addition to promulgating companion legislation to provide
national standards for insuring prescription drugs and home care, we
would like to amend the CHA to cover all medically necessary diagnostic services such as magnetic resonance imaging (MRI) and genetic
testing that, with advances in technology, need not be delivered within
hospital walls or under the supervision of a physician. Clearly, if a
two-tier system developed for diagnostic services, then people who
could afford to purchase diagnostic services in the private sector
would also be able to gain quicker access to publicly funded hospital
and physician services that require the prior use of diagnostic tests.

Integration of Funding and Delivery of Care
Part of the problem in not providing full public funding for prescription drugs and home care services is that this results in different
sources of funding for health care services, which leads to separate
standards in delivering care and opportunities for cost-shifting (e.g.,
cash-strapped decision-makers in the public system will, if feasible,
shift costs to others). The funding and delivery of the full range of
health care goods and services (hospital, physician, drugs, diagnostic
services, home and community care) must be integrated into budgets
held by appropriate decision-making bodies (regional health authori-

ties, hospitals, and primary care teams). The CHA may only require 100 per cent of 'medically necessary' hospital and 'medically required' physician services to be publicly funded, but it does not preclude provincial governments from integrating this spending with other public funding for programs such as prescription drugs and home care. For example, experiments with integration through regionalization cannot be completed until funding for physicians and prescription drugs are included in these regional budgets (Lomas 1999). In our opinion, the CHA could help break the lock of physicians opposed to regional authorities holding budgets for physician services. This could be done by requiring the provinces to integrate funding for publicly funded health care services (whether covered by the CHA or not) and ensure that such funding is held by the appropriate level of decision-maker.

Recommendations

- The CHA require provinces to establish transparent, democratic, and accountable processes for determining which services and goods should be covered by medicare.
- The CHA stipulate that, in general, provinces give priority to publicly funding services of proven effectiveness.
- Companion legislation to the CHA should provide national standards for public insurance of prescription drugs and home care. It is imperative that companion legislation provide for access standards, for example, maximum income levels below which user charges may not be imposed. This proposal is discussed more fully in the second section of the chapter.
- The CHA be amended to provide protection for all 'medically necessary' diagnostic services, wherever provided.
- The CHA should require provinces to integrate *all* public funding for health care services (whether covered by the CHA or not) and ensure that such funding is held by the appropriate level of decision-maker.

Accessibility, Extra-billing, and User Charges

Accessibility is a fundamental component of any insurance program, as having insurance coverage is an empty right without access to services. Section 12 requires provinces to ensure that Canadians have 'reasonable access' to services that physicians are paid 'reasonable compensation' for services 'rendered,' and that hospitals are paid for 'the costs of insured health services.' In addition to section 12, sections 18 and 19 ensure access to health care on the basis of need and not the ability to pay by prohibiting extra-billing and user charges.

Do the Provisions of the CHA Prevent Innovative Health Care Reform?
We first address whether the accessibility criterion and the prohibitions on extra-billing and user charges prevent innovation in health care reform. The CHA appropriately prevents experimentation with private financing through the prohibitions on user charges and extra-billing but it *neither impedes nor encourages* reform or innovation in the *delivery* of health care. We think the CHA should be reformed to actively encourage innovation and evidence-based reform in the delivery of care.

One of the most consistent criticisms of the Canadian system is its reliance on physicians who work solo and are paid on a fee-for-service basis. Report after report has spoken of the need for 'primary care reform' that would require physicians to work in teams with other health care providers, such as nurses, to provide continuous primary care.[5] These reports also recommend changing the way doctors are paid to eliminate the financial incentive in the existing system to focus on the quantity rather than the quality of care. The language in section 12 – 'reasonable compensation' for services 'rendered' by physicians – implies indemnity insurance (where all costs incurred are covered without question), with physicians reimbursed on a fee-for-service model. However, it is important to note that while the CHA *assumes* a certain model of insurance and payment, it does not require it. Thus, there is flexibility within the CHA for provinces to employ different payment mechanisms. The CHA has certainly not prevented every province in Canada, over the course of the 1990s, from experimenting with different payment arrangements in primary care (Hutchinson, Abelson, and Lavis 2001, 121). The slow rate of progress in this regard is not attributable to the CHA but to other factors, such as lack of political will, lack of accountability for good governance and management, and resistance on the part of some in the medical profession.

As we discuss further below under extra-billing and user charges, the most important sections of the CHA are those that prohibit private financing for necessary medical and hospital services. There is, however, no prohibition in the CHA to prevent health care reform in the *delivery* of health care services.

'Reasonable Access'
As with the term 'medically necessary,' the CHA does not define what 'reasonable access' is. There are no explicit statements about what 'reasonable access' means, such as guidelines for ratios of patients to physicians or distance from hospitals. What is 'reasonable' depends, of course, on a number of factors, including the resources available to society, societal values, the type of health care need, and changes in technology. As these factors change over time, it is fruitless to attempt to provide a substantive definition of 'reasonable access' within the CHA. As with comprehensiveness, the path forward is for the CHA to require provinces to account for the processes that they have in place to ensure that all residents of the province have reasonable access to health care goods and services.

No Specific Commitment to 'Timely' Treatment
There is no explicit requirement in the CHA for Canadians to have access to 'timely' care, although this could be inferred from the term 'reasonable access.' Timeliness of care and concerns about waiting lists have received considerable media attention. Growing waiting times impose greater private costs on Canadian patients in terms of days off work, lost productivity, and so on. As these costs are not covered by the public purse, there may not be sufficient incentives within the public system to control them. That being said, compared with other countries like the United Kingdom and New Zealand (which allow extra-billing and a two-tier system), Canada has a significantly smaller proportion of its population on waiting lists (Tuohy, Flood, and Stabile 2001) and, on average, patients have to wait for a much shorter time for treatment. For example, one study compared waiting times for coronary bypass between New Zealand in 1994–95 and Ontario in the same period, and found that the New Zealand mean and median waiting times (232 and 106 days, respectively) were significantly longer than the Canadian mean and median (34 and 17 days, respectively) (Jackson, Doogue, and Elliot 1999). It is also unclear how serious the waiting list and time problems truly are in Canada (O'Brien 1998).

Nonetheless, the existing data, as flawed as they may be, do suggest that waiting times are increasing (Walker and Wilson 2001). Perhaps more importantly, Canadians themselves are convinced that they have to wait longer for care – a 2001 survey found that 52 per cent of Canadians thought that waiting times were either slightly or much longer than they had been five years before (PriceWaterhouseCoopers 2001).

Canadians are accustomed to speedy and efficient service in all other spheres of life; they can be expected to demand it in health care as well. As Michael Decter (2000) writes, '[I]n every walk of life the consumer's desire for speed has brought about a transformation, be it fast food or fast entertainment' (7). If Medicare does not respond to Canadians' concerns regarding timeliness of treatment, support for it will be undermined and pressure for privately financed options will increase.

In our opinion, accessibility means little unless we speak of access to timely care. The CHA criterion of accessibility should be broadened to read something like 'reasonable access in a reasonable time frame, given the nature of the health need.' Again, the meaning of 'reasonable time frame' cannot and should not be rigidly defined in the CHA. Instead, the CHA should require the provinces to account for the processes they have in place to determine what is 'reasonable.'

Extra-billing and User Charges
In addition to the criterion of 'accessibility' provided for in section 12, the CHA also seeks to ensure accessibility through sections 18 and 19. Respectively, these sections require provincial plans to prohibit 'extra-billing' and 'user charges' to qualify for federal contributions. A 'user charge' is a charge made to a patient that the patient must pay out of his or her own pocket to cover a portion or the entire price of health services. So, for example, if patients were required to pay $10 every time they consulted a physician, this would amount to a user charge. 'Extra-billing' is a concept closely related to user charges where a physician (or any other health care provider) supplements his or her income by billing the patient or the patient's private insurance company for publicly insured health services *in addition to* receiving sums from the government (Flood 1999).

Extra-billing and a Two-tier System: Sections 18 and 19 of the CHA are largely what make Canada unique in how it allocates health care and reflects a communitarian ideal (we are all in this together) (Flood 2000a, chap. 2). In many countries, physicians and hospitals are free to bill patients covered by public insurance plans for amounts above and beyond those laid down in the government fee schedule. Moreover, they are also free to provide services on an entirely private basis that are covered by the public system but for which there may be lengthy waiting lists. This capacity allows a two-tier system to flourish, in which physicians are allowed to work in the public sector and to top up their incomes by working in the privately financed sector. In countries such as the United Kingdom and New Zealand, some people have supplementary private insurance that provides coverage for (a) extra-billing in connection with publicly insured services, (b) purchasing private health care services that are also available in the public system but for which there are queues, or both.

In Canada, provinces have taken a variety of regulatory approaches, all designed with a view to creating strong disincentives against (if not outright prohibiting) a private system that requires cross-subsidization from the public system (Flood and Archibald 2001). In all provinces, physicians can opt out of the public system and operate wholly in the private sector – but they cannot work in both. The result is that private markets for health care in Canada only distribute services that receive no public funding at all, such as cosmetic surgery and in vitro fertilization. Unlike in the United Kingdom, Australia, or New Zealand, people in Canada do not have the choice of buying a service such as a hip operation from the private system in order to jump the waiting list in the public system.

There is ongoing debate about the equity and efficiency of extra-billing and whether or not a two-tier system should be allowed in Canada. After reviewing the international evidence, Tuohy, Flood, and Stabile (2001) recently concluded that a two-tier system would reduce equity. They saw no evidence that a parallel private system would reduce pressure on the public system by, for example, reducing waiting lists. In fact, countries with two-tier systems such as the United Kingdom and New Zealand recorded much longer waiting lists and timelines than Canada. There was also no evidence that increased private financing would relieve any of the other problems that beset the Canadian health care system and others around the globe.

User Charges: In any debate addressing the validity of user fees, it is important to establish what the goal is. Is the goal to act as a brake on use of services and reduce overall health care spending, or to generate additional private funds for health care? If the goal is the latter, the experience in the United States amply demonstrates that more private financing does not result in a better system per se, measured either by equity or efficiency.

The imposition of user charges on patients does not take into account the fact that it is primarily *physicians* who make recommendations to patients about what care is needed and that patients rely on their physicians' advice. If this assumption is generally true, then user charges may not result in more appropriate use of services. If a patient faced with a user fee attempted to self-diagnose, he or she might believe – mistakenly – that the condition is not serious and not seek appropriate treatment, which could result in a crisis and greater costs later on. Also, if the goal is to decrease spending by reducing use, user charges will not be effective if private insurance completely covers the cost of the user charge.[6] Finally, total health spending will not decline if physicians in a fee-for-service system respond to a decline in demand by simply providing more services to those patients who can afford them or who have private insurance (Epp et al. 2000; Rice and Morrison 1994; Stoddart et al. 1993; Flood 1996, 1–3; Hutton 1989; and Deber 2000a, 2000b).

From an equity and fairness perspective, user charges are obviously of concern, as they are contrary to the core principle that access to needed health care services should be distributed on the basis of need and not the ability to pay. A regime of user charges could satisfy this principle only if generous safety nets were constructed so that people on low incomes were not deterred from seeking the care they need; otherwise, there would be concern about the adverse impact on the health of low-income people (Tamblyn et al. 2001). Any province that wanted to impose a system of user charges would have the heavy burden of demonstrating that the charges would not prevent people from receiving the care they really need.

Recommendations

- The criterion of access in the CHA be changed to 'reasonable access in a reasonable time frame, given the nature of the health need.'
- The CHA require the provinces to account for the processes that they have in place to ensure that all residents of the province have reasonable access to health care goods and services in a reasonable time frame.
- The prohibition on extra-billing remain in place.
- The prohibition on user charges remain in place.

Enforcement of the CHA

The federal government can enforce the terms of the CHA by withholding federal funding from the provinces. There are two enforcement tracks. The discretionary enforcement track applies to the five criteria, and provides that the federal government *may* (but need not) deduct monies from provincial transfer payments for violations of the criteria (CHA 1985, ss. 14–15). Even if the federal government decides to make a deduction, the amount is that which '... the Governor General considers to be appropriate, having regard to the gravity of the default' (CHA sec. 15(1)(a)). The mandatory enforcement track applies to the specific bans on extra-billing and user fees, and provides, pursuant to section 20, that the minister of health *must* deduct, on a dollar-for-dollar basis, the amounts paid as extra-billing or user charges for services that should be freely available.

Enforcement efforts have been checkered (Choudhry 1996; 2000; Flood 1999). The discretionary enforcement track has never been used despite the Auditor General's finding in 1999 that there were several cases of ongoing non-compliance with the five criteria of the CHA (Office of the Auditor General 1999, chap. 29, paras 29.45–29.49). For example, Quebec remains in breach of the portability requirement because it has refused to reimburse patients for care received in other provinces at the amount that the other province would normally pay. Another study, relying on media reports and Hansard, suggests that many alleged violations of the CHA have not prompted a public response by the federal government (Choudhry 2000). Despite this, the federal government has not exercised its right to impose financial penalties.

In contrast, under the mandatory enforcement track, approximately $245 million was withheld from the cash contributions to seven provinces between 1984 and 1987. As provided for in the CHA, this money was returned to the provinces once they had eliminated the user charges. From 1992 to 1995, $2 million was deducted from transfer payments to one province that permitted extra-billing. Pursuant to the federal policy on private clinics (Marleau 1995), a total of approximately $6 million has been withheld since November 1995 from four provinces where patients were charged a 'facility fee' for 'medically necessary' services. One province is still not in compliance and is being penalized in the amount of $4,780 per month. Pursuant to section 20(6), the federal government could withhold additional sums beyond the amount of the facility fees; however, to date it has not chosen to do so (Office of the Auditor General 1999, chap. 29, paras 29.45–29.49).

Why Is the CHA Not Enforced More Vigorously?

Why is the CHA not enforced more vigorously? Why, for example, does the federal government refrain from using its discretionary powers to impose heavier financial penalties in the case of extra-billing or user charges where deductions on a dollar-for-dollar basis do not result in provinces moving quickly to eradicate these activities? Also, why has the federal government *never* penalized a province financially for failing to comply with the CHA's five criteria?

Lack of Deductions Does Not Necessarily Mean Lack of Enforcement
The fact that few deductions are being made does not necessarily mean that the CHA is not being enforced through alternative means. The Auditor General notes that the federal government tries to resolve issues of non-compliance through political negotiation rather than penalizing the provinces through financial sanctions. Over the last five years, six cases of non-compliance have been resolved using this approach. However, the Auditor General was concerned about delay in resolution, as four cases had taken between fourteen and forty-eight months to be resolved, and two cases had continued for as long as five years without penalty (Office of the Auditor General 1999, chap. 29, para. 29.46). In sum, there is a lack of transparency here, making it extremely difficult to draw a definitive conclusion regarding the extent of federal enforcement activity.

Inherent Difficulty of Enforcing Criteria
Although the federal government has withheld funding where provinces have allowed extra-billing or user charges, it has never withheld funds under its discretionary powers for breach of one of the five criteria. This is likely due in part to the difficulty in determining whether any of these criteria have been substantively breached. Whether or not a province has complied with the criteria of comprehensiveness or accessibility, for example, is easily debatable. As discussed earlier, these criteria are couched in general terms and their definitions are circular – comprehensiveness, for example, means that all insured services must be insured. This definition begs the question of what, at a minimum, must be covered. We advocate that the primary approach to the CHA should not be one of enforcing criteria as goals in themselves but of asking provincial governments to account for the processes they have in place to achieve these goals.

Reductions in Federal Contributions in the 1990s

It is widely thought that the federal government's ability to enforce compliance with the CHA's criteria has been seriously diminished by reductions in federal *cash* transfers (Choudhry 2000). At the inception of medicare, the federal government contributed 50 per cent of all costs. The provincial and territorial ministers of health report that the federal share of provincial health costs was, on average, 10.2 per cent in 1998–99, although one-time federal transfers in 1999–2000 and 2000–2001 brought the federal cash contribution up to 13.8 per cent (Provincial and Territorial Ministers of Health 2000, 19). The federal government argues that its contribution is actually higher than this, approximately 30 per cent, if tax-point transfers are taken into account.

Apart from the *quantity* of the federal contribution, another significant concern for the provinces has been to ensure the *stability* of federal funding in provincial insurance plans.[7] Rapid reductions in federal funding undoubtedly caused significant hardships for the operation of provincial insurance plans in the early to mid-1990s, because, of course, funding reductions are not mirrored by reductions in health care needs or patient and provider expectations.

The turmoil over funding, and the resulting tense and bitter federal-provincial relations that have ensued, must to some extent have had an impact on the willingness and capacity of the federal government to impose its own vision of medicare upon the provinces. Increasingly, a number of provinces are saying that the federal government has failed to show leadership in health care issues, and that, in the absence of significant financial contributions, it can no longer count itself a significant player in charting the future direction of medicare in Canada. This state of affairs is completely unsatisfactory, and it is imperative to rebuild and restore a functional relationship between the federal and provincial governments.

Sophisticated governance is fundamental to solving many of the challenges that Canada's health care system faces. The present situation is characterised by blame, cost shifting, and 'sterile, childish bickering' (Institute for Research in Public Policy 2000). Governance in health care is in a state of paralysis, as both provincial and federal governments find it more politically expedient to blame each other for Canadians' concerns about medicare than do something about it. How unsatisfying and difficult the health portfolio has become is arguably reflected in the high turnover of health ministers. The Canadian Institute for Health Information (2001) reports that since 1990, 75 health ministers have served at the federal, provincial, or territorial levels across the country with an average median term varying from a low of thirteen months in the Northwest Territories to 41.5 months in Alberta (54).

We now turn to proposing new methods of institutional oversight that could revitalize federal-provincial relations in this critical area.

Institutional Oversight

The allocation of institutional responsibility for the oversight of national standards lies at the heart of the federal-provincial conflict over the future of medicare. Currently, the responsibility lies exclusively with the federal government. The advantage of the current arrangement is that final responsibility for enforcement lies with the federal cabinet, which, in theory, can impose a significant financial sanction to elicit corrective action on the part of a province. The federal cabinet also has discretion to fine-tune the sanction and tailor it to political realities. However, as we noted earlier, the federal government has never used its discretionary power to withhold funds for the breach of any of the five criteria.

Even though the federal government's powers of enforcement lie largely unused, the provinces oppose the vesting of this responsibility with the federal government, for a variety of reasons:

- Unilateral federal enforcement is out of keeping with the quasi-contractual nature of conditional grants.
- The enforcement of standards has been selective, uneven, and political, and has stymied innovation in health care reform.
- Provinces enjoy a comparative institutional advantage over the federal government in contextualizing the meaning of national standards in light of each province's needs and capacities.
- Federal enforcement has lost legitimacy following reductions to transfers in the early 1990s, which have arguably made it more difficult for provinces to satisfy national standards.

Whatever the merit of the arguments, most observers would agree that the unilateral reduction of federal transfers in 1995 poisoned the well of federal-provincial goodwill that is required to ensure the successful governance of medicare. In our view, breaking the present impasse requires reconceptualizing national standards, and redesigning the institutions that oversee them. In brief, we propose that:

- with respect to the criteria of accessibility and comprehensiveness, and the suggested criterion of public governance and accountability, the emphasis be on encouraging provinces to establish transparent and democratic processes to specify provincial goals for these criteria, rather than laying down a common standard for all of Canada;
- the establishment of a national Medicare Commission, the members of which would be appointed by the provincial and federal governments, with the mandate of providing both intellectual capital and federal financial support for provincial initiatives to redesign health care delivery that have the goal of better meeting the criteria of the CHA; and
- the establishment of a permanent and publicly transparent procedure to settle disputes (including citizen complaints) over the interpretation of national standards in the CHA under the Social Union Framework Agreement.

Provincial Processes to Specify Accessibility, Comprehensiveness, and Public Administration

Although the CHA provides for a single set of national standards that all provincial health insurance plans must satisfy, the reality on the provincial ground is different. There is variation across provinces in the extent to which services are accessible, and to a lesser but growing extent, in the range of services that provincial health insurance plans cover. Interprovincial variation reflects, in part, the fact that the criteria of comprehensiveness and accessibility are open-ended and have not been specified either by the federal government or the courts. The decision not to mandate a specific set of services or standards for accessibility in the CHA reflects the reality that provinces have access to better information regarding the health care needs and institutional capacities of their own systems, and that these needs and capacities differ from province to province.

However, this rationale for federal deference to the provinces still requires provinces to grapple with the national standards of comprehensiveness and accessibility. The fact that national standards can be satisfied by a variety of means (or provincial health insurance plans), should not render the standards devoid of content. Rather, the emphasis should be on the provinces establishing democratic processes to specify provincial goals for these criteria. The federal government could ask the provincial governments to demonstrate the *processes* they have in place to specify and comply with these five criteria – in particular, the criteria of comprehensiveness and accessibility, and the suggested criterion of public governance and accountability – on an annual basis.

The CHA should be amended to require provincial governments to engage their respective citizens in processes to fulfill the five criteria. This is the best way to ensure that the criteria are viewed by the provinces and by the citizens of Canada as fair and the best way to give them substantive content. This kind of provincial undertaking could spark an important public debate within each province over what citizens can reasonably expect of their health care systems (Daniels 2000). In this way, one of the democratic benefits of a federal system – the potential for meaningful citizen participation through decentralized decision-making – is realized.

Reconceptualizing national standards as we propose would have many benefits. It would shift the focus of federal-provincial relations away from disputes over enforcement towards a partnership between governments. It would recognize that the application of the five criteria of the CHA might lead to different results in different communities. The latter, of course, might be viewed as a disadvantage, as it could lead to an increase in interprovincial variation. This variation would undermine the 'citizenship' rationale of national standards. However, as discussed above, this variability could also be a strength, as a one-size-fits-all approach is appropriate to the goals the system should strive for but not the various means of achieving those goals.

Medicare Commission

A second component of reforming the structure of federal-provincial relations in medicare concerns the institutions that govern it (Choudhry 2000). At present, to the extent that we can speak of a national medicare system, it is governed exclusively by the federal or provincial governments. As a consequence, medicare has fallen prey to politics and has become one of the principal arenas for federal-provincial conflict. To be sure, it would be both impossible and undesirable, from the point of view of democratic accountability, for elected governments to extricate themselves from the business of governing medicare. However, there is a real need for a non-partisan national body, protected from day-to-day politics, and with a longer-term view than is possible for elected government. This national body should ensure that additional federal funding in health care is used to promote reform in accordance with the five criteria of the CHA.

What we propose is the creation of a Medicare Commission. The commission would be an expert, independent body. Its members would be appointed by provincial and federal governments and its funding secured from the federal government. We address the function, funding, and membership of this body in turn.

Function
The role of the Medicare Commission would be:

- to determine specific performance indicators to help provinces achieve the national standards set out in the CHA. For example, the commission might issue performance metrics for 'reasonable access' that are tailored to particular contexts of treatment (e.g., specialist services, primary care, emergency services);
- to publish (in conjunction with the Canadian Institute for Health Information) annual reports on the performance of provincial health insurance systems according to these performance indicators and how provinces are measuring up to their own identified goals;
- to identify programs that constitute 'best practices,' by drawing on both research and experiences in Canada and abroad. If followed, these practices would yield improvements according to standard performance indicators (e.g., best practice standards in primary care and best practice models in primary care reform);
- to provide financial assistance to those provinces that undertake to implement the processes or programs identified by the commission; and
- to work with provinces to establish processes to better satisfy the criteria of public governance and democratic accountability, accessibility, and comprehensiveness (e.g., processes that best incorporate technical evidence and public values in determining which hospital and physicians services should be publicly funded).

Funding
The commission's funding would have to be stable and guaranteed. The funding would be separate from federal transfers for health care and would be adjusted for inflation and population growth each year.

This new federal money would pull together all one-off payment initiatives the federal government has currently undertaken in primary care and other areas. *To ensure its legitimacy and credibility, it is crucial that the commission receive a significant sum of federal funds.*

Membership and Terms of Office
The commission would have to have both expertise and independence, the latter being achieved through security of tenure and financial security. To ensure that the provincial governments recognize the legitimacy of the commission, the commission would need to be appointed jointly by the provincial and federal governments. One possible method of composition would be for each province to appoint one commissioner and the federal government to appoint five, for a total of fifteen. Commissioners would serve full time. They could not be federal or provincial civil servants, consult independently or hold private sector employment. Moreover, to be effective, the commission must be non-partisan and, to the extent possible, non-politicized. The commissioners would select a chief commissioner from among them. All decisions would require a two-thirds majority, meaning that federal commissioners would require support from a majority of provincial commissioners for any decision. An expert staff of health service researchers would assist the commission. Finally, the commission would make its reports publicly available, including specific findings on the compliance of provincial health care plans with national standards.

Procedures for Settling Disputes

Disputes will, unfortunately, continue to arise over provincial compliance with the CHA, although, we would argue, with less frequency and with less bitterness should the reforms we propose be implemented. Nonetheless, we think it important to establish procedures under the Social Union Framework Agreement (SUFA) for settling disputes (Choudhry 2000). The need for procedures was evident during the dispute over Alberta's Bill 11, which ultimately turned on competing interpretations of the CHA. The need for procedures has become all the more pressing given the stated desire of some provinces to experiment with public-private partnerships and to delist services that are currently publicly insured.

Article 6 of SUFA establishes a general framework for creating procedures to settle disputes. Within this framework, negotiations should be premised on joint fact-finding, which may be conducted by a third party and would be made public if one party so requests. In addition, negotiations may be accompanied by mediation; again, mediation reports would be made public if one party so requests. Also according to SUFA, mechanisms for dispute resolution must respect a list of general principles. They must be 'simple, timely, efficient, effective and transparent'; allow for the possibility of non-adversarial solutions; be appropriate for the specific sectors in which the disputes arise; and provide for the expert assistance of third parties.

The federal and provincial ministers of health on 24 April 2001 announced the establishment of a dispute settlement mechanism for disagreements regarding the interpretation of the CHA. The full details of the proposal have not been released to the public. A Government of Alberta News Release (2002) explains that if the federal government and a provincial government are in a dispute over the interpretation of the CHA, then either party may refer the matter to a third-party panel: 'The panel will be composed of one representative appointed by the federal government, one representative appointed by the province or territory and a chairperson agreed to by each government. It will have the ability to provide non-binding advice and recommendations. To ensure an open process, the panel's final report will be made public.'

This initiative on the part of the federal and provincial governments is an important step towards facilitating good governance of medicare. Our reservations are that it is not clear from this proposal whether or not the panels that are constituted will be permanent or ad hoc. We think the creation of one permanent national panel is by far the best way to build up expertise and consistency regarding interpretation of the CHA. We also would argue that citizens should be able to invoke the process, as federal and provincial governments may lack the incentive to enforce the law.[8] If a Medicare Commission were created, the regime for settling disputes could be tied to the commission's work. For example, the commission might produce fact-finding reports that could serve as the basis for mediations or negotiations and be introduced as evidence in hearings. Finally, we would note that *any* dispute resolution mechanism will remain a hollow protection unless and until the federal government takes a stronger role in enforcing the criteria of the CHA.

Expanding the Envelope of Publicly Insured Services

As discussed earlier, there is a need for the creation of national insurance programs for pharmacare and home care, with national standards. These standards need not, however, be the same criteria or standards as those presently in the CHA. In particular, it may be appropriate to levy user charges on people who can afford to pay for certain aspects of home care that bridge the divide between medical and social services (housekeeping services, for example). The prospect of user charges and extra-billing for these services does not raise concerns of the magnitude as are raised in the case of medically necessary physician and hospital services. There is also not the same level of concern about human resources (particularly physicians' labour) being siphoned off by patients willing to pay amounts above and beyond those covered by public health insurance. Moreover, some provinces may wish to follow Quebec's model of managed care in providing for provincial drug plans that cover all citizens and regulate the operation of private insurers as opposed to nationalizing the insurance function. In the eyes of some, this may be seen to be in breach of the public administration criterion as presently configured. Thus, in our opinion, it would be appropriate to provide for national standards for pharmacare and home care by way of separate legislation.

Under our proposal, the federal government would have two policy instruments available to create and implement national standards for prescription drugs and home care: a new federal-provincial shared-cost statute (the 'Canada Pharmacare and Home Care Act'); and federally created and administered prescription drugs and home care programs (via the federal Crown's contracting power).

A Federal-Provincial Shared-Cost Statute

The most obvious solution is to create a new shared-cost statute whereby the federal government would make transfers to the provincial governments in exchange for upholding certain national standards for insuring prescription drugs and home care programs. Because these programs would be created through separate legislation, there would be no need to amend the CHA. The funding arrangements for this new shared-cost statute would be identical to those under the CHA – block funding – and could be incorporated into the new 'Canada Health

Transfer' that we propose above. The national standards of public administration, comprehensiveness, universality, portability, and accessibility would also still apply, subject to the clarifications and changes discussed earlier. However, we do not think the specific bans on extra-billing and user fees should be included in this new act; at least in the short term. The legislation would, however, have to specify, at a minimum, national standards regarding the income level below which user charges are unacceptable (that takes into account interprovincial variations in the cost of living). Ideally we think it should also provide that care which if not provided in the home or community would result in the patient being hospitalized be provided free of any user charge.

There are disadvantages to this option. First, it would require a significant new federal funding commitment. Second, given the experience surrounding the introduction of the CHST, provinces may be reluctant to launch new public programs without a long-term funding commitment from the federal government or increases in federal cash transfers for CHA-covered programs. Even if the federal government were willing to make such commitments, short of constitutional amendment, a federal government with a majority in Parliament is always free to alter the level of its financial contributions. This option would become more attractive, though, if combined with both the proposals for a Medicare Commission and procedures for settling disputes. Those institutions would restrict federal power (albeit not with respect to levels of funding) and could be viewed accordingly as a quid pro quo for new provincial responsibilities.

Direct Federal Pharmacare and Home Care Programs

If the federal government possesses the resources but the provinces are unwilling to enter into new shared-cost arrangements for insuring pharmacare and home care, a second option would be for the federal government to create and administer such programs directly. For example, the provinces may be willing to hand over responsibility for the prescription drug budget, given the increasing proportion of total health care costs absorbed by drugs (Canadian Institute for Health Information 2001). For this very reason, however, the federal government may also be reluctant to take on board such a program, as it would require a significant new funding commitment.

Should direct federal programs be politically viable, the next question is the legal means by which such programs could be created.

While the text of the Constitution is silent on jurisdiction over social insurance, the courts have stated that publicly operated insurance schemes that seek to safeguard persons against the risk of illness lie outside federal jurisdiction. Consequently, direct federal regulation of health insurance has been thought to be unconstitutional. This line of analysis seems to preclude the creation of federal insurance programs for prescription drugs and home care without making a constitutional amendment similar to the one that transferred jurisdiction over employment insurance from the provinces to the federal government in 1951. It is exceedingly unlikely that the Constitution could be reopened for such a narrow amendment, given the broad range of unresolved issues the federation already faces and the rise of 'mega-constitutional' politics during the Canada Round in the early 1990s.

There is reason, however, to question the thinking behind this premise. A good constitutional argument can be made that Parliament holds the right to legislate health insurance as part of its jurisdiction over the peace, order, and good government of Canada (Choudhry 2002; contra see Jackman 1996, 6; 2000). In the current political climate, however, such a frontal challenge to provincial jurisdiction would exact enormous political costs, and its constitutionality would likely be challenged in the courts.

An alternative would be for the federal government to use its contractual power (Choudhry 2002). This power is not mentioned by name in the Constitution. Its source is the common law rule that the Crown (including the federal Crown) possesses all the powers and privileges of a private individual. Like a private person, the Crown can enter into contracts and, under those contracts, acquire and dispose of its property, including its money. The federal Crown can enter into contracts with individuals or institutions such as corporations or hospitals. Those contracts may contain terms that provide for federal payments to the contracting party in exchange for compliance with certain conditions. When exercising this power, the federal Crown is not constrained by the division of powers. This means that it can enter into contracts in areas outside of federal jurisdiction. Moreover, Parliament has the jurisdiction to legislate with respect to contracts made by the federal Crown, such as laying down the conditions that attach to those payments.

Contracting power has considerable advantages over its spending power (the federal Crown's central policy instrument in health care). The principal limitation of spending power is that conditions are *not* legally enforceable against the recipient in court. The federal Crown's only remedy for non-compliance is to withhold funds. In contrast, once entered into, contracts are legally binding and enforceable in court. However, contracts share one major limitation of conditional grants – unlike legislation, contracts cannot impose legal obligations without the agreement of both contracting parties.

Although federal housing policy through the Canada Mortgage and Housing Corporation uses contracts, federal health policy does not, but it could. The federal government's contractual jurisdiction could be used in a variety of ways. We sketch out here, in rudimentary fashion, two examples involving pharmaceuticals. The details of any such initiatives would obviously need to be more fully fleshed out than is possible here.

In the first case, the federal government could set itself up as a provider of pharmaceutical insurance, operating in a manner nearly identical to that of a private insurer. A private pharmaceutical insurer enters into contracts to regulate its relationships with a variety of parties – beneficiaries (who pay premiums in exchange for receiving coverage) and providers such as pharmacies (who agree to provide pharmaceuticals for a fee set out in a schedule and bill insurance companies directly). If it wished to do so, the federal Crown could enter into a similar set of contractual relationships with beneficiaries and providers. If its terms of coverage were sufficiently attractive, the federal drug plan could coexist or compete with private plans and replace them in the marketplace. As a variation, the federal Crown could contract directly with pharmaceutical companies over its fee schedule, using its purchasing power to contain costs.

In the second case, the federal government could facilitate not only access to prescription drugs but also cost-effective prescribing by physicians. The central contractual relationship would be between the federal Crown and group practices of primary care physicians. The contracts would provide for a fixed, per capita payment to the group practice (altered for case-mix). In exchange, the group practice would agree to manage this budget and pay for pharmaceuticals out of it. Because it would be at risk for pharmaceutical expenditures, the group practice would have the incentive to contain costs.

The two options on the table for expanding program coverage – a new shared-cost statute or the creation of federally governed programs – each have advantages and disadvantages from the vantage points of federal-provincial relations and democratic accountability. At this point in time, we would recommend the former option – a new shared-cost statute, modelled on the CHA, but with modifications regarding extra-billing and user fees – as part of the overall package of proposals outlined in this chapter. Provinces would more likely accept this package if it adhered to the shared-cost model in the CHA and did not introduce direct federal programs into the mix.

Summary of Recommendations

Three goals drive our recommendations: first, how to modernize the five criteria of the CHA and expand its scope to better reflect the needs of contemporary society; second, how to give content to the criteria in the act, cast as they are in very general terms; and, third, how to overhaul federal-provincial relations in the health care sector.

Modernizing the Criteria

With regard to the five criteria, we recommend the following:

- *Universality*: The criterion of universality is a fundamental principle and should be maintained for hospital and physician services and expanded specifically into diagnostic services. Through separate legislation there should also be universal coverage for prescription drugs and home care. The criterion of universality does not necessitate funding from general tax revenues but, rather, that funding is progressive (i.e., based on ability to pay). New national programs for home care and prescription drugs could be funded, for example, by compulsory social insurance.
- *Portability*: Out-of-country coverage is not core to medicare. The criterion of portability should be amended so that provinces are not in breach of the CHA if they do not pay for out-of-country treatment.
- *Public Administration*: The criterion of public administration should be recast as 'public governance and democratic accountability' to emphasize the importance of good governance and accountability of decision makers at all levels in medicare. The federal government should monitor the growth of health care delivery by for-profit firms but acknowledge that the CHA does not preclude their participation, *provided services are fully publicly funded*.
- *Comprehensiveness*: The CHA should require provinces to establish transparent and democratic *processes* to determine on an ongoing

basis which services and goods should or should not be publicly funded. It should also require that provinces give priority to publicly funding services of proven effectiveness. As well, the scope of services protected by the CHA should be expanded to include all medically necessary diagnostic services (e.g., MRIs). Consideration should be given to requiring provinces to integrate funding for *all* publicly funded health care services (whether protected by the CHA or not) and held by the appropriate level of decision-maker.

• *Accessibility*: If medicare does not respond to Canadians' concerns regarding timeliness of treatment, support for it will be undermined and pressure for privately financed options will increase. The criterion of accessibility in the CHA should be changed to read 'reasonable access in a reasonable time frame, given the nature of the health need,' in order to incorporate a guarantee of timely access. The CHA should require the provinces to account for the processes they have in place to ensure that all residents of the province have reasonable access to health care goods and services in a reasonable time frame.

Extra-billing and User Charges

To prevent the emergence of two-tier health care and queue jumping, the prohibition on extra-billing should remain in place. Extra-billing would allow wealthier Canadians to queue-jump. There is no evidence from any country that allowing extra-billing will reduce waiting lists in public hospitals. On the contrary, countries like New Zealand and the United Kingdom that allow extra-billing and queue jumping have longer waiting lists and times in their public hospitals. Evidence shows that user charges for hospital and physician services may deter both unnecessary and necessary use of care. Thus the prohibition on user charges should remain in place unless a province could establish that a proposed regime of user charges would not deter Canadians from seeking the care they need but only unnecessary care.

The CHA appropriately prevents experimentation with private financing through the prohibitions on user charges and extra-billing *but neither impedes nor encourages* reform or innovation in the *delivery* of health care. We think the CHA should be reformed to actively encourage innovation and evidence-based reform in the delivery of care.

Processes for Giving Content to the Criteria of the Act

Currently, the five criteria in the CHA are statements of the values that Canadians want to see reflected in provincial insurance systems across the country. There is, however, no substantive definition provided for crucial phrases such as 'medically necessary' and 'reasonable access.' This is understandable, given that these kinds of requirements must vary over time and between provinces. To give real content to the values articulated in the CHA, the CHA should require provinces to demonstrate the *processes* they have in place to define and comply with the criteria on an annual basis. We believe that this approach would shift the focus of federal-provincial relations away from disputes over enforcement and pervasive acrimony towards a partnership between the federal and provincial governments. By shifting towards a system that focuses primarily on accountability for processes, we recognize that a one-size-fits-all approach is appropriate to the *values* the system strives for but not the various *means* of realizing those values.

Overhauling Federal-Provincial Relations in Health Care

Federal-provincial relations in health care are in desperate need of repair. To this end, medicare requires the creation of two sets of joint federal-provincial institutions to govern it. First, we propose the establishment of a jointly appointed, non-partisan and expert Medicare Commission to work with the provinces to establish processes to better satisfy the criteria of comprehensiveness, accessibility, and public governance and accountability. The commission would reward provinces that meet objective performance indicators or that implement those reforms the commission identifies as worthwhile. To effect real change in the system, the commission would have to receive a significant sum of federal funds above and beyond existing transfer payments. Second, we propose the creation of permanent procedures under the Social Union Framework Agreement to deal with disputes over the interpretation of the CHA. Disputes would be heard by specialist panels. Moreover, in addition to being triggered by government complaints, the machinery could also be invoked directly by citizens.

National Programs for Prescription Drugs and Home Care

Separate legislation is required to provide for national standards for insuring prescription drugs and home care. This legislation will likely have to take the form of a new shared-cost statute similar to the CHA, but with national standards for access rather than an outright prohibition on user charges. We believe that some user charges may be appropriate in a national home care system as home care straddles the medical care and social services sector, for example, homemaking services may appropriately attract a user fee. In the case of prescription drugs, it is vital that Canadians not be deterred from obtaining necessary prescription drugs because of fees. But, for example, the imposition of a user charge upon a brand name drug as opposed to a generic drug would seem acceptable.

Conclusion

The Canada Health Act has served Canadians extremely well since 1984. However, to continue to realize the values that lie behind the Act, some changes are necessary. Instead of regarding the CHA as a quasi-constitutional document that should be altered with great reluctance, the statute should be regarded as a delivery vehicle for public health care policy that from time to time must be adapted to changing circumstances. In other words, the act is a means, not an end in itself. At this critical juncture, to view it in any other way would be dangerous because it would make the CHA an obstacle to necessary change in the structure and governance of medicare as opposed to a facilitator of those changes. Underlying and uniting the specific reforms we propose, is a broader call for dramatic change in the mindset that governs the legal and governance framework for medicare. For medicare to survive into the twenty-first century, it must be both effective and legitimate. And to be both of these things, it must be flexible and adaptable. Canadians deserve no less.

NOTES

We would like to thank Pat Baranek, Michael Decter, Bob Rae, and Terry Sullivan for their comments on earlier drafts of this paper; two anonymous reviewers for their comments; Monique Bégin, Charlyn Black, Dale McMurchy, and Carolyn Tuohy for the various discussions we had over our proposals; Susan Zimmerman for her research assistance work; and Margaret Williams for her proofreading and editorial comments. All opinions, errors, and omissions remain the authors'.

1 'Extended health care services' are defined as nursing home intermediate care, adult residential care, home care, and ambulatory health care services. To obtain a federal contribution for extended health care services, the provinces need only comply with section 13. This section requires provinces to provide information to the federal government and formally recognize the latter's contributions in promotional material and public documents.

2 Thus, for example, the Australian government has reciprocal agreements with eight countries: the United Kingdom, New Zealand, Finland, Italy, Ireland, Malta, the Netherlands and Sweden. In these countries, Australians are provided with urgent or emergency medical treatment. See http://www.hic.gov.au/yourhealth/services_for_travellers/tofa.htm.

4 We are grateful to Carolyn Tuohy for this point.

5 Any process to decide which services to include is a complex one that must incorporate societal values in achieving different kinds of health states, technical evidence about the efficacy of different means of achieving these states, and economic evidence of the cost of those, given the value as a society we put on achieving different health care outcomes and responding to different needs.

6 In 2000, provincially appointed committees in Quebec (the Clair Commission) and Saskatchewan (the Fyke Commission) reported, both calling for primary care reform (see Quebec, Ministry of Health, Commission on Medicare. *Emerging Solutions: Report and Recommendations*. Quebec: Commission on Medicare, 2001. Available at http://www.cessss.gouv.qc.ca/pdf/en/01–109–01a.pdf); Saskatchewan, Department of Health, Commission on Medicare. *Caring for Medicare: Sustaining a Quality System*. Regina: Commission on Medicare, 2001. Available at http://www.legassembly.sk.ca/hcc). In 2001, a provincially appointed committee in Alberta (the Mazankowski Commission) required a raft of controversial reforms, but included among these reforms is yet a further call for primary care reform – see http://www.premiersadvisory.com.

6 Thus, any province that imposes user charges should prohibit private insurance coverage if the goal is truly to control total health care costs and utilization. This is what Australia does for physician services.

7 There have been several initiatives designed to meet the need for security in terms of the amount of federal funding. In 1996, following the recommendations of the National Forum on Health, the federal government further amended the Federal-Provincial Fiscal Arrangements Act to provide a floor of $11 billion per year for the cash component of the CHST, and in 1997–8, this floor was increased to $12.5 billion.

8 To guard against frivolous and vexatious complaints and ensure that novel issues reach panels, a screening body such as a permanent secretariat would

need to investigate complaints. It is also important to ensure that this process would not be captured by health care providers and used as a means to resolve disputes over compensation and working conditions.

REFERENCES

Canada Health Act (CHA). R.S.C. 1985, c. C-6.

Canada National Forum on Health. 1997. 'Creating a Culture of Evidence-Based Decision Making in Health.' In *Canada Health Forum: Building on the Legacy.* Volume 2: *Synthesis Reports and Issues Paper.* Sainte-Foy: Éditions MultiMondes.

Canada Royal Commission on New Reproductive Technologies. 1993. *Proceed with Care: Final Report of the Royal Commission on New Reproductive Technologies.* Ottawa: Minister of Government Services Canada.

Canadian Institute for Health Information. 2001. 'Health Care in Canada 2001.' http://ecomm.cihi.ca/ ec/product.asp?code=01HCR%28HC%29PDF.

– 2000. 'National Health Expenditure Trends, 1975–2000, Report.' http:// www.cihi.ca/medrls/11dec2000execsumm.shtml (21 October 2001).

Caulfield, Timothy A. 1996. 'Wishful Thinking: Defining "Medically Necessary" in Canada.' *Health Law Journal* 4: 63–87.

Choudhry, Sujit. 2002. 'Recasting Social Canada: A Reconsideration of Federal Jurisdiction over Social Policy.' *University of Toronto Law Journal* 52: 163–252.

– 2000. 'Bill 11, the Canada Health Act and the Social Union: The Need for Institutions.' *Osgoode Hall Law Journal* 38: 39–97.

– 1996. 'The Enforcement of the Canada Health Act.' *McGill Law Journal* 41: 461–508.

Coutts, Jane. 1998. 'Too Many Hysterectomies Performed in Ontario Report Says,' *Globe and Mail*, 26 February, A4.

Daniels, Norman. 2000. 'Accountability for Reasonableness in Private and Public Health Insurance.' In *The Global Challenge of Health Care Rationing*, ed. Angela Coulter and Chris Ham, 89–106. Philadelphia: Open University Press.

Deber, Raisa B. 2000a. 'Thoughts before Rethinking: Some Thoughts about Babies and Bathwater.' *HealthcarePapers* 1(3): 25–31.

– 2000b. 'Getting What We Pay For: Myths and Realities About Financing Canada's Health Care System.' *Health Law in Canada* 21(2): 9–56.

Decter, Michael B. 2000. *Four Strong Winds: Understanding the Growing Challenges to Health Care.* Toronto: Stoddart.

Devereaux, P.J., et al. 2002. 'A Systematic Review and Meta-analysis of Studies

Comparing Mortality Rates of Private For-profit and Private Not-for-profit Hospitals.' *CMAJ* 166(11): 1399–1406.

Epp, Michael J., et al. 2000. 'The Impact of Direct and Extra-Billing for Medical Services: Evidence from a Natural Experiment in British Columbia.' *Social Science and Medicine* 51: 691–702.

Epps, Tracey, and Colleen M. Flood. 2002. 'The Implications of the NAFTA for Canada's Health Care System: Have We Traded Away the Opportunity for Innovative Health Care Reform?' *McGill Law Journal* 47(4): 747–90.

Evans, Robert G., et al. 2000. 'Private Highway, One-Way Street: The Deklein and Fall of Canadian Medicare.' http://www.chspr.ubc.ca/hpru/pdf/2000-3d.PDF.

Flood, Colleen M. 2000a. *International Health Care Reform: A Legal, Economic and Political Analysis.* London: Routledge.

– 2000b. 'Accountability, Flexibility and Integration: How to Fix Medicare.' *Policy Options* 21(4): 17–19.

– 1999. 'The Structure and Dynamics of the Canadian Health Care System.' In *Canadian Health Law and Policy,* ed. Jocelyn Downie and Timothy Caulfield, 5–50. Toronto: Butterworths.

– 1996. 'Will Supplementary Private Insurance Reduce Waiting Lists?' *Canadian Health Facilities Law Guide* 11: 1–3.

Flood, Colleen M., and Tom Archibald. 2001. 'The Illegality of Private Health Care in Canada.' *CMAJ* 164(6): 825–30.

Flood, Colleen M., Mark Stabile, and Carolyn H. Tuohy. 2002. 'The Borders of Solidarity: How Countries Determine the Public/Private Mix in Spending and the Impact on Health Care.' *Health Matrix* 12(2): 297–355.

Government of Alberta News Release. 2002. 'Provinces Accept Federal Proposal on Disputes Resolution Mechanism.' http://www.gov.ab.ca/acn/200204/12223.html (24 April).

Hirschman, Albert O. 1970. *Exit, Voice, and Loyalty: Responses to Decline in Firms, Organizations, and States.* Cambridge, MA: Harvard University Press.

Hutchinson, Brian, Julia Abelson, and John Lavis. 2001. 'Primary Care in Canada: So Much Innovation, So Little Change.' *Health Affairs* 20(3): 116–45.

Hutton, Susan M. 1989. 'Physicians' Freedom of Contract in Ontario: An Economic Justification for the Ban on Extra-Billing with Some Recommendations for Structural Change.' *University of Toronto Faculty of Law Review* 47: 780–824.

Institute for Research in Public Policy. 2000. *IRPP Taskforce on Health Policy, Recommendations to First Ministers.* Montreal: IRPP.

Jackman, Martha. 2000. 'Constitutional Jurisdiction over Health in Canada.' *Health Law Journal* 8: 95–120.

– 1996. 'The Constitutional Basis for Federal Regulation of Health.' *Health Law Review* 5(2): 3–10.

Jackson, N.W., M.P. Doogue, and J.M. Elliot. 1999. 'Priority Points and Cardiac Events While Waiting for Coronary Artery Bypass Surgery.' *Heart* 81: 367–73.

Jacobs, Lawrence, Theodore Marmor, and Jonathan Oberlander. 1999. 'The Oregon Health Plan and the Political Paradox of Rationing: What Advocates and Critics Have Claimed and What Oregon Did.' *Journal of Health Politics, Policy and Law* 24(1): 161–80.

Jacobzone, S. 2000. 'Pharmaceutical Policies in OECD Countries: Reconciling Social and Industrial Goals.' *Labour Market and Social Policy: Occasional Papers*, No. 40, 1–62. Paris: OECD.

Klein, Ralph. 2001. *Premier's Advisory Council on Health for Alberta.* http://www.premiersadvisory.com.

Laghi, Brian, and Rod Mickleburgh. 2002. 'Premiers Threaten to Act Alone on Health,' *Globe and Mail*, 25 January, A1.

Lomas, Jonathan. 1999. 'The Evolution of Devolution: What Does the Community Want.' In *Health Reform: Public Success, Private Failure*, ed. D. Drache and T. Sullivan, 169–85. London: Routledge.

Marleau, Dianne, Federal Health Minister. 1995. Letter to All Provincial and Territorial Ministers of Health. 6 January. Copy on file with authors.

Naylor, C. David. 1999. 'Health Care in Canada: Incrementalism under Fiscal Duress.' *Health Affairs* 18(3): 9–26.

O'Brien, Bernard J., McMaster University, Faculty of Health Sciences. 1998. 'Parallel Public/Private Finance and Waiting Lists.' Paper presented at the Centre for Health Economics and Policy Analysis, Shifting Involvements: Private and Public Roles in Canada Health Care: Eleventh Annual Health Policy Conference, 28–29 May, Hamilton, Ontario.

OECD. 2001. *OECD Health Data 2000: A Comparative Analysis of 29 Countries.* Paris: Organisation for Economic Co-operation and Development.

Office of the Auditor General. 1999. 'Federal Support of Health Care Delivery.' In *Report of the Auditor General of Canada to the House of Commons*, 29.1–29.30. Ottawa: Auditor General's Office.

PriceWaterhouseCoopers. 2001. *HealthInsider, Survey Number Five*. Toronto: PriceWaterhouseCoopers.

Provincial and Territorial Ministers of Health. 2000. 'Understanding Canada's Health Care Costs: Final Report.' http://www.scics.gc.ca/pdf/850080012e.pdf (August).

Reed, Marie C., and Ha T. Tu. 2002. 'Triple Jeopardy: Low Income, Chronically Ill and Uninsured in America.' http://www.hschange.org/CONTENT/411/ (February).

Rice, Thomas, and Kathleen R. Morrison. 1994. 'Patient Cost Sharing for Medical Services: A Review of the Literature and Implications for Health Care Reform.' *Medical Care Review* 51: 235–87.

Roos, Noralou P., and Leslie L. Roos. 1994. 'Small Area Variations, Practice Style, and Quality of Care.' In *Why Are Some People Healthy and Others Not?* ed. Robert G. Evans, Morris L. Barer, and Theodore R. Marmor, 231–46. New York: De Gruyter.

Stabile, Mark. 2001. 'Private Insurance Subsidies and Public Health Care Markets: Evidence from Canada.' *Canadian Journal of Economics* 34(4): 921–42.

Stoddart, Greg L. et al. 1993. *Why Not User Charges? The Real Issues: A Discussion Paper.* Ontario: Premier's Council on Health, Well-being and Social Justice.

Tamblyn, Robyn, et al. 2001. 'Adverse Events Associated with Prescription Drug Cost-Sharing among Poor and Elderly Persons.' *JAMA* 285(4): 421–9.

Willison, Don, M. Wiktorowicz, P. Grootendoorst, B. O'Brien, M. Levine, R. Deber, and J. Hurley. 2001. 'International Experience with Pharmaceutical Policy: Common Challenges and Lessons for Canada.' CHEPA Working Papers Series 01-08 (Hamilton: Centre for Health Economics and Policy Analysis, McMaster University). Available from http://www.chepa.org/research/01-08.pdf.

Tuohy, Carolyn H. 1999. *Accidental Logics: The Dynamics of Change in the Health Care Arena in Britain, the United States and Canada.* New York: Oxford University Press, 1999.

Tuohy, Carolyn. H., Colleen M. Flood, and Mark Stabile. 2001. 'How Does Private Finance Affect Health Care Systems: Marshalling the Evidence from OECD Nations.' http://www.law.utoronto.ca/ healthlaw /index.htm (1 June).

Walker, Michael, and Greg Wilson. September 2001. 'Waiting Your Turn: Hospital Waiting Lists in Canada, 2001.' http://www.fraserinstitute.ca/shared/readmore.asp?sNav=pb&id =206 (September).